W9-ASO-419

NUTRITIONAL CONCERNS in RECREATION, EXERCISE, and SPORT

Edited by
Judy A. Driskell
Ira Wolinsky

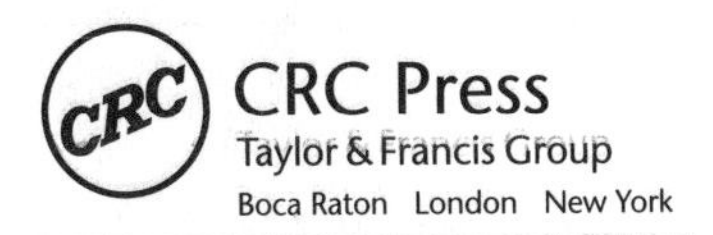

CRC Press is an imprint of the
Taylor & Francis Group, an **informa** business

CRC Press
Taylor & Francis Group
6000 Broken Sound Parkway NW, Suite 300
Boca Raton, FL 33487-2742

Printed in the United States of America on acid-free paper
10 9 8 7 6 5 4 3 2 1

International Standard Book Number: 978-1-4200-6815-3 (Hardback)

Library of Congress Cataloging-in-Publication Data

Nutritional concerns in recreation, exercise, and sport / Judy A. Driskell, Ira Wolinsky, editors.
p. cm.
Includes bibliographical references and index.
ISBN 978-1-4200-6815-3 (hardcover : alk. paper)
1. Athletes--Nutrition--Requirements. 2. Physical fitness--Nutritional aspects. 3. Exercise--Nutritional aspects. 4. Energy metabolism. 5. Dietary supplements. I. Driskell, Judy A. (Judy Anne) II. Wolinsky, Ira. III. Title.

TX361.A8N895 2009
613.2'024796--dc22 2009016173

Visit the Taylor & Francis Web site at
http://www.taylorandfrancis.com

and the CRC Press Web site at
http://www.crcpress.com

Dedication

This book is dedicated to the experts who wrote the chapters.

Contents

Preface

Through our books and research, we are pleased to have played a small part in the recent rapid growth of the science of sports nutrition. Taken together, our series of monographs and edited books form an exhaustive and comprehensive corpus on the subject. These books have been very well received and we are proud of them. You have in your hands the latest book on the subject, *Nutritional Concerns in Recreation, Exercise, and Sport.* In it are in-depth discussions of important topics of interest to health and nutrition professionals as well as the motivated layman and the weekend athlete. This volume covers a wide span of interests in sports nutrition and brings you the latest authoritative information from experts. As such, it can be used as a resource and will also find use as a textbook.

Judy A. Driskell

Ira Wolinsky

The Editors

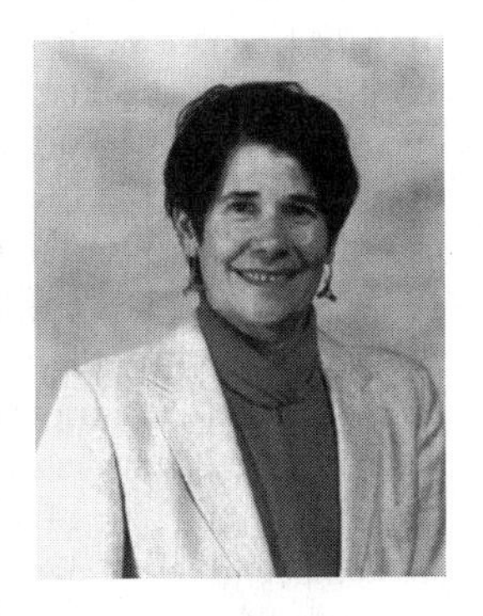

Judy Anne Driskell, PhD, RD, is Professor of Nutritional Science and Dietetics at the University of Nebraska. She received her BS degree in Biology from the University of Southern Mississippi in Hattiesburg. Her MS and PhD degrees were obtained from Purdue University. She has served in research and teaching positions at Auburn University, Florida State University, Virginia Polytechnic Institute and State University, and the University of Nebraska. She has also served as the Nutrition Scientist for the U.S. Department of Agriculture/Cooperative State Research Service and as a Professor of Nutrition and Food Science at Gadjah Mada and Bogor Universities in Indonesia.

Dr. Driskell is a member of numerous professional organizations including the American Society for Nutrition, the American College of Sports Medicine, the International Society of Sports Nutrition, the Institute of Food Technologists, and the American Dietetic Association. In 1993 she received the Professional Scientist Award of the Food Science and Human Nutrition Section of the Southern Association of Agricultural Scientists. In addition, she was the 1987 recipient of the Borden Award for Research in Applied Fundamental Knowledge of Human Nutrition. She is listed as an expert in B-complex vitamins by the Vitamin Nutrition Information Service.

Dr. Driskell co-edited the CRC book *Sports Nutrition: Minerals and Electrolytes* with Constance V. Kies. In addition, she authored the textbook *Sports Nutrition* and co-authored the advanced nutrition book *Nutrition: Chemistry and Biology*, both published by CRC. She co-edited *Sports Nutrition: Vitamins and Trace Elements, first and second editions*; *Macroelements, Water, and Electrolytes in Sports Nutrition; Energy-Yielding Macronutrients and Energy Metabolism in Sports Nutrition*; *Nutritional Applications in Exercise and Sport*; *Nutritional Assessment of Athletes*; *Nutritional Ergogenic Aids*; *Sports Nutrition: Energy Metabolism and Exercise*; and the current book *Nutritional Concerns in Recreation, Exercise, and Sport*, all with Ira Wolinsky. She also edited the books *Sports Nutrition: Fats and Proteins* and *Nutrition and Exercise Concerns of Middle Age,* published by CRC Press. She has published more than 165 refereed research articles and 18 book chapters as well as several publications intended for lay audiences, and has given numerous presentations to professional and lay groups. Her current research interests center around vitamin metabolism and requirements, including the interrelationships between exercise and water-soluble vitamin requirements.

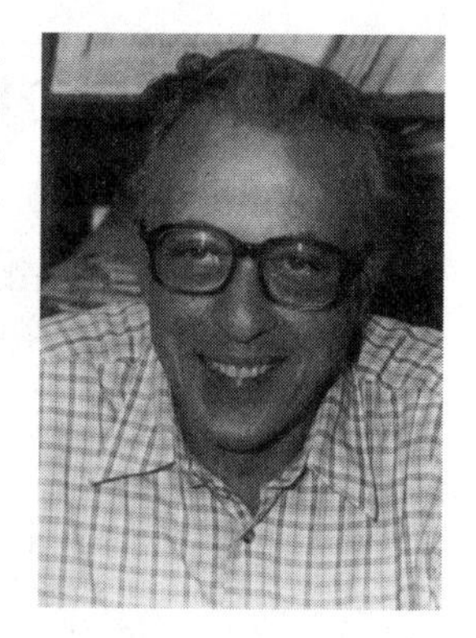

Ira Wolinsky, PhD, is Professor Emeritus of Health and Human Performance at the University of Houston. He received his BS degree in Chemistry from the City College of New York and his MS and PhD degrees in Biochemistry from the University of Kansas. He has served in research and teaching positions at the Hebrew University, the University of Missouri, The Pennsylvania State University, and the University of Houston, as well as conducted basic research in NASA life sciences facilities and abroad.

Dr. Wolinsky is a member of the American Society for Nutrition, among other honorary and scientific organizations. He has contributed numerous nutrition research papers in the open literature. His major research interests relate to the nutrition of bone and calcium and trace elements and to sports nutrition. He has been the recipient of research grants from both public and private sources. He has received several international research fellowships and consultantships to the former Soviet Union, Bulgaria, Hungary, and India. He merited a Fulbright Senior Scholar Fellowship to Greece in 1999.

Dr. Wolinsky has co-authored a book on the history of the science of nutrition, *Nutrition and Nutritional Diseases*. He co-edited *Sports Nutrition: Vitamins and Trace Elements, first and second editions; Macroelements, Water, and Electrolytes in Sports Nutrition; Energy-Yielding Macronutrients and Energy Metabolism in Sports Nutrition*; *Nutritional Applications in Exercise and Sport*; *Nutritional Assessment of Athletes*; *Nutritional Ergogenic Aids*; *Sports Nutrition: Energy Metabolism and Exercise*; and the current book *Nutritional Concerns in Recreation, Exercise, and Sport*, all with Judy Driskell. Additionally, he co-edited *Nutritional Concerns of Women*, two editions, with Dorothy Klimis-Zacas, *The Mediterranean Diet: Constituents and Health Promotion* with his Greek colleagues, and *Nutrition in Pharmacy Practice* with Louis Williams. He edited three editions of *Nutrition in Exercise and Sport*. He also served as the editor for the CRC Series on *Nutrition in Exercise and Sport*, the CRC Series on *Modern Nutrition*, the CRC Series on *Methods in Nutrition Research*, and the CRC Series on *Exercise Physiology*.

Contributors

Barry Braun, PhD
Department of Kinesiology
University of Massachusetts
Amherst, Massachusetts

Ellen J. Coleman, MA, MPH, RD, CSSD
The Sport Clinic in Riverside California
Riverside, California

Judy A. Driskell, PhD, RD
Department of Nutrition and Health Sciences
University of Nebraska
Lincoln, Nebraska

Tom J. Hazell, MS
Exercise Nutrition Research Laboratory
The University of Western Ontario
London, Ontario

Douglas S. Kalman, PhD, RD, CCRC, FACN
Miami Research Associates
Miami, Florida

Mark Kern, PhD, RD, CSSD
School of Exercise and Nutritional Sciences
San Diego State University
San Diego, California

Young-Nam Kim, PhD
Department of Nutrition and Health Sciences
University of Nebraska
Lincoln, Nebraska

Susan M. Kleiner, PhD, RD, FACN, CNS, FISSN
High Performance Nutrition
Mercer Island, Washington

Richard B. Kreider, PhD, EPC, FACSM, FASEP, MX, FISSN
Department of Health and Kinesiology
Texas A&M University
College Station, Texas

Peter W.R. Lemon, PhD
Department of Kinesiology
University of Western Ontario
London, Ontario

Chris M. Lockwood, MS
Department of Health and Exercise Science
University of Oklahoma
Norman, Oklahoma

Benjamin F. Miller, PhD
Department of Health and Exercise Science
Colorado State University
Fort Collins, Colorado

Fiona E. Pelly, PhD
School of Health and Sport Sciences
University of the Sunshine Coast
Moroochydore, Queensland, Australia

Peter R.J. Reaburn, BHMS, PhD
Department of Health and Human Performance
Central Queensland University
Rockhampton, Queensland, Australia

Abbie E. Smith, MS, CSCS
Department of Health and Exercise Science
University of Oklahoma
Norman, Oklahoma

Jeffrey R. Stout, PhD, FNSCA, FACSM, FISSN
Department of Health and Exercise Science
University of Oklahoma
Norman, Oklahoma

Sarah E. Tobkin, MS, CSCS
Department of Health and Exercise Science
University of Oklahoma
Norman, Oklahoma

Stella L. Volpe, PhD, RD, LDN, FACSM
Division of Biobehavioral and Health Sciences
University of Pennsylvania School of Nursing
Philadelphia, Pennsylvania

Colin D. Wilborn, PhD, CSCS, ATC
Department of Exercise and Sport Science
University of Mary Hardin-Baylor
Belton, Texas

Ira Wolinsky, PhD
Department of Health and Human Performance
University of Houston
Houston, Texas

1 Energy Requirements

Benjamin F. Miller and Barry Braun

CONTENTS

I. INTRODUCTION

There is an ever-increasing focus on preventing over-nutrition by reducing energy intake in the general population. However, in athletes, a strategy based on simple calorie cutting may be detrimental. Athletes require sufficient energy to maintain muscle mass, sustain metabolic flux, and achieve optimal performance. On the other hand, an energy surplus that raises body fat, even slightly, can impair performance. In response, athletes often tend to underemphasize ("food is just fuel, eat, burn it, get some more") or overemphasize ("each mouthful of food that enters my body must conform to rigid requirements") the importance of nutrition to exercise performance.

Making sound nutritional choices does not guarantee athletic prowess, but consistently making poor choices is almost certainly detrimental, as adequate nutrition is essential to take advantage of the cellular signals put into motion by exercise training.[1] From the 1920s studies on exercise performance by Krogh and Lindhard[2] of high-carbohydrate versus high-fat diets to the 1970s glycogen supercompensation studies of Bergstrom and Hultman[3] to the more recent studies of post-exercise protein feeding on muscle protein synthesis,[4] it is clear that total energy and the macronutrient (i.e., carbohydrate, fat, protein) composition of the diet modulate acute exercise performance and adaptations to training.

The foci of this chapter are understanding how energy is stored and produced, how it is used during exercise, and the variations in energy and macronutrient requirements across sports and environmental conditions. Our goal is to outline these basic principles of energy metabolism and introduce the concepts that will be reviewed in more depth in later chapters.

II. ENERGY BALANCE AND ITS COMPONENTS

A. What Is Energy?

The sun is the ultimate source of all energy required for human life, as its thermonuclear energy is converted to chemical-bond energy in plants and animal tissues. When humans consume plant and animal tissues as food, the energy contained in chemical bonds is liberated and used immediately or stored. Free energy changes from the disruption of chemical bonds are used to perform all the tasks that require energy: e.g., circulating blood, moving ions across membranes, exercise, etc. In a sense, human energy metabolism is similar to an internal combustion engine in which energy substrates (food or gasoline) go in, are combusted, and heat and work are produced. Metabolic energy is expressed in kilocalories (kcal, 1000 calories) in the United States and kilojoules (kJ, 1000 joules) or megajoules (MJ, 1000 kJ = 239 kcal) everywhere else.

Because energy can neither be created nor destroyed, the energy that is not immediately needed from food intake is stored as chemical bonds in triglyceride (fat), glycogen (carbohydrate) and, arguably, skeletal muscle (protein). The human system, as well as the systems of most other taxa, has devised mechanisms to efficiently store energy. The storage of energy frees the body from the demands of continuously adding energy to the system. Changes in storage are primarily reflected, at least over the long term, by increases or decreases in body fat. Of course, in reality, the flow of energy is a bit more complicated.

B. Energy Intake

Total energy intake is made up of contributions from the four energy-yielding macronutrients; carbohydrate, fat, protein, and (optional) ethanol. Each macronutrient has a different energy density (i.e., energy contained per unit weight of the nutrient). Digestible carbohydrates, e.g., simple sugars such as sucrose and fructose, and complex carbohydrates such as starch contain approximately 4 kcal/gram of carbohydrate. Indigestible carbohydrates, i.e., dietary fiber such as cellulose and pectin, do not contain useable energy (not strictly true because intestinal bacteria can partially process these compounds to short-chain fatty acids that can be absorbed and used for energy, but quantitatively, the caloric value is negligible). Dietary fats, mainly composed of triglyceride, are considerably more energy dense, containing on average 9 kcal/gram of fat. Dietary protein contains 5.25 kcal/gram of protein but, after accounting for incomplete digestibility (averaging 92–95%) and inability for humans to extract energy from the amino nitrogen group (0.85 kcal/gram), the useable energy density for protein is 4 kcal/gram. Ethanol (beer, wine, mixed drinks) is not typically a large component of the athlete's habitual diet, but contains 7 kcal/gram and so can be a significant source of dietary energy when consumed in more than limited quantity.

C. Energy Expenditure

Total daily energy expenditure (TDEE) can be roughly divided into three categories: resting metabolic rate (RMR), diet-induced thermogenesis (DIT), and physical activity (PA). Resting metabolism represents the energy demand during sitting or lying down and is used for maintenance of general body functions such as circulation, respiration, brain activity, etc. The RMR is largely determined by skeletal muscle mass, which represents a considerable source of energy demand because of energy consuming processes such as protein synthesis, ionic regulation, and heat generation. For non-athletes, RMR is often the largest component of energy expenditure (more than 50%), but for athletes in hard training, RMR may represent less than 1/3 of TDEE. This is not to say that RMR in non-athletes exceeds that of athletes though, as athletes have a higher mass-specific RMR.[5]

Diet-induced thermogenesis represents the cost of processing and storing nutrients and depends mainly on energy intake. Because DIT is difficult to measure reliably in humans, it is usually estimated as representing 10% of TDEE. This expenditure can vary somewhat with the macronutrient composition of the diet, with diets high in protein increasing the DIT above 10% whereas diets high in fat lower it. Even with these slight variations, DIT is the lowest contributor to TDEE.

Physical activity traditionally represents energy expenditure attributed to voluntary movement and is the most variable component of TDEE. Physical activity increases energy expenditure because, among other things, there are energy costs associated with actin/myosin cross-bridge cycling, ion pumping, hormone synthesis, etc. Of note is a relatively new concept termed non-exercise activity thermogenesis

(NEAT), which has been coined to include very low intensity activity like fidgeting or simple standing, and is incorporated into measurements of physical activity.[6]

III. HOW TO ASSESS INTAKE AND EXPENDITURE IN ATHLETES

It is possible to make calculations of the amount of energy needed to perform a bout of work. This can be on a scale as small as the number of adenosine-5′-triphosphate (ATP) needed for twitch activity or the amount of work performed over a 30-second test of maximal bicycling capacity. For longer time periods, the measurement of oxygen consumption (VO_2), known as indirect calorimetry, is a convenient tool for making lab-based measurements of energy demand. These studies are most frequently performed at rest or during steady-state exercise over a defined period of time. Assuming energy is derived from oxidation of carbohydrate and fat in about a 50:50 ratio, for every kJ of aerobic energy production, approximately 50 mL of oxygen is required (or 20.2 kJ/L). Therefore, multiplying VO_2 (L/min) by the energy equivalent of oxygen (20.2 kJ/L) will provide a reasonable estimate of the rate of energy expenditure (kJ/min). By measuring both O_2 consumption and CO_2 production (VCO_2) respiratory exchange ratio ((RER) = VCO_2/VO_2) can be calculated. This calculation allows for more accurate measurements of the proportion of carbohydrate and fat (ignores protein) being used as fuels at that time. A ratio near 0.8 indicates primarily fat oxidation, while a ratio near 1.0 indicates primarily carbohydrate oxidation. Obvious limitations of indirect calorimetry are that it can account only for aerobic energy production and ignores non-aerobic energy production, measurements are generally confined to a laboratory environment (although the accuracy of smaller units that can be used in the field is improving), and long-term measurements (anything longer than a few hours) of energy consumption are not practical. Measurements of energy expenditure up to about 24 hours can be made using room calorimeters in the few facilities where they are available.

For longer assessment (days to weeks), the doubly labeled water technique is the gold standard. The method is expensive, but getting cheaper, and easy to administer. Subjects drink what looks to be an ordinary glass of water that contains known amounts of a stable isotopic "label" on both the hydrogen and oxygen. The labeled hydrogen equilibrates with the body water pool only, while the labeled oxygen equilibrates with the body water pool and CO_2. Knowing the initial dose of the labels, and measuring the difference in the excretion rates in the body water pool between the two labels, one can calculate the excretion rate of the unmeasured CO_2 pool. Knowing CO_2 production and estimating VCO_2/VO_2 from the composition of the habitual diet (food quotient, FQ), energy expenditure can be calculated. The biggest advantage of this technique is that subjects can be free living, with only a couple of urine samples needed after the initial consumption of the water.

Finally, for truly long-term measures (weeks to years), changes in dietary intake and body weight can estimate energy demand. This measurement is based on the First Law of Thermodynamics. When dietary energy intake exceeds energy expenditure, the excess energy will be stored. Over time, energy storage equates to greater body weight. So, by this relatively crude, but reliable and valid, form of energy expenditure assessment, weight gain means that energy intake is exceeding energy demands and weight loss means that energy intake is insufficient for energy demands.

IV. CHALLENGES OF MATCHING SUPPLY WITH DEMAND

A. Matching ATP Production with ATP Requirements

Matching energy supply to energy demand requires several components:

1. A way to assess energy stores and send that information out to the rest of the body
2. A processing center to integrate information and direct an appropriate response
3. Systems to change intake and expenditure in the appropriate directions
4. A signal to the processing center reflecting the new state

In meeting the need to match energy supply to energy demand, relevant time spans can range from seconds to years (Figure 1.1). On the period of seconds, limited stores of ATP and phosphocreatine (PCr) are taxed and must be replenished as other energy producing pathways are activated. Progressing further, exercise bouts of 5 min, 30 min, 1 hr, 4 hr, and 8 hr will all have different supply and demand considerations due to finite energy stores. Finally, over the periods of days, weeks, and years, the matching of supply and demand is dependent on habitual physical activity patterns and dietary habits.

During hard exercise, energy demand can increase by more than 20-fold over the resting metabolism of about 4.2 kJ/min (1 kcal/min), or roughly equivalent to a 100W light bulb. Neural, biochemical and hormonal changes that accompany (and even precede) muscle contraction are signals for the change in demand, and energy provision is initiated. For example, the rapid increase in inorganic phosphate (Pi) and ADP in the muscle increases the activity of creatine kinase (CK) to regenerate ATP

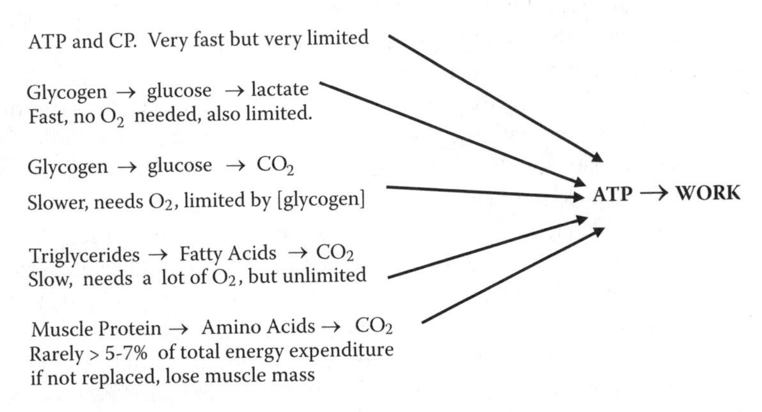

FIGURE 1.1 Schematic drawing showing highlights of the systems used to generate the ATP required to accomplish cellular work.

from PCr hydrolysis and also accelerates glycolysis. Simultaneously, activation of the sympathetic nervous system and an increase in blood catecholamines (flight-or-fight response) cause glycogen breakdown in muscle and liver as well as triglyceride breakdown in adipose tissue (and maybe intramuscular triglycerides). So, stored carbohydrate and fat are catabolized to increase the available pool of glucose and fatty acids. A key point is that the matching of supply to demand is almost instantaneous in terms of the magnitude of the response (i.e., there is excellent matching between the kJ required and the kJ provided) but the blend of energy sources is skewed toward the rapidly activated "local" sources in the first few minutes of exercise. Much of the energy early in exercise is derived from PCr and muscle glycogen in order to meet the energetic needs while the other systems are "titrated" into play. As exercise continues, the supply of glucose derived from glycogen, blood glucose, adipose-derived fatty acids, intramyocellular fatty acids, and amino acids is continually changing to meet demand. The precise regulation of these interconnected pathways is a topic of much research and certainly has implications for pre-, during, and post-exercise nutritional strategies.

B. Exercise Intensity and Duration

No discussion of the consequences of a mismatch between energy supply and demand is fruitful without considering the appropriate time scale. During very high intensity exercise, the rapid demand for ATP may exceed the ability to resynthesize it from PCr, which can be depleted rapidly (within seconds). Thereafter, the stores have to recover during rest periods or a transition to less intense aerobic exercise for replenishment. PCr storage has been demonstrated to respond favorably to supplementation and the increase in storage can enhance high-intensity exercise performance,[7,8] which in itself is indirect evidence that PCr stores are limiting in short-duration intense activity. During steady-state exercise, resynthesis of ATP between contractions by PCr, glycolysis and oxidative phosphorylation of carbohydrate and fat is usually adequate to keep intracellular ATP concentration from dropping. During very prolonged steady-state exercise, the capacity to completely recycle ATP between contractions can be compromised and ATP concentrations begin to fall. The fall in ATP has been associated with fatigue and inability to maintain exercise performance, however, the idea that fatigue is "caused" by a fall in cellular ATP concentration is a dramatic oversimplification of the complex process of fatigue. Nonetheless, it is clear that an inability to match demand with the appropriate supply will force the individual to reduce exercise intensity to a level that can be sustained with the available energy supply, or even to stop exercise entirely.

The substrates for anaerobic glycolysis are blood glucose and muscle glycogen. Although in most cases blood glucose can be sustained by liver glycogenolysis and gluconeogenesis, muscle glycogen supply is limiting to exercise performance. Like PCr, glycogen satisfies the criteria for being considered limited in supply; exercise in a glycogen-depleted state will decrease exercise performance, whereas increasing glycogen concentration (supercompensation) will usually enhance exercise performance. Exactly why fatigue is so closely associated with low muscle glycogen is not entirely clear because complete glycogen depletion is not observed even when study subjects fatigue and can no longer maintain exercise.[9] Speculation exists that some minimal concentration of glycogen is "protected" and resistant to use during exercise, perhaps to ensure that some fuel is spared in case of dire necessity (e.g., to keep from becoming dinner as in our primitive ancestors' case).

The recent work by Schulman and colleagues suggesting that glucose entering the muscle cell is incorporated into glycogen before being shunted into glycolysis, especially when glycogen stores are low,[10] supports but does not prove that theory. Also, it is possible that the spatial arrangement of glycogen is important in that there is local depletion of stores or mechanical disruption of sarcoplasmic reticulum calcium cycling.[11] The close connection between glycogen stores and exercise performance has made carbohydrate supplementation before, during, and after exercise one of the best studied areas of exercise nutrition. In addition, the role of glycogen depletion in exercise performance has crossed into new areas such as energy sensing,[12] cellular signaling,[13] and training-induced adaptations.[14]

For all practical purposes fat supply is never limiting to exercise demand. An extremely large supply of fat energy is stored in the body, even in very lean people (e.g., a person weighing 50 kg with 10% body fat has more than 40,000 kcal of stored fat energy), and the capacity for working muscles to derive energy from fat during exercise at more than low-moderate intensity is limited. There has been great interest in trying to "train" the athlete to rely more on fat energy by feeding high-fat diets to increase the enzymes required for fat oxidation. While it is possible to induce some of the appropriate metabolic adaptations that increase fat utilization, these interventions do not enhance exercise performance.[15] Thus, as opposed to PCr and glycogen, fat supply does not deplete. Rather, it is the capacity to use fat that is limiting, not the supply itself, and supplementation does not improve exercise capacity.

C. Multiple Bouts of Exercise

The matching of energy intake and expenditure is especially relevant to performance in an event requiring extremely high energy outputs extended over multiple days or weeks, such as the Tour de France bicycle race. Researchers from Holland performed the first measurements of energy intake and output during that race.[16,17] The cyclists in their research group consumed 24.7 MJ/day (5,900 cal/day), with the highest average value for a single day being 32.4 MJ (7,750 kcal). On average, the cyclists expended 29.4–36.0 MJ/day (7020–8600 cal/day). In other words, energy expenditure roughly matched energy intake even though energy expenditure was 3.6–5.3 times the resting metabolic rate. A report by Kirkwood demonstrated that across mammals and birds the maximum possible sustainable energy expenditure was 4–5 times RMR.[18] Therefore, these cyclists at the Tour de France were operating right at the proposed maximum energy expenditure. An intriguing question then emerges as to whether food intake is limiting to exercise performance in such an event. In other words, it may just be extremely difficult to eat more than 30 MJ/day and therefore, the upper limit to sustainable energy expenditure is 30 MJ/day. Recently, there was an effort in another 3-week cycling race, the Vuelta a España, to shorten stages to make such races more humane and to discourage doping. Rather than take advantage of the "easier" conditions, the riders simply rode faster over the shorter courses.[19] Therefore, even though the stage race was shorter in distance, the athletes were expending the same amount of energy as a longer-distanced stage race. It may be that these athletes are capable of pushing themselves to the physiological limits of energy expenditure no matter how long or short the event is. Further, since the ability to produce energy day after day is dependent on being able to get that energy back into the system, it may be that physiological performance at a race is limited by how much food can be properly eaten and digested.

D. Quantity vs. Quality of Energy Requirements

A final point regarding the matching of the supply and demand during an acute bout of exercise distinguishes between the quantity and quality of fuels. The consequences of mismatching the *quantity* of energy required results in fatigue, or the inability to maintain the desired force output. On the other hand, the consequences of mismatching the *quality* of the energy required are more subtle. For example, too much carbohydrate utilization will allow maintenance of high exercise intensity but will cause rapid glycogen depletion and fatigue. Too little carbohydrate utilization will spare precious glycogen reserves but, by forcing greater reliance on fatty acid oxidation, will constrain exercise to a relatively low intensity. Therefore, the body systems designed to sense, integrate, and deliver the appropriate energy to match demand must be sensitive to the quality of the energy required as well as the quantity.

E. Long-Term Mismatch of Energy Supply and Demand

1. Excessive Intake Relative to Demand (Energy Surplus)

Energy supply can be mismatched to demand with no acute loss of function, but over the long term (days/weeks/months) there are deleterious consequences on body composition and exercise performance. Excess energy intake or deficient energy expenditure results in an energy surplus. Energy surplus, extended over weeks or months, leads to a gain of body mass, which inhibits performance of most exercise tasks. Decrements in exercise performance will be especially profound if the excess mass is stored as adipose tissue, because this tissue does not directly contribute to mechanical work.

2. Insufficient Intake Relative to Demand (Energy Deficit)

Chronic energy shortage has profound effects on exercise performance in many different ways. An important advancement in this area is the distinction between inadequate energy intake as opposed to high energy expenditure. Based on pioneering work by Anne Loucks and others,[20,21] the cluster of symptoms (disordered eating, amenorrhea, low bone mineral density) that are often described as the "female athlete triad" is now believed to be more closely related to energy shortage rather than to excess training or low body fat.[20] It has also been observed that chronic energy deficit can alter hormone profiles,[21] cause loss of muscle mass,[22] and change substrate oxidation patterns.[23]

V. ENERGY DEFICIT FOR WEIGHT LOSS

In most cases, a desirable outcome is selective loss of body fat while maintaining (or when possible, even increasing) muscle mass. Without using illegal performance enhancing agents such as anabolic steroids and (possibly) human growth hormone, the ability to concurrently lose body fat and gain muscle mass in trained athletes is a "holy grail" that is rarely attainable. As has known for decades, energy deficit leading to fat loss almost unavoidably causes at least some loss of lean tissue. The challenge is to combine diet and training to maximize fat loss while minimizing concurrent loss of lean tissue. Continued high levels of physical activity are important because whether the energy deficit is induced solely by decreased caloric intake or by increased energy expenditure may have functional consequences. Caloric restriction in the absence of physical activity lowers all three components of TDEE. Therefore, all three components of TDEE respond to caloric restriction in a direction that conserves expended energy and minimizes fat loss:

	RMR	+ DIT	+ PA	= TDEE
Caloric restriction energy deficit:	↓	↓	↓	↓↓

Severe restriction of total energy intake or carbohydrate increases the need to use functional protein stores to provide the carbon skeletons for glucose production and to maintain the capacity for oxidative energy production. In addition, protein synthesis is an energetically expensive process requiring the highest proportion of RMR[24] and, in times of negative energy balance, skeletal muscle protein synthesis is compromised. Therefore, low-energy diets (e.g., > 1000 kcal less than required for weight maintenance) induce rapid weight loss but greatly increase the catabolism of skeletal muscle protein for energy, causing an undesirable loss of lean tissue.

Instead of caloric restriction, energy deficit can also be induced by maintaining caloric intake and increasing energy expended by PA (exercise). Since exercise with amino acid provision helps preserve lean tissue mass, RMR may not decline, and may even increase, if there is a significant change in body composition. Since DIT is primarily determined by caloric intake, energy expended by DIT should not decrease if energy intake is not restricted. Therefore, a weight management program based on increasing energy expenditure by PA could result in a strikingly different pattern of changes to TDEE that are more likely to promote selective loss of body weight as fat and also facilitate continued weight loss:

	RMR	+ DIT	+ PA	= TDEE
Exercise energy deficit:	↔	↔	↑	↑

The response to exercise-induced energy deficit may be mediated by an endocrine response different from that observed with caloric restriction. How exercise-induced energy deficit impacts endocrine signals has not been systematically studied. In addition, sex differences in the neuroendocrine response to exercise training have been noted in rodents.[25] Data from human and animal studies indeed suggest that increased physical activity, with *ad libitum* feeding, causes loss of body weight in males but not in females.[26,27] Whether this is a true sex difference or an artifact of experimental design (to maintain the same relative exercise energy expenditure, women expend fewer absolute kJ in the training intervention because they tend to have lower baseline daily energy expenditure) remains to be elucidated.

VI. DOES IT MATTER WHEN YOU CONSUME YOUR ENERGY?

A. Acutely (Day of Competition or during Competition)

If one considers endurance exercise of more than an hour in length, timing of energy intake before, during, and after exercise can influence exercise performance. In elite endurance athletes, exercise bouts as long as a marathon are dependent almost exclusively on carbohydrate metabolism.[28] Thus, carbohydrate supplementation is of primary importance for sustaining energy over a bout of exercise, with fat and protein supplementation being less important.

An overnight fast is sufficient to deplete the liver of glycogen. Therefore, it is generally a good idea for one to replete liver (and to a lesser extent, muscle) glycogen in the period before exercise. There has been some discussion of whether consuming a carbohydrate source with a high glycemic index may inhibit exercise performance because of the resultant spike in insulin. However, it seems as though the metabolic effects of exercise overwhelm those of a transient insulin increase, so there is no detriment to exercise performance.[29]

During exercise, supplementation with carbohydrate helps maintain blood glucose concentrations and decreases muscle glycogen use. Provision of exogenous glucose increases the oxidation of exogenous carbohydrate, thus decreasing oxidation of endogenous stores. The rates of exogenous carbohydrate oxidation can exceed 1.3 g/min, which requires a substantial carbohydrate intake of 1.8 g/min.[30] For practical purposes, it is unlikely that an individual will be able to exceed maximum exogenous oxidation rates, so the more carbohydrate an athlete can consume during a prolonged exercise bout, the better.

The timing of carbohydrate intake after exercise impacts the time course of glycogen repletion in athletes. When carbohydrate is given immediately post-exercise, glycogen resynthesis is more rapid than when carbohydrate feeding is delayed by 2 hours.[31] These and other data suggest that glycogen resynthesis is most effective immediately post-exercise (coincides with maximal activation of enzymes involved in glycogen synthesis) and that delaying carbohydrate feeding may result in less complete glycogen resynthesis. Delaying carbohydrate feeding, however, apparently has no effect on glycogen concentration when measured after longer time frames (e.g., 24 hours post-exercise) despite the slower initial rate of resynthesis.[31,32]

In addition to differences in glycogen resynthesis rates observed with delayed carbohydrate/energy refeeding, meal timing also likely influences the substrate and hormonal environment, which may have an impact on the magnitude and persistence of post-exercise metabolic adaptations. In the aforementioned study by Ivy et al.,[31] when carbohydrate feeding was delayed 2 hours post-exercise, blood glucose concentrations remained elevated longer and insulin concentrations were slower to rise and slower to decrease than with immediate post-exercise carbohydrate feeding. Stephens et al. noted that, although there was no difference in the rate at which glucose was taken up by muscle, more of the glucose was shunted to storage (i.e., glycogen storage) rather than oxidation when a meal was consumed immediately post-exercise as compared with before exercise or 3 hours after exercise.[33]

To reiterate, a discussion of the acute effects of energy feeding is really a discussion of carbohydrate feeding. An exercise bout less than 45 minutes is unlikely to deplete energy stores,[30] while exercise longer than 45 minutes may be limited by glycogen stores, but not by fat stores, diminishing fat's importance in acute feeding. Finally, although post-exercise protein nutrition is important for anabolic processes, provision of amino acids is generally not important for energy metabolism.

B. Chronically

Theoretically, certain eating patterns over time could affect the storage or utilization of energy. For instance, circadian hormone release could direct food consumed early in the day toward oxidation while the same food consumed later in the day could be directed toward storage. Likely mediators of these effects could be gut peptides such as leptin or glucagon-peptide-1 (GLP-1), or other metabolic mediators such as thyroxin or insulin. When regulating weight, lay advice is to not consume food before going to bed because it will be directed to storage. Insight into eating before bed can be gained from a condition termed "night-eating syndrome" in which individuals eat little in the morning and consume the greatest portion of their calories (greater than 50%) after the evening meal, and even through the night. While studying this condition it has been determined that there is no association between those who eat the majority of their calories at night and weight gain.[34] Further, it seems as though the body can buffer changes in meal timing if a person is on an abnormal circadian rhythm (e.g., shift workers).[35] However, an important point is that in these studies the subjects were otherwise in energy balance. Therefore, if one maintains energy balance, *when* the food is consumed will have little effect on weight gain over time. Finally, it is worth mentioning again that athletes managing body composition during periods of heavy training should concentrate their nutrient intake, including energy, during and around the training bout because of other anabolic factors.

VII. RANGE OF INTAKES IN VARIOUS SPORT SITUATIONS

For a discussion of energy expenditure, it is useful to consider an American football offensive lineman, a gymnast, and an ultra marathoner. For an offensive lineman, the requirements for a high absolute power output and to offer considerable resistance to movement by external forces make it advantageous to maintain a large muscle mass. Because of this, this athlete will have prodigious resting energy expenditure. Given the intermittent nature of his training (practice or weight lifting) and competition, the energy expenditure due to activity will be less significant than resting energy expenditure. This athlete can consume large amounts of energy because it is balanced by his huge resting energy expenditure, and the fact that excess mass will not have negative consequences. For a gymnast, a large muscle mass is advantageous, but excess mass is not. A gymnast will also have high resting energy expenditure due to a large lean body mass, although not nearly as high as the offensive lineman. Again, given the intermittent nature of a gymnast's activity, energy expenditure due to physical activity will probably not equal resting energy expenditure. This athlete will have to closely monitor energy intake and expenditure since there is a negative consequence for any added mass that is not working skeletal muscle. Finally, an ultra marathoner must maintain a low lean mass, because any excess mass, even skeletal muscle, is a clear disadvantage in the sport. In this situation, where prolonged aerobic exercise requires considerable energy output, energy expenditure due to physical activity will likely exceed resting energy expenditure (although the low body fat in marathon runners causes them to have a higher resting energy expenditure than a comparably sized sedentary individual).

Exercise increases total energy needs due to a rise in the PA component of TDEE. As discussed above, competitive events such as the Tour de France put huge demands on energy intake. Insight regarding the energy demands in a variety of sports was obtained by using 4- to 7-day diet records in Dutch athletes.[36] Average dietary intake varied from 110 kJ/kg/day (26 kcal/kg/day) in female body builders and 157 kJ/kg/day (38 kcal/kg/day) in female top-level gymnasts to 272 kJ/kg/day (65 kcal/kg/day) in male triathletes and 347 kJ/kg/day (83 kcal/kg/day) in Tour de France cyclists. In general, sports that emphasized aesthetics had the lowest intake, team sports were intermediate, and endurance sports the highest. It is important to note, however, that these were reported intakes and were not confirmed by objective assessment of energy expenditure. From these data, it is apparent that energy intake for aesthetic-type athletes is far below the 9.6–13.0 MJ/day (2300–3100 kcal/d) recommended for a healthy adult. Conversely, a single day in the Tour de France bike race can have an energy expenditure of close to 37.5 MJ (9,000 kcal),[17] or three to four times average energy intake.

Better methods to assess energy expenditure (e.g., doubly labeled water) allow a more complete record of the energy expenditure involved in a variety of activities. Recent publications have demonstrated energy expenditures of 14.7 MJ/day (3500 kcal/day) in soccer players,[37] 14.7 MJ/day (3500 kcal/day) in elite Kenyan runners,[38] 16.5 MJ/day (3950 kcal/day) in female lightweight rowers,[39] 19.2 MJ/day (4600 kcal/day) and 20.5 MJ/day (4900 kcal/day) for forest-wildfire suppression,[40] and 23.5 MJ/day (5600 kcal/day) in elite female swimmers.[41] It is interesting that when self-reported energy intakes are compared with energy outputs calculated from doubly labeled water, it appears that many of these athletes should be in energy deficit. Although it may be true that some athletes maintain a chronic energy deficit, it is also likely that some athletes are underreporting actual dietary intake. A recent report on elite Kenyan runners indicates that in the period leading up to competition, these athletes may indeed be in a negative energy balance.[38] Support for the latter possibility comes from the variety of sources showing that underreporting intake is common in nutritional surveys. As doubly labeled water measurements and carefully controlled studies of dietary intake become more feasible, we should achieve a better understanding of energy status (deficit, balance, surplus) in different physical activities.

VIII. ENERGY EFFICIENCY

A. Do Athletes Become More Energetically Efficient?

There is a notion that athletes become more "energetically efficient" with training. Whether this is true depends on the definition of the term. Typically, efficiency is defined as gross efficiency, which equals work accomplished divided by energy expended; net efficiency, which subtracts out resting energy expenditure from energy expended; or delta efficiency, which is the change in work divided by the change in energy expended. It is generally accepted that trained runners have a greater efficiency than their novice counterparts. That is, a highly trained runner will require less oxygen consumption at a given running speed (termed economy) than their novice counterparts. Interestingly, this does not seem to be the case in cycling.[42] However, if the idea that cycling efficiency does not change has been challenged by a case study in a Tour de France champion that reports that changes in performance were due to changes in efficiency with a potential fiber type transition.[43]

When discussing energy efficiency, the quantity and quality of mitochondria is also important. Indeed, it has been known for some time that endurance exercise training increases mitochondria density[44] and that this is one of the primary adaptations of endurance exercise training. An increase in mitochondria quantity leads to an increase in efficiency of energy production (less glycolytic, more aerobic) and perhaps an increase use of fat as a substrate. However, strictly speaking, carbohydrate is still a more oxygen-efficient fuel source, and at a given relative exercise intensity carbohydrate is used in the same percentage whether trained or untrained.[45] Regarding the quality of mitochondria, it has been demonstrated that an endurance exercise-training program can increase State 3 respiration (ADP-stimulated), but not the ratio of inorganic phosphate to oxygen (P/O ratio).[46] Therefore, although mitochondrial respiratory capacity increases, efficiency at the level of the electron transport chain does not.

B. Is There a Conservation of Energy?

If an athlete is in a prolonged energy deficit, energy-conserving mechanisms may result. These mechanisms are likely detrimental to performance because anabolic and repair mechanisms are down regulated. The preponderance of data related to the area of energy conservation has been collected in previously overweight or obese subjects losing weight (see Hill[47]) and indicates that the body tries to protect a set weight in the face of negative energy balance. How these concepts apply to athletes is not well explored. However, it is apparent that exercise-associated menstrual disorders related to the female athlete triad may indeed stem from energy conserving mechanisms.[48] An evolutionary perspective helps put these energy-conserving mechanisms in context.

An individual has limited energy that can be directed toward two main processes, reproduction and somatic repair. If one has a shortage of energy, indicating a period of low energy availability, reproduction is often compromised because the conditions are not right for child bearing. Instead, the individual invests available energy into somatic repair to help maintain a healthy body until conditions are again ready for reproduction. This framework has been used to explain why lifelong caloric restriction increases life span.[49] Although this serves well to explain why prolonged negative energy balance may cause menstrual disorders, whether negative energy balance actually increases somatic repair is still a contentious issue.

IX. ENVIRONMENTAL FACTORS AND SPECIAL POPULATIONS

A. Altitude

In response to hypoxia, a shift in substrate use to favor greater dependency on glucose and less utilization of lipid has been reported in a variety of experimental models.[50,51] In young men, both whole-body and leg glucose uptake rose sharply upon acute exposure to hypobaric hypoxia (4300 meters on Pikes Peak in Colorado) and remained elevated above sea level values even after 18 days of acclimatization.[51] In other studies, however, exposure to hypobaric hypoxia has not resulted in a greater dependency on glucose. In one of the first studies to systematically evaluate substrate utilization at high altitude, Young et al. reported the opposite, i.e., reduced dependence on carbohydrate and greater use of fat after several weeks' acclimatization.[52] The discrepancy between these results and those from Brooks and colleagues is likely a result of different energy states. Depressed energy intake and elevated resting metabolism, both common responses to hypobaric hypoxia, cause energy deficit and weight loss.[53] A shift to more fat utilization and muscle glycogen conservation are typical responses to energy deficit. In contrast, energy balance was maintained and weight loss prevented in the studies by Brooks and colleagues to deliberately isolate the impact of hypoxia from energy deficit.[51] The fact that energy deficit can obscure the effects of "true" hypoxia suggests that it is a more potent metabolic stimulus. Taken together, these data have led to novel research directly testing the independent effects of hypoxia and energy deficit[54] and also provided key insights that inform practical recommendations for nutrition at altitude.

B. Climate

Several environmental factors also change fuel preferences. It is often the case that with a new Olympic cycle, a new environmental factor gets increased attention. Before the high altitude of Mexico City, research on exercise at altitude was popular, whereas the Sydney and Athens games stimulated research on exercise in the heat. In general, exercise in both heat and cold increases glycogen use.[55] A legitimate concern for the 2008 Olympics in Beijing was air quality. Although it is not clear whether air pollutants alter substrate use, it is possible that medications used to treat asthma, such as Clenbuterol, do change fuel preference.[56]

C. Masters Athlete

Although there is a steady physiological decline with aging, chronic exercisers maintain higher function throughout their lifespan. For example, life-long exercise training does not attenuate the rate of decrease of such performance variables as VO_2max, but life-long exercisers maintain a higher VO_2max across ages.[57] Therefore, masters athletes maintain a higher capacity to use energy. It appears that for running, masters athletes do not decrease exercise economy when compared with young individuals[58] and this is likely due in part to the fact that muscle fiber type changes little in older athletes compared with young.[59] At the level of the mitochondria, masters runners can have enzyme activities that exceed young runners,[60] thus maintaining mitochondrial efficiency. Finally, a recent study in older, lifelong exercisers (at least 25 years of training) indicated that at a given relative exercise intensity, the lifelong exercisers used more fat for oxidation than their sedentary counterparts.[61] This finding is in contrast to short-term training programs in younger individuals that do not shift substrate preference at a given relative intensity. Perhaps this shift in fuel preference is unique to lifelong training.

D. Diabetic Athlete

People with diabetes have successfully competed at the highest level in sport, and in many cases, like Gary Hall, Jr., an Olympic gold medalist in swimming, have succeeded. How people manage exercise and diabetes is dependent on whether they are insulin dependent (IDDM) or non-insulin dependent (NIDDM). It has been demonstrated that when compared to control subjects, individuals with IDDM use slightly more fat as a fuel source during moderate intensity exercise, but use similar fuels during high intensity exercise.[62] Conversely, in NIDDM, there seems to be a shift to a greater reliance on carbohydrate metabolism at any given exercise intensity when subjects are compared with age-, weight-, and activity-matched control subjects.[63] Mitochondrial abnormalities and their contribution to or causation of NIDDM is a hot topic in metabolism.[64] It has been demonstrated that mitochondrial efficiency is decreased in diabetics,[65] although this has recently been challenged.[66] Importantly, these studies were done in obese NIDDM subjects. However, it has been demonstrated that this mitochondrial deficiency can be restored to normal levels with exercise training,[67] indicating that energy production should not be impaired in those with diabetes undergoing regular exercise training. An important point of consideration is that the majority of studies performed in those with well-controlled diabetes are in those with controlled diabetes. Certainly the diabetic athlete has to take preventive measures to ensure controlled glucose concentrations during exercise training, something that regular exercise training may actually improve.

E. Sex Differences

For many years, all of the examples used in the field of exercise metabolism were based on observations from the standard 70-kg male. With increased participation of women in sport through Title IX and The Women's Health Equity Act of the 1990s, physiologists and biochemists began to investigate sex-based differences in women and men. Presumably because the experiments were initially done on men, femaleness (and the physiological effects of the ovarian hormones estrogen and progesterone) is still treated as the "experimental" condition and males the "control." Most well-controlled studies show that at any given relative exercise intensity, men oxidize more carbohydrate and less fat than do women.[27,68] It appears that the differences between the patterns of relative fuel use in men and women are due to circulating female hormones rather than male hormones or the relatively greater proportion of type I fibers in women than men.[26,27,69]

IX. FUTURE RESEARCH NEEDS

As discussed, a great number of studies have quantifed the energetic needs of various sports, including both acute bouts of exercise and short-term training or competition. However, these measurements have been in sports that are amenable to the laboratory setting. Obtaining good field-based measurements of energy expenditure is still relatively difficult. And, although the doubly labeled water technique has provided some insight, it still remains a relatively blunt tool by measuring accumulated changes that do not account for the different components of energy expenditure. Similarly, the second component of energy balance, energy intake, is limited by the accuracy of self-report, or in limited publications, weighed-diet records. Even when weighed-diet records are employed, one should consider the influence the recording process has on "real" intake. Therefore, there still remains a need for quantifying the actual energy intake and use of real athletes. The development of "nanotechnology" may significantly advance field-based measurement of energy flux.

In addition, it is now apparent that cells respond to energetic signals. Changes in ATP, or more accurately the ratio of adenosine monophosphate (AMP) to ATP, can initiate adaptive changes in the cell.[70] An important next step is to determine how the athlete can design his or her training to maximize the positive adaptive responses of this pathway or others. One interesting study design has subjects exercising in the glycogen-depleted versus glycogen-replete state.[14,71] The findings from these studies will certainly stimulate more studies exploring the cellular signals of sport adaptation.

Finally, scientists must go beyond describing what athletes do and continue to question established paradigms of exercise training by introducing novel strategies. For example, recent studies document similar endurance-training adaptations from multiple high-intensity exercise bouts as from prolonged submaximum exercise.[72] These studies challenge the long-held notion that long-duration exercise is needed for increased aerobic exercise performance. However, these studies also open an opportunity to examine how one might address issues of energy balance when performing such a small absolute volume of exercise.

X. CONCLUSIONS

Complex biologic systems monitor energy demand and meet that demand by precisely releasing stored energy in the appropriate quantity and "quality" (blend of fuel sources). These mechanisms adhere to the basic principles of thermodynamics and function to preserve the top metabolic priorities: providing glucose for the central nervous system, maintaining adequate muscle glycogen stores to facilitate physical activity required to catch (or avoid becoming) dinner, and storing sufficient energy to survive periods of extended fasting. Athletes and other active individuals must conform to the same physical laws, but test the boundaries of the metabolic systems because of their high energy and carbohydrate flux, obligating considerably higher rates of energy and carbohydrate replacement.

Energy requirements vary by sport, age, and environmental conditions. In addition, the components of energy expenditure can vary as well, depending on body composition or training volume. It is difficult to consider energy requirements in isolation without considering macronutrient intake. Those athletes wishing to maintain or decrease weight must balance macronutrient requirements within the confines of energy balance, while those wishing to gain weight must do so with macronutrient intakes that lead to the accretion of muscle rather than metabolically inactive tissue. Although a good number have described what athletes do, more studies must continue to determine how one might take advantage of the signaling put in motion in response to energetic and macronutrient manipulation. These key discoveries will enable sport nutritionists to craft optimal dietary strategies that maximize athletic performance.

REFERENCES

1. Miller, B. F., Human muscle protein synthesis after physical activity and feeding, *Exerc Sport Sci Rev* 2007, 35, (2), 50–5.
2. Krogh, A., Lindhard, J., The relative value of fat and carbohydrate as sources of muscular energy: With appendices on the correlation between standard metabolism and the respiratory quotient during rest and work, *Biochem J* 1920, 14, (3–4), 290–363.
3. Bergstrom, J., Hermansen, L., Hultman, E., Saltin, B., Diet, muscle glycogen and physical performance, *Acta Physiol Scand* 1967, 71, (2), 140–50.
4. Tipton, K. D., Ferrando, A. A., Phillips, S. M., Doyle, D. Jr., Wolfe, R. R., Postexercise net protein synthesis in human muscle from orally administered amino acids, *Am J Physiol* 1999, 276, (4 Pt 1), E628–34.
5. Bell, C., Seals, D. R., Monroe, M. B., Day, D. S., Shapiro, L. F., Johnson, D. G. Jones, P. P., Tonic sympathetic support of metabolic rate is attenuated with age, sedentary lifestyle, and female sex in healthy adults, *J Clin Endocrinol Metab* 2001, 86, (9), 4440–4.
6. Zderic, T. W., Hamilton, M. T., Physical inactivity amplifies the sensitivity of skeletal muscle to the lipid-induced downregulation of lipoprotein lipase activity, *J Appl Physiol* 2006, 100, (1), 249–257.
7. Harris, R. C., Soderlund, K., Hultman, E., Elevation of creatine in resting and exercised muscle of normal subjects by creatine supplementation, *Clin Sci (Lond)* 1992, 83, (3), 367–74.
8. Greenhaff, P. L., Casey, A., Short, A. H., Harris, R., Soderlund, K., Hultman, E., Influence of oral creatine supplementation of muscle torque during repeated bouts of maximal voluntary exercise in man, *Clin Sci (Lond)* 1993, 84, (5), 565–71.
9. Bergstrom, J., Hultman, E., Synthesis of muscle glycogen in man after glucose and fructose infusion, *Acta Med Scand* 1967, 182, (1), 93–107.
10. Shulman, R. G., Glycogen turnover forms lactate during exercise, *Exerc Sport Sci Rev* 2005, 33, (4), 157–62.
11. Duhamel, T. A., Perco, J. G., Green, H. J., Manipulation of dietary carbohydrates after prolonged effort modifies muscle sarcoplasmic reticulum responses in exercising males, *Am J Physiol Regul Integr Comp Physiol* 2006, 291, (4), R1100–1110.
12. Rauch, H. G., St. Clair Gibson, A., Lambert, E. V., Noakes, T. D., A signalling role for muscle glycogen in the regulation of pace during prolonged exercise, *Br J Sports Med* 2005, 39, (1), 34–8.

13. Wojtaszewski, J. F., MacDonald, C., Nielsen, J. N., Hellsten, Y., Hardie, D. G., Kemp, B. E., et al., Regulation of 5'AMP-activated protein kinase activity and substrate utilization in exercising human skeletal muscle, *Am J Physiol Endocrinol Metab* 2003, 284, (4), E813–22.
14. Hansen, A. K., Fischer, C. P., Plomgaard, P., Andersen, J. L., Saltin, B., Pedersen, B. K., Skeletal muscle adaptation: Training twice every second day vs. training once daily, *J Appl Physiol* 2005, 98, (1), 93–9.
15. Burke, L. M., Kiens, B., "Fat adaptation" for athletic performance: The nail in the coffin? *J Appl Physiol* 2006, 100, (1), 7–8.
16. Westerterp, K. R., Saris, W. H., van Es, M., ten Hoor, F., Use of the doubly labeled water technique in humans during heavy sustained exercise, *J Appl Physiol* 1986, 61, (6), 2162–7.
17. Saris, W. H., van Erp-Baart, M. A., Brouns, F., Westerterp, K. R., ten Hoor, F., Study on food intake and energy expenditure during extreme sustained exercise: The Tour de France, *Int J Sports Med* 1989, 10 Suppl 1, S26–31.
18. Kirkwood, J. K., Minireview. A limit to metabolisable energy intake in mammals and birds, *Comp Biochem Physiol A* 1983, 75, (1), 1–3.
19. Lucia, A., Hoyos, J., Santalla, A., Earnest, C., Chicharro, J. L., Tour de France versus Vuelta a Espana: which is harder? *Med Sci Sports Exerc* 2003, 35, (5), 872–8.
20. Loucks, A. B., Energy availability, not body fatness, regulates reproductive function in women, *Exerc Sport Sci Rev* 2003, 31, (3), 144–8.
21. Loucks, A. B., Verdun, M., Heath, E. M., Low energy availability, not stress of exercise, alters LH pulsatility in exercising women, *J Appl Physiol* 1998, 84, (1), 37–46.
22. Todd, K. S., Butterfield, G. E., Calloway, D. H., Nitrogen balance in men with adequate and deficient energy intake at three levels of work, *J Nutr* 1984, 114, (11), 2107–18.
23. Jebb, S. A., Prentice, A. M., Goldberg, G. R., Murgatroyd, P. R., Black, A. E., Coward, W. A., Changes in macronutrient balance during over- and underfeeding assessed by 12-d continuous whole-body calorimetry, *Am J Clin Nutr* 1996, 64, (3), 259–66.
24. Rolfe, D. F., Brown, G. C., Cellular energy utilization and molecular origin of standard metabolic rate in mammals, *Physiol Rev* 1997, 77, (3), 731–58.
25. *Dietary Guidelines for Americans 2005*; U.S. Department of Health and Human Services and the U.S. Department of Agriculture: 2005; pp 1–73.
26. Braun, B., Gerson, L., Hagobian, T., Grow, D., Chipkin, S. R., No effect of short-term testosterone manipulation on exercise substrate metabolism in men, *J Appl Physiol* 2005, 99, (5), 1930–7.
27. Braun, B., Horton, T., Endocrine regulation of exercise substrate utilization in women compared to men, *Exerc Sport Sci Rev* 2001, 29, (4), 149–54.
28. O'Brien, M. J., Viguie, C. A., Mazzeo, R. S., Brooks, G. A., Carbohydrate dependence during marathon running, *Med Sci Sports Exerc* 1993, 25, (9), 1009–17.
29. Febbraio, M., Keenan, J., Angus, D. J., Campbell, S. E., Garnham, A. P., Preexercise carbohydrate ingestion, glucose kinetics, and muscle glycogen use: Effect of the glycemic index, *J. Appl. Physiol.* 2000, 89, 1845–1851.
30. Jeukendrup, A. E., Jentjens, R., Oxidation of carbohydrate feedings during prolonged exercise: Current thoughts, guidelines and directions for future research, *Sports Med* 2000, 29, (6), 407–24.
31. Ivy, J. L., Katz, A. L., Cutler, C. L., Sherman, W. M., Coyle, E. F., Muscle glycogen synthesis after exercise: Effect of time of carbohydrate ingestion, *J Appl Physiol* 1988, 64, (4), 1480–1485.
32. Parkin, J. A., Carey, M. F., Martin, I. K., Stojanovska, L., Febbraio, M. A., Muscle glycogen storage following prolonged exercise: Effect of timing of ingestion of high glycemic index food, *Med Sci Sports Exerc* 1997, 29, (2), 220–224.

33. Stephens, B. R., Sautter, J. M., Holtz, K. A., Sharoff, C. G., Chipkin, S. R., Braun, B., Effect of timing of energy and carbohydrate replacement on post-exercise insulin action, *Appl Physiol Nutr Metab* 2007, 32, (6), 1139–47.
34. Andersen, G. S., Stunkard, A. J., Sorensen, T. I., Petersen, L., Heitmann, B. L., Night eating and weight change in middle-aged men and women, *Int J Obes Relat Metab Disord* 2004, 28, (10), 1338–43.
35. Holmback, U., Lowden, A., Akerfeldt, T., Lennernas, M., Hambraeus, L., Forslund, J., et al., The human body may buffer small differences in meal size and timing during a 24-h wake period provided energy balance is maintained, *J Nutr* 2003, 133, (9), 2748–55.
36. van Erp-Baart, A. M., Saris, W. H., Binkhorst, R. A., Vos, J. A., Elvers, J. W., Nationwide survey on nutritional habits in elite athletes. Part I. Energy, carbohydrate, protein, and fat intake, *Int J Sports Med* 1989, 10 Suppl 1, S3–10.
37. Ebine, N., Feng, J. Y., Homma, M., Saitoh, S., Jones, P. J., Total energy expenditure of elite synchronized swimmers measured by the doubly labeled water method, *Eur J Appl Physiol* 2000, 83, (1), 1–6.
38. Fudge, B. W., Westerterp, K. R., Kiplamai, F. K., Onywera, V. O., Boit, M. K., Kayser, B., Pitsiladis, Y. P., Evidence of negative energy balance using doubly labelled water in elite Kenyan endurance runners prior to competition, *Br J Nutr* 2006, 95, (1), 59–66.
39. Hill, R. J., Davies, P. S., Energy intake and energy expenditure in elite lightweight female rowers, *Med Sci Sports Exerc* 2002, 34, (11), 1823–9.
40. Ruby, B. C., Shriver, T. C., Zderic, T. W., Sharkey, B. J., Burks, C., Tysk, S., Total energy expenditure during arduous wildfire suppression, *Med Sci Sports Exerc* 2002, 34, (6), 1048–54.
41. Trappe, T. A., Gastaldelli, A., Jozsi, A. C., Troup, J. P., Wolfe, R. R., Energy expenditure of swimmers during high volume training, *Med Sci Sports Exerc* 1997, 29, (7), 950–4.
42. Moseley, L., Achten, J., Martin, J. C., Jeukendrup, A. E., No differences in cycling efficiency between world-class and recreational cyclists, *Int J Sports Med* 2004, 25, (5), 374–9.
43. Coyle, E. F., Improved muscular efficiency displayed as Tour de France champion matures, *J Appl Physiol* 2005, 98, (6), 2191–6.
44. Holloszy, J. O., Biochemical adaptations in muscle. Effects of exercise on mitochondrial oxygen uptake and respiratory enzyme activity in skeletal muscle, *J. Biol. Chem.* 1967, 242, (9), 2278–2282.
45. Brooks, G. A., Mercier, J., Balance of carbohydrate and lipid utilization during exercise: The “crossover” concept, *J Appl Physiol* 1994, 76, (6), 2253–61.
46. Tonkonogi, M., Walsh, B., Svensson, M., Sahlin, K., Mitochondrial function and antioxidative defense in human muscle: Effects of endurance training and oxidative stress, *J Physiol* 2000, 528, (2), 379–388.
47. Hill, J. O., Understanding and addressing the epidemic of obesity: An energy balance perspective, *Endocr Rev* 2006, 27, (7), 750–61.
48. Williams, N. I., Lessons from experimental disruptions of the menstrual cycle in humans and monkeys, *Med Sci Sports Exerc* 2003, 35, (9), 1564–72.
49. Kirkwood, T. B., Understanding the odd science of aging, *Cell* 2005, 120, (4), 437–47.
50. Holden, J. E., Stone, C. K., Clark, C. M., Brown, W. D., Nickles, R. J., Stanley, C., Hochachka, P. W., Enhanced cardiac metabolism of plasma glucose in high-altitude natives: Adaptation against chronic hypoxia, *J Appl Physiol* 1995, 79, (1), 222–228.

51. Brooks, G. A., Butterfield, G. E., Wolfe, R. R., Groves, B. M., Mazzeo, R. S., Sutton, J. R., et al., Increased dependence on blood glucose after acclimatization to 4,300 m, *J Appl Physiol* 1991, 70, (2), 919–27.
52. Young, A. J., Evans, W. J., Cymerman, A., Pandolf, K. B., Knapik, J. J., Maher, J. T., Sparing effect of chronic high-altitude exposure on muscle glycogen utilization, *J Appl Physiol* 1982, 52, (4), 857–62.
53. Butterfield, G. E., Maintenance of body weight at altitude. In search of 500 kcal/day. In *Nutritional Needs in Cold and High Altitude Environments*, National Academy Press: Washington D.C., 1996; pp 357–378.
54. Barnholt, K. E., Hoffman, A. R., Rock, P. B., Muza, S. R., Fulco, C. S., Braun, B., et al., Endocrine responses to acute and chronic high-altitude exposure (4,300 meters): modulating effects of caloric restriction, *Am J Physiol Endocrinol Metab* 2006, 290, (6), E1078–88.
55. Febbraio, M. A., Alterations in energy metabolism during exercise and heat stress, *Sports Med* 2001, 31, (1), 47–59.
56. Hunt, D. G., Ding, Z., Ivy, J. L., Clenbuterol prevents epinephrine from antagonizing insulin-stimulated muscle glucose uptake, *J Appl Physiol* 2002, 92, (3), 1285–92.
57. Tanaka, H., Desouza, C. A., Jones, P. P., Stevenson, E. T., Davy, K. P., Seals, D. R., Greater rate of decline in maximal aerobic capacity with age in physically active vs. sedentary healthy women, *J Appl Physiol* 1997, 83, (6), 1947–53.
58. Allen, W. K., Seals, D. R., Hurley, B. F., Ehsani, A. A., Hagberg, J. M., Lactate threshold and distance-running performance in young and older endurance athletes, *J Appl Physiol* 1985, 58, (4), 1281–4.
59. Trappe, S. W., Costill, D. L., Fink, W. J., Pearson, D. R., Skeletal muscle characteristics among distance runners: A 20-yr follow-up study, *J Appl Physiol* 1995, 78, (3), 823–829.
60. Coggan, A. R., Spina, R. J., Rogers, M. A., King, D. S., Brown, M., Nemeth, P. M., Holloszy, J. O., Histochemical and enzymatic characteristics of skeletal muscle in master athletes, *J Appl Physiol* 1990, 68, (5), 1896–1901.
61. Boon, H., Jonkers, R. A., Koopman, R., Blaak, E. E., Saris, W. H., Wagenmakers, A. J., Van Loon, L. J., Substrate source use in older, trained males after decades of endurance training, *Med Sci Sports Exerc* 2007, 39, (12), 2160–70.
62. Raguso, C. A., Coggan, A. R., Gastaldelli, A., Sidossis, L. S., Bastyr, E. J., 3rd, Wolfe, R. R., Lipid and carbohydrate metabolism in IDDM during moderate and intense exercise, *Diabetes* 1995, 44, (9), 1066–74.
63. Ghanassia, E., Brun, J. F., Fedou, C., Raynaud, E., Mercier, J., Substrate oxidation during exercise: Type 2 diabetes is associated with a decrease in lipid oxidation and an earlier shift towards carbohydrate utilization, *Diabetes Metab* 2006, 32, (6), 604–10.
64. Petersen, K. F., Dufour, S., Befroy, D., Garcia, R., Shulman, G. I., Impaired mitochondrial activity in the insulin-resistant offspring of patients with type 2 diabetes, *N Engl J Med* 2004, 350, (7), 664–671.
65. Kelley, D. E., He, J., Menshikova, E. V., Ritov, V. B., Dysfunction of mitochondria in human skeletal muscle in type 2 diabetes, *Diabetes* 2002, 51, (10), 2944–50.
66. Boushel, R., Gnaiger, E., Schjerling, P., Skovbro, M., Kraunsoe, R., Dela, F., Patients with type 2 diabetes have normal mitochondrial function in skeletal muscle, *Diabetologia* 2007, 50, (4), 790–6.
67. Toledo, F. G., Menshikova, E. V., Ritov, V. B., Azuma, K., Radikova, Z., DeLany, J., Kelley, D. E., Effects of physical activity and weight loss on skeletal muscle mitochondria and relationship with glucose control in type 2 diabetes, *Diabetes* 2007, 56, (8), 2142–7.

68. Horton, T. J., Braun, B., *Sex-Based Differences in Substrate Metabolism*, Elsevier: Amsterdam, 2004; Vol. 34, p 209–228.
69. Staron, R. S., Hagerman, F. C., Hikida, R. S., Murray, T. F., Hostler, D. P., Crill, M. T.,et al., Fiber type composition of the vastus lateralis muscle of young men and women, *J Histochem Cytochem* 2000, 48, (5), 623–9.
70. Hardie, D. G., Hawley, S. A., Scott, J. W., AMP-activated protein kinase—development of the energy sensor concept, *J Physiol* 2006, 574, (Pt 1), 7–15.
71. De Bock, K., Derave, W., Eijnde, B. O., Hesselink, M. K., Koninckx, E., Rose, A. J., et al., Effect of training in the fasted state on metabolic responses during exercise with carbohydrate intake, *J Appl Physiol* 2008, 104, (4), 1045–1055.
72. Gibala, M. J., McGee, S. L., Metabolic adaptations to short-term high-intensity interval training: A little pain for a lot of gain? *Exerc Sport Sci Rev* 2008, 36, (2), 58–63.

2 Carbohydrates and Fats

Mark Kern

CONTENTS

I. INTRODUCTION

As the major providers of energy during physical activity, carbohydrates and fats are critical nutrients for exercisers and athletes. These nutrients should be considered from performance-related perspectives as well as for their implications in promoting wellness of active individuals. Dietary sources of carbohydrate and fat as well as endogenous stores are contributors to human metabolism; therefore, effects of both acute (particularly with regard to carbohydrates) and chronic dietary intake of these key nutrients are of prime importance. Research performed to date allows us to predict to at least some degree how consumption of various carbohydrates, fats, and nutrients that affect metabolism will influence fuel utilization, risk factors for chronic diseases, and athletic performance.

II. CARBOHYDRATES

A. Classifications and Dietary Sources

Carbohydrates are macronutrients composed of carbon, hydrogen, and oxygen atoms that can be divided into many categories based on their structure (i.e., monosaccharides, disaccharides, polysaccharides, and non-digestible polysaccharides) as well as their metabolic effects (e.g., digestibility, glycemic responses, etc.). The term "saccharide" describes a molecule that is a sugar or sweet and is often used as a synonym for "carbohydrate." These nutrients are typically the most abundantly consumed components of our diets. Many foods from each of the five major food groups, as wells as sweets and foods specifically developed for athletes such as sports drinks, bars, and gels, can provide significant amounts of carbohydrate in the diet. Some examples of carbohydrate-rich foods and their carbohydrate contents in 100-gram servings are provided in Table 2.1. Although many of the foods on the list appear to be rather low in carbohydrates, most of those foods have a high or very high water content, which can be misleading as the values are expressed relative to the weights of the foods rather than as a percentage of energy content provided by carbohydrate, which is high for all of the foods listed.

Carbohydrates are often classified structurally as either simple sugars (typically monosaccharides and disaccharides) or complex carbohydrates (i.e., polysaccharides or starches). Monosaccharides are carbohydrates composed of a single monomeric unit, while disaccharides include two monosaccharides linked by a glycosidic bond. Mono- and disaccharides are often referred to collectively and sometimes individually as sugars or simple sugars, although the term "sugar" is often used to refer to carbohydrates in general or specifically to table sugar (sucrose) or blood sugar (glucose). The major dietary monosaccharides are glucose, fructose, and galactose, while sucrose (glucose + fructose), lactose (glucose + galactose), and maltose (glucose + glucose) compose the key disaccharides of the diet.

Sugars are found in a variety of naturally occurring and processed foods. Glucose is a hexose found abundantly in various forms in an array of foods. Free glucose is found in many fruits, honey, corn syrup, sports drinks and numerous other foods. Glucose is also a component of most other carbohydrates including, but not limited

TABLE 2.1
Typical Carbohydrate Content of 100-Gram Servings of Selected Foods and Sports Products Rich in Carbohydrate

Food	Carbohydrate Content (g)
Bread, Cereal, Rice, and Pasta Group	
Bagels (plain)	50–55
Brown rice (cooked)	24
Cooked cereal (prepared with water)	10–20
Corn Tortillas (unfried)	47
Crackers (saltine)	72
English muffins	46
Flour Tortillas	56
Noodles (egg, cooked)	25
Pancakes	37
Pasta	25–30
Pretzels	79
Ready-to-eat cereal (dry)	80–90
Waffles	33
White bread or toast	50–55
White rice	29
Whole wheat bread or toast	47–51
Vegetable Group	
Corn	20
Peas	16
Potatoes (baked)	21
Yam (boiled)	28
Fruit Group	
Canned fruits	5–30
Dried fruits	60–80
Fruit juices	10–15
Raw fruits	15–25
Milk, Yogurt, and Cheese Group	
Cheese (fat free, processed)	13
Chocolate milk (lowfat)	10
Ice cream (fat free)	30
Milk (fat free)	5
Yogurt (fat free with fruit)	19
Meat, Poultry, Fish, Dry Beans, Eggs, and Nuts Group	
Chestnuts (roasted)	53
Dry beans (boiled)	23–27
Lentils	20
Sweets	
Candy	80–98
Candy bar	60–70

(*Continued*)

TABLE 2.1 (CONTINUED)
Typical Carbohydrate Content of 100-Gram Servings of Selected Foods and Sports Products Rich in Carbohydrate

Food	Carbohydrate Content (g)
Cookies (lowfat/fat free)	70–80
Honey	82
Jam/preserves	69
Maple syrup	67
Soft-drinks	10–11
Table sugar	100
Sports products*	
Sports bars	65–75
Sports drinks	5–7
Sports gels	70–80

* Usually low nutrient density

Source: Information obtained from USDA National Nutrient Database for Standard Reference, Release 16-1; from Kern, M. *CRC Desk Reference for Sports Nutrition.* CRC Press. Boca Raton, FL. 2005. pp. 28–29.

to, starches, sucrose, lactose, and maltose. Any foods rich in these nutrients ultimately provide the body with significant amounts of glucose. Furthermore, the other primary dietary monosaccharides fructose and galactose are ultimately converted to glucose or glucose derivatives after absorption. Because most carbohydrate can be converted into glucose eventually, it is an extremely important nutrient physiologically, as will be discussed. Glucose can be made available for the body from more than dietary carbohydrates, however. Many amino acids, glycerol, and pyruvic and lactic acids can be used to produce glucose. The monosaccharide fructose is also a hexose. It is primarily found in food in either its simple form or bound to glucose as part of the disaccharide sucrose. Foods rich in this monosaccharide as the hexose monomer include many fruits and honey, although much of the fructose in the diet is consumed in processed foods such as soft drinks, sports drinks, baked goods, etc., that are sweetened with high fructose corn syrup. Because one half of the sucrose molecule is fructose, foods rich in sucrose also provide much of the fructose in the diet. Another major hexose consumed in the diet is galactose, which is found predominately in food as part of the disaccharide lactose. Other foods containing galactose include peas, lentils, some legumes, organ meats, cereals, and some fruits and vegetables. Some sports foods contain galactose as well, which will be discussed in more detail later. Other monosaccharides, including pentoses such as ribose and xylose, are found in the diet in small quantities as well. Ribose, commonly consumed as a part of nucleic acids, is produced metabolically from glucose through the hexose monophosphate shunt.

Three major disaccharides, sucrose, lactose and maltose, are also found in most individuals' diets. Sucrose is present at high levels in sugar cane and sugar beets, from which it is extracted to produce table sugar. It is also found in lower amounts in many fruits as well as vegetables and grains. Several sports foods are sweetened with sucrose. Lactose is a disaccharide produced from the monosaccharides glucose and galactose and is the primary sugar found in milk. Maltose is found in malted milk products as well as sweet potatoes, pears, and in lower amounts in other fruits, vegetables, grain products, and honey.

"Complex carbohydrate" usually describes digestible polysaccharides made up of many glucose monomers. Digestible polysaccharides are found in a variety of plant foods and are often richest in foods such as grains and grain-based foods (e.g., pasta, breads, cereals, etc.), potatoes, beans, and peas, etc. Non-digestible polysaccharides (i.e., fiber) are also made of saccharide units (not always glucose), but are resistant to digestion by human enzymes. The most prevalent examples of complex carbohdyrates in the human diet are amylose and amylopectin, both of which are considered starches. Amylopectin comprises a higher percentage (typically 70–80%) of the starch in foods containing complex carbohydrate. Glucose polymers or maltodextrins are also typically considered complex carbohydrates. These molecules are relatively short chains of glucose units linked by glycosidic bonds in a manner similar to amylose and are produced by partial hydrolysis of starch molecules.

Many nutritionists have used the term "complex carbohydrate" simply to refer to foods that are rich in starches. These foods typically provide many nutrients other than the glucose that composes the starches and have long been considered to provide a nutritional advantage over simple sugars. Historically, this advantage has been used as a basis for suggesting that the diets of exercisers and athletes be rich in complex carbohydrates. While many foods rich in complex carbohydrates are also rich in other nutrients, this is not always the case. Foods rich in complex carbohydrate as well as fiber (e.g., whole grain breads, etc.) are prime examples of nutrient-rich foods that should form the basis of a healthy diet.

Fiber is a group of non-digestible polysaccharides found in plant foods as well as lignin, which is primarily associated with the structural components of plants. Although fibers are not digestible by enzymes of the human intestinal tract, colonic bacteria possess the ability to partially ferment some fiber, not lignin, thereby producing short-chain fatty acids that can be absorbed by the colonic epithelium and provide some energy to the body. Therefore, while the term non-digestible is accurate regarding human digestion, some fiber digestion does occur within the human body through the assistance of our colonic microflora. Fibers are usually classified as those that are soluble in water and those that are insoluble in water. Water-soluble fibers that are common in the diet include pectins, gums, mucilages, algal polysaccharides, beta-glucans, pysllium, resistant starches, and inulin. Water-insoluble fibers include cellulose, some hemicelluloses, and lignin. The potential impact of fiber consumption on exercise performance has not been directly studied; however, for meals consumed prior to or during competition, most sports dietitians recommend foods relatively low in fiber to avoid gastrointestinal discomfort, which may negatively impact performance. Most practitioners also recommend that the typical diet of an athlete contain similar amounts of fiber to those recommended to the general population (usually approximately 20–35 grams per day). Research does not necessarily support the notion that consumption of moderate amounts of fiber will adversely affect performance during competition. In fact, as described in the section on glycemic index, consumption of some fiber-containing foods has produced a lower glycemic response with pre-exercise feedings, which translated to improvements in performance. Other studies have not demonstrated such performance improvements but also do not report decreases in performance. Until solid research regarding alternative recommendations is available, the amount of fiber that an athlete should consume before competition depends on how well the individual can tolerate foods that contain fiber and must be determined on a case-by-case basis.

The Acceptable Macronutrient Distribution Range established by the Institute of Medicine when determining the Dietary Reference Intakes is 45–65% of total energy intake. Research on dietary intake of various athletes suggests that most are consuming carbohydrates at rates that are within this range. For example, one group of researchers demonstrated that the average intake of U.S. collegiate cyclists during training was 58 ± 8% of energy.[1] Similar data were obtained for Australian national-level triathletes and runners who respectively consumed 60 ± 8% and 52 ± 5% of energy from carbohydrate[2] and U.S. swimmers and divers who consumed 65 ± 7% of energy from carbohydrate at season's end.[3] At the extreme, elite male Kenyan runners have been demonstrated to eat as much as 607 ± 57 grams of carbohydrate per day during training, accounting for approximately 77% of energy intake on average.[4]

B. Digestion and Absorption

Ingestion of carbohydrates other than monosaccharides requires digestion prior to absorption. When starches are consumed, the final product of digestion will ultimately be glucose units. While a limited degree of starch digestion begins in the oral cavity by the action of salivary amylase secreted into the mouth, most starch digestion will occur in the small intestine by the glycosidic cleavage capacities of pancreatic amylase and various brush border saccharidases. Amylase is primarily responsible for digesting starches into shortened saccharides in the duodenum, where it enters along with other pancreatic secretions. It does so by cleaving starches at their α-1,4 glycosidic bonds. The products of the digestive effects of amylase on amylose are primarily maltose and maltotriose, which is made up of three glucose units linearly connected, and a limited amount of glucose. Since amylopectin also possesses α-1,6 glycosidic bonds, amylase activity will produce branched oligosaccharides called α-limit dextrins, usually possessing five or six glucose units, in addition to maltose and maltotriose. Complete digestion of the saccharides produced from starch digestion requires other enzymes including maltase-glucoamylase, isomaltase, and sucrase. The resulting glucose is now available for absorption into the enterocyte.

Other non-monosaccharides must be digested as well prior to absorption of their respective monomers. Glucose polymers and maltodextrins are digested in a manner similar to that described for amylose. Sucrose is digested to the monosaccharides glucose and fructose primarily by the enzyme sucrase, which is secreted at the brush border of the small intestine. Lactose is digested to its complementary monosaccharides by the enzyme lactase, which is also secreted at the brush border of the small intestine. If inadequate amounts of lactase are produced by the body to appropriately digest this sugar, lactose intolerance occurs, which makes it difficult for an individual to tolerate large (or sometimes even small) amounts of lactose. As described above for maltose that is produced from the breakdown of starches, dietary maltose is primarily digested to form glucose monomers by the brush border enzymes maltase-glucoamylase and sucrase. Although a less common dietary constituent, the disaccharide trehalose must be digested to two molecules of free glucose by the enzyme trehalase. Therefore, the final digestive products of dietary carbohydrates are typically glucose, fructose, and galactose, which can be absorbed by cells of the small intestine.

Glucose and galactose are absorbed along with sodium by a common transporter referred to as sodium-glucose cotransporter 1 (SGLT1). This is an active transport process in which energy is provided for the exit of Na^+ by the Na^+K^+-ATPase. Glucose is exported from the enterocyte across the basolateral membrane by the GLUT2 transporter for entry into the portal circulation by which the hexoses make their way to the liver. Fructose is absorbed into the gut cell by a facilitated diffusion process involving the transporter GLUT5 and also exported across the basolateral membrane by GLUT2. This absorption mechanism is highly saturable, meaning that the rate of fructose absorption is limited, which produces absorption at a relatively slow rate. Because it is absorbed more slowly than other monosaccharides, particularly when consumed in the absence of other carbohydrates, it produces a lower glycemic response, which in turn produces a lower insulinemic response. This slower absorption has been considered a cause for concern for athletes, because large amounts of fructose residing in the gut for an extended period of time can produce gastrointestinal distress including cramping and diarrhea. However, as described later, foods producing a lower glycemic response may be beneficial for performance as pre-exercise feedings when compared with those that produce a higher glycemic response. In contrast, recent research has demonstrated that because fructose is absorbed by a transporter different from that which allows for glucose absorption, when consumed with a source of glucose, total exogenous carbohydrate bioavailability during exercise may be enhanced.

In summary, when a carbohydrate is ingested, it must be broken down by digestion to its simplest form prior to absorption, as the gut prefers to allow only the monosaccharides into the bloodstream. The blood circulating around the intestinal tract is directed first to the liver. The liver is instrumental in converting non-glucose saccharides into glucose derivatives that can either be metabolized further by the liver or released to the general circulation. The vast majority of carbohydrate that is found within the blood is glucose, which provides a source of energy to most tissues of the body and is especially preferred by the red blood cells and tissues of the central nervous system. Furthermore, much of the energy produced within the skeletal and heart muscle is from glucose. When energy production is not required, glucose can be stored as glycogen within the body for future use, particularly in the muscle cells and liver.

C. Carbohydrate Metabolism

The metabolic processes that are ultimately responsible for the eventual production of energy from glucose include glycogenolysis, glycolysis, the pyruvate dehydrogenase complex, Krebs cycle, and the electron transport chain. Complete catabolism of glucose for energy yields adenosine triphosphate (ATP), carbon dioxide, and water. Along with that provided by fat catabolism, the energy produced by carbohydrate metabolism is critical for the metabolic processes and muscle contraction needed during the performance of exercise.

1. General Metabolic Processes of Carbohydrate Metabolism

Carbohydrate for metabolism comes from a variety of sources. These include the diet, via absorption through the intestinal mucosa, glycogen stored primarily in the liver and muscle, and glucose produced from non-glucose precursors via gluconeogenesis. A very limited supply of glucose is also found in the circulation at any given time; however, the concentration of glucose in the bloodstream must be kept relatively constant, so while the glucose present is a critical source of energy for working muscles, it is not a large depot for storage.

Glucose serves as a primary fuel for the body and a highly preferred fuel for many cells including the central nervous system and red blood cells. The catabolism of glucose to pyruvate for energy in these cells and all others is called glycolysis. When athletes need to rapidly produce energy from glucose during very strenuous exercise that can last for only a short time, a large proportion of that glucose will be metabolized anaerobically to produce ATP and the final product, lactic acid (lactate). Lactate is obtained by an anaerobic reaction catalyzed by lactic acid dehydrogenase, which converts pyruvate to lactate. During exercise of a lower intensity, aerobic glucose metabolism will predominate, and although ATP will be produced less rapidly, the final product of glycolysis will be pyruvic acid, which can undergo further metabolism via the pyruvate dehydrogenase complex, followed by Krebs cycle and ultimately the electron transport system to produce additional ATP. If the glucose to be catabolized is found in its storage form as glycogen, the glycogen must first be broken down to glucose derivatives via glycogenolysis.

When pyruvate is produced from glucose during aerobic glycolysis, it must first be converted to acetyl CoA prior to further metabolism via Krebs cycle. The pyruvate dehydrogenase (PDH) complex is responsible for this conversion, which along with glycolysis occurs in the cytosol of a cell. The PDH complex requires many enzymes and cofactors to accomplish this process. Cofactors involved include coenzyme A, which includes pantothenic acid as part of its structure, nicotinamide adenine dinucleotide (NAD^+, a coenzyme form of niacin), flavin adenine dinucleotide (FAD, a coenzyme form of riboflavin), thiamin diphosphate (TDP, coenzyme form of thiamin) as well as magnesium and lipoic acid. During the series of reactions, carbon dioxide is eliminated and $NADH + H^+$ (reduced NAD) is produced, which can be used for ATP synthesis through the electron transport system.

Krebs cycle, also known as the citric acid cycle or the tricarboxylic acid (TCA) cycle, is a metabolic pathway that is instrumental in obtaining energy from all macronutrients. In this cyclic pathway, oxaloacetate, produced from pyruvate, accepts the two carbons of acetate from acetyl CoA (produced primarily from carbohydrates and fats via glycolysis and beta-oxidation, respectively) yielding the 6-carbon molecule citrate. Following several intermediate steps, citrate is ultimately converted back to the 4-carbon molecule oxaloacetate with the loss of two carbons as carbon dioxide. The oxaloacetate is now available to accept two more carbons from acetyl CoA and continue the cycle. Also produced in Krebs cycle is guanosine triphosphate (GTP) and the energy producing equivalents NADH + H^+ and $FADH_2$ (reduced FAD). Like ATP, GTP possesses a high energy bond that when cleaved can produce free energy similarly to that of ATP. NADH + H^+ and $FADH_2$ are further metabolized via the electron transport system to produce ATP.

The electron transport system (ETS) accounts for the vast majority of ATP production in the body. The role of the "chain" of molecules in the ETS is to shuttle electrons from one component in the inner mitochondrial membrane to another via a series of oxidation-reduction reactions with the ultimate production of water and ATP from ADP and inorganic phosphorus. This process has also been termed oxidative phosphorylation. Coenzyme forms of niacin and riboflavin as NADH + H^+ and $FADH_2$ are particularly instrumental in the process, since they serve as the initial electron donators. As described, these molecules are produced in the metabolism of macronutrients by several metabolic pathways including glycolysis, beta-oxidation and Krebs cycle.

Glucose that is not needed for energy production can be stored until a time for which it is needed. Glycogen, is a very compact, highly branched chain of glucose molecules linked together by both α-1,4 and α-1,6 glycosidic bonds. The majority of glycogen stored in the body is located in the muscles and liver. In times of energy need, glycogen is broken down via glycogenolysis to produce glucose or glucose derivatives. Glycogen within a muscle cell must be used for energy within that cell, since glycogenolysis continues only until the production of the molecule glucose-6-phosphate in the muscle cell, because muscles lack the enzyme glucose-6-phosphatase, which produces free glucose from glucose-6-phosphate. Glucose-6-phosphate cannot exit the cell, but can enter the glycolytic pathway within the muscle cell for the production of energy. Glycogen within liver cells can be broken down to free glucose molecules, because the liver produces glucose-6-phosphatase, which removes the phophate molecule. Free glucose can leave the liver cell and travel via the circulation to tissues requiring energy production.

During rest, glucose enters the cells via the action of glucose transporters. The GLUT4 transporter is responsible for entry of glucose into muscle cells (as well as the heart and adipose cells) and is activated by the action of the hormone insulin. When activated by insulin, GLUT4 migrates to the cellular membrane to allow for the facilitated diffusion of glucose into the cell. Exercise stimulates the function of GLUT4 transporters thereby enhancing insulin sensitivity; thus, serum concentrations of insulin usually drop during exercise when food is not eaten. Because the demand for glucose by the muscles increases during exercise, glucose is released from the liver in the circulation to allow for uptake by the tissues and production of energy.[5]

During intensive exercise, blood glucose utilization increases sharply with time and can supply up to 30% of the total energy needed by the muscle, with muscle glycogen supplying most of the remaining energy requirements.[6] During prolonged exercise, blood glucose becomes a major contributor as muscle glycogen availability is diminished. Once the liver's output of glucose fails to sustain the muscle's glucose uptake, blood glucose levels decrease significantly and might even fall to hypoglycemic values. When carbohydrate stores are depleted work capacity decreases as well.[6]

As carbohydrate stores become depleted, the production of glucose via gluconeogenesis increases. While the rate of gluconeogenesis is typically not considered to be adequate for optimal exercise performance as a sole source of glucose, it can be an important contributor to total glucose availability. Precursors of gluconeogenesis include glycerol (the 3-carbon backbone to acylglycerides such as TGs), lactic acid, pyruvic acid, and many amino acids. The rate of gluconeogenesis is stimulated during exercise to provide glucose to working muscles and other cells. The majority of gluconeogenesis occurs in the liver, as the cells of most tissues do not possess all of the enzymes needed for this process. Other tissues are important providers of gluconeogenic precursors, however. For example, muscles can provide the highly gluconeogenic amino acid alanine from protein catabolism or transamination from pyruvate and glutamate to the liver via the circulation by way of the alanine cycle, and adipose tissue provides fats that contribute glycerol to gluconeogenesis. The alanine cycle is a series of reactions in which alanine obtained in the muscle from pyruvate through a transamination (pyruvate accepts an amino group from a different amino acid) reaction enters the bloodstream and is taken up by the liver for conversion to glucose. Glucose can be secreted from the liver and then taken up by the muscle, where it again produces pyruvate through glycolysis, which is now available once again for transamination to alanine or for energy production.

2. Carbohydrate Metabolism during Exercise

Dietary carbohydrate intake as well as endogenous carbohydrate production and metabolism, particularly during exercise, are critical issues for most athletes. Those athletes who should be particularly cognizant of their carbohydrate intake are endurance athletes, but most individuals utilizing high amounts of energy during training or competition are likely to benefit from strategies regarding optimal carbohydrate consumption and metabolism. Therefore, knowledge and understanding of the influence of exercise on carbohydrate metabolism is key to determining how dietary intake of carbohydrates and nutrients related to carbohydrate metabolisms may alter athletic performance. Much of the research with this regard has been on strategies that could potentially spare glycogen stores; therefore, it is critical to understand the impact of exercise on carbohydrate utilization.

Research suggests that liver glycogen stores are the principal target through which dietary carbohydrate consumption regimens may act to prevent glycogen depletion.[7] Adequate fuel substrates for exercise are critical for preventing the fatigue that can limit exercise output. In simple terms, when muscle glycogen stores are sufficiently depleted and liver glycogen decreases during exercise, adequate production of glucose is not possible under conditions of intense physical activity; therefore, hypoglycemia ensues and fatigue occurs.

Symptoms of hypoglycemia include dizziness, muscular weakness, fatigue, and hunger. When blood glucose concentration drops below normal, glucagon is secreted, mobilizing glycogen from the liver to elevate blood glucose concentration. Glucagon is a peptide hormone synthesized in the alpha cells of the pancreas. A primary function of glucagon is in the regulation of blood glucose, in which it most notably raises blood glucose by simulating gluconeogenesis and glycogenolysis. During exercise, glucagon production and secretion is typically enhanced to provide glucose to working muscles.

In rare cases, hypoglycemia can be a chronic condition, but more often, hypoglycemia is a transient phenomenon. During exercise, particularly prolonged vigorous exercise, demands for carbohydrate for fuel is high. While the liver and muscle can initially supply a relatively large amount of glycogen for physical activity, during prolonged exercise those supplies can be depleted and gluconeogenesis (synthesis of glucose from non-carbohydrate sources) cannot occur at a rate sufficient to replenish the blood glucose. Ultimately, without adequate exogenous carbohydrate, hypoglycemia and fatigue will occur. For this reason it is imperative for endurance athletes to consume a diet containing adequate amounts of carbohydrates to provide sufficient or perhaps optimal stores of glycogen. Likewise, it is important to consume adequate amounts of carbohydrates before or during exercise to prevent glycogen loss and hypoglycemia.

Under some conditions, consumption of a pre-exercise carbohydrate-rich meal (usually 15–60 minutes before exercise) can produce a sharp elevation in blood sugar. This increase results in enhanced production and release of insulin, which has a glucose-lowering effect. When exercise begins, the blood sugar concentration can be further decreased by enhanced tissue uptake of glucose. If the decrease is sufficiently extreme, a transient hypoglycemia referred to as reactive hypoglycemia occurs. Because hypoglycemia can induce feelings of fatigue, exercise performance can be diminished in some athletes.[8,9] While this has been demonstrated in some research, other studies have failed to detect either hypoglycemia or impaired endurance performance with similar protocols. As described later, some but not all research suggests that feedings of lower glycemic index foods may be optimal as pre-exercise feedings within this timeframe and serve as a solution for providing food if preferred by the athlete during this critical period while minimizing the risk of reactive hypoglycemia.

Consumption of exogenous carbohydrate before or during exercise has long been used to spare glycogen and prevent exhaustion from occurring prematurely during exercise. Many other supplements and dietary strategies have been promoted as glycogen-sparing as well. Although evidence has supported the use of some of these, others have not been demonstrated by research to be effective. In some cases, glycogen-sparing has been shown to occur but subsequent enhancements in performance were not detected. When that is the case, it is possible that the exercise protocol utilized failed to produce sufficient glycogen loss in control trials that could produce fatigue; therefore, the potential efficacy of those techniques may be recognized only under other exercise conditions.

Researchers have suggested that carbohydrate-sparing may be important not only from the perspective of preserving energetic precursors, but through mechanisms related to amino acid metabolism and the central nervous system as well. Scientists have theorized that when branched chain amino acids (BCAA) are used extensively for energy production by muscle tissue during exercise, the subsequent drop in plasma concentrations of BCAA combined with the displacement of tryptophan from albumin caused by a concomitant increase in the concentration of free fatty acids results in perceived exertion and thus premature fatigue. This occurs because tryptophan more readily enters the brain when the ratio tryptophan to BCAA in the blood is elevated, and serotonin production increases when tryptophan enters the brain. Serotonin (also called 5-hydroxytryptamine) is a neurotransmitter produced in the brain from tryptophan with 5-hydroxytryptophan as an intermediate in the pathway. It produces changes in mood that can include feelings of sleepiness and mellowness and may produce the sensation of fatigue, thereby decreasing an individual's ability to send a signal from the brain to the muscle for contraction.[10] This process has been referred to as the central fatigue theory. Central fatigue is most likely to occur when levels of glycogen become depleted because this depletion increases the body's reliance on BCAA and free fatty acids as fuels for working muscles. Many researchers have attempted to improve performance by limiting central fatigue through BCAA supplementation. Research, however, better supports the notion that the consumption of carbohydrate prior to and during exercise is the most effective means of delaying central fatigue and improving performance. That likely occurs due to the effectiveness of these techniques in sparing glycogen and producing less BCAA uptake as well as somewhat blunting the release of free fatty acids from the adipose tissue, so less tryptophan is displaced from albumin.[10]

D. Carbohydrates and Exercise Performance

Several studies have indicated that exogenous (dietary) carbohydrate provides an alternate fuel source that can spare the utilization of the body's glycogen reserves, thus enhancing performance and prolonging time to fatigue. This is particularly important given the relatively low amount of energy (~2000 kcal) that can be stored within the muscle and liver as glycogen.[11] A review by Jacobs and Sherman[11] summarizes much of the research regarding the efficacy of carbohydrate in optimizing endurance performance. Sports activities that are most likely to be affected include (1) rigorous endurance events lasting approximately an hour or longer, (2) events that include intermittent bursts of high intensity activity, and (3) events performed in cold environments. Much of the carbohydrate strategies that have been studied can be categorized into research assessing temporal (intake timing) issues, research on the form in which the carbohydrate is consumed, the type of carbohydrate studied, and dietary supplements that alter carbohydrate metabolism.

1. Temporal Issues

Dietary intake of carbohydrate should be considered during training as well as prior to, during, and after an event or rigorous exercise session. Research has demonstrated that adequate carbohydrate intake before or during an event is particularly effective in enhancing performance. While some studies have failed to detect endurance performance improvements with carbohydrate feedings before[12–16] and during[17–19] exercise, many examples of studies exist in which performance was improved for prolonged endurance events,[20–24] relatively short endurance trials,[25,26] and high-intensity intermittent activities as well as associated sports skills.[27–30]

A variety of consumption regimens have produced positive effects. Research by Sherman and his colleagues has demonstrated that intake of carbohydrate can improve performance even when it is consumed well in advance of exercise. One study demonstrated that consumption 4 hours prior to exercise improved performance,[31] while another showed that performance was improved with carbohydrate intake 1 hour in advance of exercise.[32] Other research has demonstrated that consumption immediately prior to exercise can also be effective in enhancing endurance.[20] Much research has also focused on carbohydrate consumption during exercise. Coyle and his colleagues[25,33] have demonstrated significant improvements in endurance in well designed studies evaluating the roles of carbohydrate feedings during exercise in optimizing performance. When carbohydrate was fed both prior to and during exercise, performance was improved to a degree greater than when either feeding protocol was followed alone.[22] Many studies assessing the influence of carbohydrates on performance have taken advantage of this effect and utilized protocols combining carbohydrate feedings immediately before and during exercise.

Some research has also suggested that incorporating protein or essential amino acids into the foods consumed during exercise may further enhance the benefits of carbohydrate feeding.[34,35] Palatability of sports beverages is typically lower when protein is incorporated, however, which may diminish beverage consumption.

Carbohydrate intake after exercise also appears to be important from the perspective of maximizing restoration of muscle and liver glycogen stores. Research suggests that an adequate intake of carbohydrate-rich foods soon after exercise can help to maximize the rate of glycogen synthesis.[36] Furthermore, some research also suggests that incorporating protein or amino acids into the post-exercise meal will stimulate additional glycogen synthesis[37]; however, not all studies are in agreement.[38] Interestingly, the combination of intake of carbohydrate and either proteins or essential amino acids after exercise may also help to stimulate muscle synthesis after resistance exercise,[39] thereby providing a second benefit to consumption of both carbohydrate and protein during the recovery period. Recent research has suggested that an effective recovery food does not need to be an expensive commercial formula. Karp et al.[40] demonstrated that chocolate milk consumed between exhausting bouts of exercise improved endurance for the second bout of exercise.

Adequate habitual carbohydrate intake is important for maintaining the body's glycogen stores during periods of training,[41] suggesting that a high carbohydrate diet will promote optimal performance; however, all research is not in agreement that performance is affected by regular consumption of a high carbohydrate diet. Some research has even suggested that a usual diet rich in fat may improve performance more than a diet richer in carbohydrate.[42] If this is true, it may be possible that adaptation to a fat-rich diet during training and then a shift to a carbohydrate-rich diet for competition could prove to be optimal. This concept has been an active area of investigation for the past few years and is described later in this chapter.

Although carbohydrate requirements vary by sport or event, timing of intake relative to competition or training, and individual athlete's preferences, a summary of basic guidelines for intake have been published in a text by Williams.[43] These guidelines apply most specifically to events or training sessions that are prolonged and rigorous in nature. A basic recommendation for carbohydrate consumption in a meal prior to an event is to consume 4–5 g/kg about 4 hours before the event begins. Individual athletes should experiment with different food sources to determine which foods will work best to achieve their goal intake level and optimal performance.

These foods could include a mixture of natural wholesome foods as well as commercial carbohydrate-rich sport foods. When carbohydrate is consumed in a closer time-gap to the event or exercise session, approximately 1–2 g/kg can be consumed 1 hour prior to the event to improve performance, and feedings of 50–60 g immediately prior to the event appears sufficient to prolong endurance. During an event, the rule of thumb is for athletes to consume approximately 8 ounces (~240 mL) of a 5–10% carbohydrate solution every 15 minutes. This consumption schedule is clearly not possible for all sports and events and should be adjusted for individual athletes in a manner that is appropriate for his or her particular competition.

2. Carbohydrate Loading

Carbohydrate loading, also known as glycogen loading or glycogen supercompensation, is a temporally related technique that has been demonstrated to provide an advantage for performance for some athletes participating in prolonged endurance events. As the name implies, carbohydrate loading is a process in which the athlete consumes very high levels of dietary carbohydrate in the days preceding an event in order to promote supercompensation of glycogen stores. This process maximizes the storage of carbohydrate (glycogen) in the muscle and liver. A recommended technique for achieving the goal of loading the muscle and liver with glycogen includes tapering the volume of exercise in the days preceding the event. During that time, dietary carbohydrate should compose approximately 70% of energy intake. The durations of the regimens have varied considerably. While most regimens last a few days, one study has suggested that a single day of carbohydrate loading during exercise restriction effectively optimized glycogen stores.[44] Restricting energy intake during carbohydrate loading regimens is not advised, as the total grams of carbohydrate consumed would likely be insufficient to maximize glycogen storage. Additionally, classical regimens for carbohydrate loading that required a period of carbohydrate restriction and glycogen-depleting exercise in the period prior to loading are not recommended, because the final outcome of carbohydrate loading is similar between the two methods and the risk of adverse effects such as hypoglycemia are greater when incorporating a depletion phase.

Carbohydrate loading effectively increases muscle glycogen content and can enhance endurance in events of a prolonged nature[45,46] or perhaps even in events that are shorter and performed at very high intensities.[47] Carbohydrate loading for events performed for shorter periods is typically not expected to produce performance enhancements, however.[48]

Tarnopolsky et al.[46] demonstrated that men who followed a 4-day carbohydrate loading regimen consisting of 75% dietary carbohydrate had a 41% increase in muscle glycogen and a 45% improvement in time to fatigue, but similar effects did not occur for women. Subsequent research has demonstrated that carbohydrate loading regimens can be effective for female athletes as well when special attention is paid to obtaining adequate energy intake.[49]

Some concern has been expressed that a fat-restricted diet can reduce intramuscular TG concentrations,[50] which may impair optimal performance. Recent research, however, has demonstrated that a decrease in intramuscular TG concentrations does not necessarily impair performance.[51] That research also demonstrated that blood lipid profiles were negatively affected by just a 3-day fat restriction, which could serve as a health concern for athletes.

Athletes should experiment during training to determine if carbohydrate loading works for their particular sport rather than first attempting the regimen for an actual event. Some athletes have reported minor side effects that can be unpleasant or may even impair performance. Symptoms include gastrointestinal discomfort, weight gain, sluggishness, cramping, and related effects. Weight gain that occurs with glycogen loading is primarily due to increased retention of water that is stored along with the glycogen in the tissues. Approximately 3 grams of water are stored with each gram of glycogen. Additionally, although no research exists on carbohydrate loading regimens in bodybuilders, some athletes have claimed that extra water storage that accompanies higher carbohydrate intake increases muscle volume, providing a larger appearance. Other athletes have suggested that the water retention can cause the muscles to appear less defined and smoother, which may produce a negative result in bodybuilding competitions. Overall, it is up to the individual athlete to determine whether carbohydrate loading is beneficial or detrimental to their performance.

Sports dietitians, coaches, athletic trainers, and other practitioners should be aware of the foods and commercial products that can best provide the athlete with the carbohydrates needed to achieve this level of dietary intake. In general, nutrient-dense foods from the grains, fruits, and vegetables groups should be the focus of dietary intake during carbohydrate loading. Table 2.1 provides a specific list of a several sources of carbohydrate-rich foods that can be incorporated into the athlete's diet during a loading regimen.

3. Food Forms

While most researchers assessing the influence of carbohydrate consumption at various times related to performance have utilized commercial foods or researcher-produced formulas, some research has assessed the potential roles of naturally occurring foods that are typically widely available and more economical in meeting the needs of athletes for optimal performance. Research by Paddon-Jones et al.[52] demonstrated the cost-effectiveness of food compared with a commercial sports supplement when consumed during exercise. Furthermore, Kern et al.[53] demonstrated that a commercial sports gel produced no performance advantage over raisins when consumed 45 minutes prior to 1 hour of vigorous exercise. In another study, honey promoted at least equal endurance and tended to enhance performance in comparison with a commercial sports gel when fed throughout exercise.[54] While commercial sports foods offer a convenient source of readily available energy, particularly from carbohydrate, naturally occurring foods may offer the advantage of promoting a more optimal dietary intake of other key nutrients that can contribute to overall wellness. Furthermore, some foods provide a more palatable alternative to commercial sports foods. However, it is likely that the complex composition of naturally occurring foods could limit their application as sports foods under some conditions.

The metabolic responses to various sources of carbohydrates selected to enhance performance is likely a secondary factor for most athletes in comparison with their practical significances in terms of food choice. While most research suggests that the type of carbohydrate has relatively little impact, some research indicates that different sources may produce varying effects on the body's physiology and therefore may differentially impact performance. For example, as just described, foods that promote a slower uptake of carbohydrate from the gut may be effective in enhancing performance relative to higher glycemic-index foods when eaten in the potentially critical period of about 15–60 minutes before exercise.[55,56] Some have also speculated, although adequate research is not available to support it, that foods promoting a faster entry of carbohydrate into the bloodstream may prove useful during and after an event. For the most part, more research is needed to determine what types of carbohydrate sources are best for various specific occasions.

Sports drinks are typically designed to provide fluid, carbohydrate, and electrolyte replacement. As of 1999, at least 25 commercial sports drinks were available for purchase in the United States.[57] Below et al.[25] demonstrated that the carbohydrate content of a beverage confers a performance advantage for endurance exercise that is separate from and additive to its hydrating effect. Optimal sports drinks will promote consumption of fluid and nutrients through palatability and will provide appropriate ingredients to meet the athletes' needs (e.g., hydration, energy, electrolytes, etc.) for a particular event with no ingredients included that can limit intake or performance or unnecessarily add to the cost of the beverage. The formulation of the beverage will impact each of these factors.

To maximize hydration, a fluid should be palatable, which will promote its consumption. Beverages sweet in taste, flavored, and providing sodium may most enhance consumption. The fluid should also maximize water absorption by limiting the osmolality (a measure of the concentration of solute particles in a solution). Fluids too high in osmolality can produce a lower rate of water absorption; therefore, fluids should be isotonic or hypotonic, depending on the other characteristics required of the sports drink. Some evidence suggests that including sodium in a sports drink may enhance intake by providing a physiological thirst response by increasing vascular sodium concentration.[58] One factor that may limit hydration by decreasing intake is excess carbonation, which may produce a sense of fullness; however, light carbonation does not appear to decrease fluid intake and can contribute to palatability for some individuals.[59]

During training or events in which an important function of the sports drink is to provide energy, which usually includes intense activities lasting about 1 hour or longer, the formulation should provide an optimal amount of readily available energy with the least risk of malabsorption. Carbohydrate is likely the optimal macronutrient to provide the bulk of energy in a sports drink. Beverages with lower concentrations of carbohydrate are typically best absorbed. When the carbohydrate concentration surpasses 6–7%, water absorption can be limited and gastrointestinal distress can occur. Some research has suggested that carbohydrate in the form of glucose polymers may provide a benefit for fluid absorption due to providing a lower osmolality of the solution.[60] Other studies indicate that glucose, sucrose, glucose polymers (maltodextrins), or combinations of these carbohydrates with or without fructose provide relatively equal performance-related benefits. When fructose is fed as the sole carbohydrate source, it may promote gastrointestinal distress since it is absorbed by a saturable facilitated diffusion process; therefore, fructose is recommended only when in combination with other carbohydrates. In fact, recent research has suggested that the addition of fructose to a beverage containing glucose in a ratio of 2:1 (glucose:fructose) enhances exogenous carbohydrate oxidation and endurance performance relative to glucose only.[61] Furthermore, combinations of various carbohydrate sources appear to promote absorption of fluids and enhance the rate of carbohydrate availability and utilization.[61]

Electrolytes (sodium, potassium, and chloride in particular) can be important ingredients in sports drinks. Popular commercial sports drinks typically provide 55–110 mg of sodium and 30–55 mg of potassium in an 8-ounce (240 mL) serving. Although the concentrations of these electrolytes in the sweat of some athletes may exceed the concentration in these beverages, reports of hyponatremia or hypokalemia in athletes using commercial sports drinks to meet 100% of sweat losses are rare. The loss of electrolytes does not typically pose a problem during competition or training unless the exercise is of a prolonged nature or is completed in conditions of high ambient temperatures or humidity; however, as stated earlier, sodium may also be beneficial within a sports drink by virtue of its tendency to promote thirst and fluid intake. Excess sodium, on the other hand, appears to limit fluid intake either by decreasing fluid palatability or promoting increased vascular volume.[62]

Some commercial sports drinks provide ingredients aside from carbohydrate, water, and electrolytes that may or may not impact performance. Some additional ingredients commonly included are vitamins, amino acids, glycerol, caffeine, herbals, and more.

Sports bars are often convenient sources of nutrients required by athletes before, during, and after training or competition. Many types of sports bars that provide varying amounts of macronutrients and micronutrients are commercially available. Whether sports bars can impart ergogenic benefits depends upon many factors including their timing of consumption as well as their nutrient content. Few studies are available to determine if sports bars are truly effective in enhancing performance. One study actually indicated that a commercial bar containing 19 grams of carbohydrate, 14 grams of protein, and 7 grams of fat impaired performance when compared with a feeding providing an equal amount of energy from a glucose polymer.[63] Because most sports bars provide a combination of carbohydrate and protein and, typically, fat as well, their use may best be geared toward recovery.

Sports gels are carbohydrate-rich semisolids used to replenish glucose utilized during a variety of exercise activities. Some sports gels contain vitamins, amino acids, protein, glycerol, caffeine, herbals, or other constituents in addition to the carbohydrate. Commercial sports gels vary in their total carbohydrate contents and the types of carbohydrates used. The carbohydrate source is typically a form of maltodextrin, but other sources of carbohydrate are used as well. These differences can elicit varying physiological responses, as many of the carbohydrates used vary in glycemic index. As discussed, recent research has evaluated the potential efficacy of raisins and honey versus commercial sports gels and found no major differences in effectiveness. Sports gels likely provide no advantage over many whole foods or commercial sports foods. In a field study of marathon runners, Burke et al.[17] demonstrated that carbohydrate provided in the form of a sports gel may even limit endurance performance of some individuals by promoting gastrointestinal discomfort, although no difference in overall performance was detected between a trial in which gel was fed at the rate of 1.1 g of carbohydrate per kilogram body weight versus one in which a flavored placebo beverage was consumed. A recent study indicated that performance was similar regardless of whether carbohydrate was provided as a gel, a sports drink, or as sports jelly beans, and that performance was greater for each carbohydrate trial than a water-only trial.[64] Other researchers evaluated the effects of a gel containing both carbohydrate and protein on performance and postexercise muscle damage.[65] That study suggested that the addition of protein to a gel improved endurance and decreased markers of muscle damage when consumed during and immediately after exercise.

Food form or carbohydrate source in general may influence the capacity for carbohydrate to alter performance based on the foods' glycemic index (GI). Glycemic index is a measure of the effect that a food has on glycemic response. It is typically determined by comparing the 2-hour blood glucose response of 50 g of available carbohydrate from a test food with 50 g of carbohydrate from a standard food (preferably glucose but sometimes white bread). Glycemic index has been demonstrated to have potential implications in optimizing performance of endurance under specific circumstances. Burke et al.[66] summarized the theories regarding the use of GI for exercise suggesting that lower GI foods may be of greatest value when consumed prior to exercise and that higher GI foods may work best during exercise and for resynthesis of glycogen during recovery.

Relatively few studies have actually assessed the role of GI of foods consumed during exercise on physical performance. The basis that higher glycemic index foods are the best carbohydrate sources during exercise is currently founded on theory rather than empirical data. Studies of a variety of types of carbohydrate sources, typically moderate or high in GI, have demonstrated that carbohydrate consumption during exercise can improve endurance performance.[67] In one study, feeding of liquid versus solid meals resulted in differing effects of blood glucose and insulin at rest; however, during exercise, these differences were not detected and the feedings affected exercise performance in a similar fashion.[68] With that in mind, since peak oxidation of carbohydrate typically occurs approximately 1 hour after feeding,[69] foods promoting faster appearance of glucose in the blood are potentially of greatest benefit. However, many factors, including individual variation in GI response and preference of food choice, should not be discounted in the absence of strong evidence against feeding more moderate glycemic foods during exercise. Unpublished research from my laboratory comparing a high GI sports gel with raisins, which have a more moderate glycemic index, suggested no difference in cycling performance when the foods were fed during exercise. Until more well-controlled comparisons of feedings of foods of various glycemic index foods are available, recommendations regarding carbohydrate ingestion during exercise based on glycemic index are predominately unfounded.

The influence of glycemic index performance when foods are provided during pre-exercise feedings has been an area of much more comprehensive investigation. Although all research is not in agreement, likely due to differences in performance testing protocols or timing, quantity, and type of feeding, some research suggests that consumption of a lower GI food prior to exercise is more effective in enhancing performance than consumption of higher GI foods.[55,56,70,71] The explanation for the improvement in performance has been suggested to be a reduction in pre-exercise hyperglycemia resulting in less hyperinsulinemia, as well as decreases in pre-exercise blood lactate concentration and maintenance of higher blood glucose and free fatty acid concentrations after commencing exercise. However, a number of studies have yielded no performance enhancement when comparing feedings of lower versus higher GI foods.[53,72–76] It is noteworthy to mention that research by Burke et al.[77] indicates that any potential effect of pre-exercise feedings of foods of various glycemic indexes is abolished when carbohydrate is also fed during exercise. From a practical perspective, it is important to consider that most athletes participating in prolonged events consume energy both before and during exercise.

Overall, glycemic index may ultimately prove to be a useful tool for pre-event feedings used to enhance endurance performance. Its usefulness as a tool to determine which carbohydrate sources should be fed during exercise appears to be more questionable.

4. Types

In addition to feedings of different food sources of carbohydrates, individual saccharides and mixtures of different carbohydrates have been tested for their influences on metabolism and performance. Carbohydrates tested have included most mono- and disaccharides, glucose polymers and maltodextrins, amylose, and amylopectin.

a. *Fructose*

Unlike glucose and galactose, the other primary monosaccharides found in our diet, fructose is absorbed by a facilitated diffusion process. This mechanism is saturable, meaning that the rate of fructose absorption is limited, which produces absorption at a slower rate. Because it is absorbed more slowly than other carbohydrates, particularly when fed in the absence of other carbohydrates, it produces a lower glycemic response. This slower absorption has been considered a cause for concern for athletes, because large amounts fructose residing in the gut for an extended period of time can produce gastrointestinal distress including cramping and diarrhea. However, as described previously, foods producing a lower glycemic response may be beneficial for performance as pre-exercise feedings when compared to those that produce a higher glycemic response.

When consumed during exercise, there are no reported benefits of pure fructose feedings in comparison to other carbohydrates. Alternatively, because large amounts of fructose can produce symptoms of gastrointestinal distress, feedings high in fructose during exercise are often discouraged. Research has recently suggested that the true value of fructose with regard to exercise metabolism and athletic performance is related to its ability to enhance exogenous carbohydrate utilization. For example, researchers[78–81] have demonstrated that simultaneous consumption of beverages containing carbohydrates absorbed by more than one mechanism enhances exogenous carbohydrate utilization compared with feedings of individual carbohydrates. Recently, Currell and Jeukendrup[61] have demonstrated that this enhancement also yielded improvements in cycling exercise performance. The optimal amount of fructose to include in such a beverage is not known; however, a maltodextrin:fructose ratio of 0.8 enhanced exogenous carbohydrate utlization and suppressed perceptions of muscle tiredness, physical exertion, and fatigue more effectively than solutions containing ratios of the two carbohydrates of 0.5 and 1.2.[82]

b. Maltodextrin

Although most evidence suggests that glucose polymers or maltodextrins offer no advantage relative to other carbohydrates for exercise performance, they can theoretically be considered a preferred fuel for endurance athletes, because as larger particles they could provide more energy within fewer total molecules, which may provide an osmotic advantage over simpler carbohydrates. The key determinant of the osmotic load is the total amount of molecules in the solution; therefore, fewer particles of maltodextrin are needed to produce a solution containing an equal or greater amount of energy. It is expected that more energy could be fed with less risk of interfering with fluid balance and production of gastrointestinal distress. Furthermore, this could allow for more rapid absorption of water; hence, a solution containing glucose polymers/maltodextrins may have a hydrating advantage over other beverages. As summarized by Lamb and Brodowicz,[60] research has supported the notion that these glucose chains may increase the rate of gastric emptying and allow for faster glucose and water absorption in the intestinal tract.[60]

Some research has suggested that maltodextrin need not be absorbed to produce ergogenic effects. Carter et al.[83] assessed the influence of oral rinses with a 6.4% maltodextrin versus placebo every 12.5% of a cycling bout. Performance was slightly but consistently better during the maltodextrin rinse trial. The authors speculated that central drive or motivation rather than direct metabolic effects of maltodextrin were responsible. Research on other carbohydrate rinses has not yet been published, so it is not clear whether this is a property limited to maltodextrins.

Researchers have also compared the influence of consumption of various starches versus maltodextrin and glucose feedings on postexercise glycogen production and performance of a subsequent short-term exercise bout.[84] Compared with the trials assessing the influences of amylopectin, maltodextrin, or glucose consumption, glycogen resynthesis was lower following ingestion of starch with a high amylose content. No differences in time trial performance were detected, however. Therefore, starches rich in amylopectin may also be excellent choices for inclusion in a sports beverage, whereas those high in amylose may be somewhat less advantageous.

c. Galactose and Trehalose

Sports foods providing galactose or trehalose have gained popularity in the past few years despite little available evidence to support a benefit for performance in comparison with other carbohydrates. Galactose is a monosaccharide most commonly consumed as a portion of lactose. Trehalose is a disaccharide composed of two glucose molecules linked via the number 1 carbon of each of the glucose units. Trehalose is found in low levels in the diet but has been detected in foods such as mushrooms, honey, shrimp, lobster, and foods made with yeasts. One study demonstrated lower glycemic and insulinemic responses when either galactose or trehalose were fed 45 minutes prior to cycling exercise versus glucose feeding. These effects produced no difference in cycling performance, however. Another study demonstrated that galactose oxidation during 2 hours of exercise is approximately half that of glucose, which suggests that energy production from galactose is less robust and limiting relative to glucose.[85] In fact, Jentjens and Jeukendrup[86] recently demonstrated impairment in endurance performance when an 8% solution of galactose was fed before and during exercise in comparison with an 8% solution containing an equal mixture of galactose and glucose. While some merit may exist for using galactose or trehalose to limit the glycemic and insulinemic responses in pre-exercise feedings, their use as sole-source carbohydrates during exercise is clearly not recommended.

d. *Ribose*

Ribose is a 5-carbon sugar produced from glucose through the hexose monophosphate shunt for the synthesis of nucleotides. Several studies have examined the effect of ribose on ATP formation as well as exercise performance in athletes. Research to date has failed to demonstrate that ribose supplementation can improve performance of activities completed at high intensities.[87–89] Results regarding the efficacy of supplementation to produce higher concentrations of ATP in the muscle are split. One study demonstrated that ATP levels were enhanced 72 hours after exercise during ribose supplementation,[88] while another yielded no effect of oral ribose.[89] Overall, the available data do not warrant ribose supplementation for performance enhancement; however, because some research has demonstrated enhanced muscle ATP content due to ribose supplement, its potential value cannot be completely discounted.

5. Carbohydrate-Related Supplements

a. *Pyruvate*

Pyruvate, also known as pyruvic acid, is a 3-carbon intermediate of metabolism produced primarily via aerobic glycolysis from glucose and through the transamination of alanine. Pyruvate is involved in a number of processes. One function of pyruvate is energy production through the pyruvate dehydrogenase complex, which produces acetyl CoA and $NADH+H^+$ as well as the elimination of carbon dioxide. Acetyl CoA produced can enter Krebs cycle resulting in $NADH+H^+$ and $FADH_2$ formation as previously described, which, along with the $NADH+H^+$ formed in the pyruvate dehydrogenase complex can produce ATP through the electron transport system.

Given its critical role in energy production, the potential of pyruvate to serve as an ergogenic aid has been examined, but only to a limited extent. Research has demonstrated that doses of 7 grams per day are ineffective in enhancing endurance.[90] However, when pyruvate was supplemented at very high doses (25 grams) along with an additional 75 grams of dihydroxacetone, another important metabolic intermediate, it improved endurance in both arm ergometry and cycling ergometry to fatigue after a 7-day supplementation regimen.[91,92] Whether pyruvate could enhance endurance under similar situations if supplemented alone is unclear. Furthermore, the threshold dose that is required to obtain similar results is not known. This is of practical importance because regular consumption of pyruvate and dihydroxyacetone at these levels would be extremely expensive.

The potential influence of pyruvate supplementation on body composition has also been studied. Research suggests that at relatively high doses (at least 6 grams per day), pyruvate may be effective in producing weight loss.[93] This study has been criticized, however,[94] because more women were in the experimental group receiving pyruvate than in the placebo and control groups. Furthermore, no weight loss was exhibited by the placebo or control groups, which, like the experimental group, were allowed limited (2000 kcal) energy consumption and participated in a moderate exercise program, both of which would be expected to produce weight loss. More research is needed before pyruvate can be recommended as a weight loss aid for exercisers or non-exercisers.

b. Lactic Acid

Lactic acid (lactate) is the final product formed when glucose is catabolized under anaerobic conditions. It is produced in metabolism by the addition of hydrogen molecules to pyruvate from $NADH+H^+$. During exercise recovery, the enzyme lactic acid dehydrogenase reconverts lactate to pyruvate, producing $NADH+H^+$. The resulting pyruvate can be used for energy production or undergo gluconeogenesis for the production of glucose.

Lactate has also been marketed as a potential ergogenic aid. Some have theorized that chronic ingestion of lactate could produce an adaptation that would enhance performance during strenuous exercise by improving the body's ability to buffer lactate accumulation during exercise. Research has failed to support this theory, however.[95] Lactate alone or in combination with a carbohydrate as part of a sports beverage also failed to enhance performance in comparison with a carbohydrate-only trial.[96]

Lactate combined with an amino acid, referred to as polylactate, has also been studied for its ergogenic potential. Manufacturers have claimed that this supplement can enhance endurance; however, research has been equivocal regarding its usefulness. One study suggested that when included with a 7% glucose polymer solution at the rate of approximately 11% of a solution, supplementation of polylactate failed to produce significant changes in performance or performance-related physiological variables.[97] A 7% solution containing an 80:20 mixture of polylactate and lactate produced an enhancement in the blood buffering capacity; however, differences in ratings of perceived exertion were not detected and no exercise performance data were reported.[98]

c. Chromium

Chromium is a trace mineral found in a variety of foods such as mushrooms, nuts, whole grains, asparagus, and beer. Chromium functions along with niacin as a component of glucose-tolerance factor. This important complex has a critical, although not particularly well understood, role in insulin function; therefore, chromium is extremely important for normal glucose metabolism. Chromium deficiency produces decreased insulin function, which results in impaired glucose intolerance and altered lipid metabolism.

Due to its essential role in blood glucose regulation along with some research suggesting that many Americans consume inadequate amounts of chromium, some have speculated that chromium supplementation (particularly as chromium picolinate) may increase lean body mass and strength as well as promote loss of body fat.[99,100] Early research suggested increased body weight ascribed to increased lean mass during 40-day[99] and 12-week[100] training programs. In the study by Hasten et al.,[100] no effects on strength, skinfolds, or circumference measures were detected; however, a statistically significant increase in body weight in female weight lifters was reported along with no change in weight of male weight lifters. Because weight gain occurred only in women, the results of that study have been questioned.[101] The results are also questioned because the authors reported an increase in fat free mass with no concurrent increase in strength. The results of the study by Evans[99] have also been questioned because subjects were poorly controlled during the training program and no standardization regarding prior weight training experience was provided.[101]

In contrast to the early research, a review of the majority of research available in healthy active humans suggests that chromium is not effective as a fat-loss supplement.[102–108] The durations of these studies ranged from 8 to 14 weeks and included training programs along with chromium supplementation. In each case the researchers failed to detect any additional benefits from chromium over training alone. Grant and colleagues[109] reported that chromium supplementation with no concurrent exercise training may result in an increase in body weight. In that study, a group of obese women gained almost 2.0 kg of body weight over a 9-week supplementation period. When a chromium nicotinate supplement was combined with a 9-week exercise training program, the obese women lost approximately 1 kg of body weight. The researchers also reported no change in body weight, fat mass, or fat free mass in an exercising placebo group and an exercising group consuming chromium picolinate. This study was the first to report statistically significant weight loss with supplementation of chromium nicotinate. The reason for the lack of a similar effect for the chromium picolinate trial is not known. This research indicates that more research on chromium nicotinate is warranted. Overall, there is little evidence from well-designed studies that chromium increases lean body mass or decreases body fatness or that athletes require more chromium in their diets than non-athletes.

d. Glycerol

Glycerol is a water-soluble, 3-carbon alcohol molecule. It serves as an important intermediate in metabolism and can be used for the synthesis of carbohydrate and lipids as well as the production of energy. Glycerol is the 3-carbon backbone of mono-, di-, and triglycerides as well as glycerophosphatides, a group of phospholipids. Although glycerol is consumed as part of many molecules, it is not considered an essential nutrient because it is also synthesized within the body.

Because glycerol can serve as an intermediate molecule in glycolysis for energy production, its role as a fuel for exercise and potential ergogenic aid has been studied. The conversion of glycerol to glucose is typically considered to be insufficient for rapid and efficient energy production during exercise;[110] however, its supplementation has also been studied for its potential hydrating capacity. Because glycerol is an extremely hydrophilic molecule, its supplementation has been used to promote the retention of fluid within the body. While not all studies are in agreement,[111] evidence from several studies has supported the notion that consumption of exogenous glycerol can increase body water content, producing increased plasma volume compared with plain water.[112,113] Glycerol-induced hyperhydration may also blunt the thermic response to exercise in the heat.[112] Maintenance of plasma volume and prevention of dehydration through glycerol supplementation may improve endurance trial performance[113] or prolong time to fatigue.[114–116] Some studies have failed to demonstrate performance enhancement with glycerol supplementation, however.[117–119] Authors of a recent meta-analysis of glycerol supplementation in exercisers concluded that glycerol clearly enhances fluid retention, and although it commonly improves performance, more research is needed to better understand its influence on exercise capacity.[120]

The optimal dose and timing of glycerol ingestion has not yet been determined. Most researchers have provided approximately 1 gram of glycerol per kg body weight as part of the glycerol supplementation regimen. Some research participants have reported minor adverse events associated with glycerol supplementation, which are likely due to an osmotic effect. Symptoms have included headaches and gastrointestinal distress such as nausea, bloating, and cramping. Furthermore, in cases when body weight gain is undesirable for competition, this could be considered an adverse side effect for some athletes.

e. *Alanine*

Alanine is a non-essential, highly gluconeogenic amino acid. Its role in glucose production through the alanine cycle was described previously. It is oxidized for energy production at a high rate,[121,122] which suggests it may have some merit for use during exercise. Research has also demonstrated that under some conditions, alanine supplementation can spare the use of essential amino acids as energy sources.[123–125] Little research has attempted to establish an ergogenic role of alanine. Its ergogenic potential as well as its influence on plasma concentrations of amino acids and fuel substrates were evaluated recently.[126] In a double blind design, four different solutions containing 6% sucrose and 6% alanine (ALA-CHO); 6% alanine (ALA); 6% sucrose (CHO); and placebo (PLC) were tested during randomly ordered trials. Exercisers cycled for 45 min at 75% of their aerobic capacity followed by a 15-minute performance trial. Blood samples were collected prior to the initiation of exercise and again immediately before the 15-minute performance ride. The key results were that alanine supplementation with or without sucrose blunted the exercise-induced decrease in plasma concentrations of most gluconeogenic amino acids; however, it failed to enhance endurance performance. Subsequent research demonstrated no performance improvements during longer bouts of exercise, which may have been linked to increased gastrointestinal distress.[127] Future research is needed to examine the importance of the amino acid sparing influence of alanine in exercisers.

III. FAT

Fats, also known as lipids, are characterized by their tendency to dissolve in nonpolar solvents. When speaking specifically about dietary fat, most nutritionists are referring to TGs, the specific class of lipids that comprise the vast majority (>95%) of lipids in the diet. Other lipids in the diet or the body include fatty acids, monoglycerides, diglycerides, phospholipids, sterols, some vitamins, eicosanoids, lipoproteins, glycolipids, and other important molecules. Lipids in general possess an array of functions, including energy provision, serving as major structural components to cells, emulsification, molecular signaling, and participating in a multitude of important biochemical processes.

A. Classifications and Dietary Sources

Numerous lipids with biologically important functions exist in nature. These lipids can be classified by their structural characteristics. Several lipids described here make up a majority of the lipids in our diet as well as our tissues and play potentially important roles in the wellness and performance of athletes.

1. TGs

The structure of a TG, also known as a triacylglycerol, includes a 3-carbon glycerol backbone linked to three fatty acids (acyl groups) through ester bonds. Triglycerides account for the vast majority of dietary lipids and provide energy as well as essential fatty acids to the body. Fatty acids bound to glycerol differ in their structures and the effects they exert metabolically. Triglyceride is a key component of the diet in both exercisers and non-exercisers.

The Acceptable Macronutrient Distribution Range (AMDR) established by the Institute of Medicine when determining the Dietary Reference Intakes is 20–35% of total energy intake for adults. AMDR values have also been established for linoleic acid (n-6 fatty acids in general) and alpha-linolenic acid (n-3 fatty acids in general) at 5–10% of energy and 0.6–1.2% of energy, respectively. The dietary intake of total fat by athletes is typically reported to be near or within the AMDR. Using a weighed food diary approach, Jensen et al.[1] reported that fat intake of U.S. collegiate cyclists during training was 27±8% of energy. A study of Australian national-level triathletes and runners indicated that they consumed a similar amount of fat (27±7% and 32±7% of energy, respectively).[2] More recently conducted research of female collegiate swimmers and divers suggest that they consumed slightly less fat (averaging approximately 22–23% of energy) than levels reported for most athletes either at the end of the competitive season[3] or during a taper from training Ousley-Pahnke et al.[128] Other research of swimmers has reported much higher fat intake averaging in a range of 30–43% of energy or more from fat.[129–133] Elite male Kenyan runners have been demonstrated to restrict fat intake to approximately 46±14 grams per day, which averages 13% of energy intake.[4]

2. Fatty Acids

Fatty acids are lipid molecules characterized by a hydrocarbon chain linked to a carboxylic acid group. These molecules vary in many ways—structurally, nutritionally and biochemically—which has led to many classifications for fatty acids as well as fats (TGs) rich in particular classes of fatty acids.

One classification is based on fatty acid length, as determined by the number of carbon atoms in the molecule. Short-chain fatty acids are composed of 2–4 carbons. Medium-chain fatty acids are usually classified as those including 6–10 carbons, and long-chain fatty acids have 12 or more. Some references classify lauric acid, which has 12 carbons, as a medium-chain fatty acid rather than a long-chain fatty acid. Fatty acids with shorter chains tend to be more soluble in water due to the hydrophilic nature of the carboxyl end of the fatty acid. Long-chain fatty acids compose the majority of fatty acids in the human diet. In general, dietary sources of most long chain saturated fatty acids are animal foods, coconut oil, palm oil, and palm kernel oil. Monounsaturated fatty acids are found in high levels in several plant foods including canola oil, olives and olive oil, avocados, and others, and are usually found in lower amounts in animal products. Fish, nuts, seeds, and many other plant oils tend to be rich in polyunsaturated fatty acids. Although small amounts of short- and medium-chain fatty acids are obtained from foods such as dairy products and coconut oil, relatively small quantities of these fatty acids are found in a natural diet. Medium chain TG oil, produced from fractionation of coconut oil, is a rich source of medium-chain fatty acids and is commonly used in dietary supplements and formulas for medical nutrition therapy.

The degree of saturation with hydrogen atoms, which is determined by the absence or presence of double bonds between carbon atoms, is also a major classification for fatty acids. These degrees yield the classifications of saturated, monounsaturated, and polyunsaturated fatty acids. Because each carbon molecule requires four bonds, the carbons linked by a double bond have only a single hydrogen bound to them. Saturated fatty acids are "saturated" with hydrogen atoms and therefore possess no double bonds. Unsaturated fatty acids have at least one double bond and those with just a single double bond are called monounsaturated fatty acids (MUFAs). Polyunsaturated fatty acids (PUFAs) have multiple double bonds.

Unsaturated fatty acids can be further classified based on the position of the double bond within the hydrocarbon chain as well as the structure of the molecules around the double bond. If the hydrogen molecules on the double-bonded carbons are oriented on the same side of the hydrocarbon chain, the bond is considered to have a cis configuration. In this configuration, these hydrogen molecules interact to produce a bend in the hydrocarbon chain. Fatty acids with a trans configuration have hydrogen atoms oriented across from one another at the site of the double bond, which allows the hydrocarbon to take on what is considered a straighter structure. Trans fatty acids are more accurately called trans unsaturated fatty acids, because they possess at least one double bond. These differences in structure produce vastly different effects on metabolism, with most trans unsaturated fatty acids producing harmful effects relative to cis unsaturated fatty acids. Dietary sources of trans fatty acids include those industrially produced through the process of hydrogenation (i.e., shortening and other partially hydrogenated plant oils) and natural sources, particularly tissue and dairy products from ruminant animals.

The position of the double bond or bonds on the hydrocarbon chain is also important for determining the metabolic fates of unsaturated fatty acids. The system most

TABLE 2.2
Characteristics of Common Fatty Acids

Name	Chain Length	Double Bonds	Omega Class
SCFAs			
Acetate	2	0	NA
Propionate	3	0	NA
Butyrate	4	0	NA
MCFAs			
Caproate	6	0	NA
Caprylate	8	0	NA
Caprate	10	0	NA
LCFAs			
Laurate*	12	0	NA
Myristate	14	0	NA
Palmitate	16	0	NA
Stearate	18	0	NA
Oleate	18	1	9
Linoleate	18	2	6
α-Linolenate	18	3	3
γ-Linolenate	18	3	6
Arachindonate	20	4	6
Eicosapentaenoate	20	5	3
Docosahexaenoate	22	6	3

* Sometimes classified as a medium-chain fatty acid.

commonly used by nutritionists for classifying fatty acids based on double bond location is the omega classification, which is determined by the position of the first double bond when counting from the hydrocarbon end. Fatty acids with the first double bond on the third carbon are called omega-3 fatty acids. Those with the first double bond on the number 6 carbon are called omega-6 fatty acids, and so on. While the amount of energy produced from catabolism of fatty acids is similar regardless of omega classification, the position of the double bond is critical for determining other functions of fatty acids. Table 2.2 depicts the names and various classifications for many fatty acids prevalent in the diet or produced in metabolism along with further information regarding their structures.

Two fatty acids, linoleic acid and alpha-linolenic acid (the omega-3 form of linolenic acid), are additionally classified as essential fatty acids, because they are required in the human diet. Essential fatty acids are required in the diets of humans, because we lack the ability to produce them ourselves. This is because we lack the delta-12 and delta-15 desaturase enzymes that are required to produce the double bonds needed in the final steps of the synthesis of these fatty acids. Deficiencies of essential fatty acids produce clinical symptoms including dermatitis, decreased growth or weight loss, organ dysfunction, and abnormal reproductive status. Although these are the only fatty acids required in the diet, other omega-3 fatty acids such as eicosapentaenoic acid (EPA) and docosahexaenoic acid (DHA) can be consumed to meet a portion of the alpha-linolenic acid requirement, which is usually expressed as total omega-3 fatty acid needs. Rich dietary sources of linoleic acid include a variety of vegetable oils such as soybean, corn, safflower, cottonseed, sunflower seed, and peanut oil. Soybean, flaxseed, linseed, and walnut oils are particularly good sources of alpha-linolenic acid, while fatty fish are particularly good sources of EPA and DHA.

Fatty acids are extremely important to athletes for normal biochemistry and health as well as for the production of energy. Metabolism of fatty acids during exercise is described later. Many specific fatty acids and fatty acids within particular classifications have been studied for their potential ergogenic benefits and are covered later as well.

3. Phosphoplipids

Phospholipids belong to a family of molecules containing both lipid and phosphate components (e.g., glycerophosphatides, sphingolipids, etc.). In particular, glycerophosphatides consist of two fatty acids bound to carbons 1 (sn-1) and 2 (sn-2) of glycerol with a phosphate molecule, which is also linked to one of many compounds including choline, serine, ethanolamine, and inositol, bound to the carbon at the sn-3 position. Phosphatidyl choline, also known as lecithin, is a key phospholipid. Functions of phospholipids include serving as a major constituent of cellular membranes, participating in numerous biochemical reactions, and providing important structural and functional components of tissues of the central and peripheral nervous systems.

4. Cholesterol

As a member of a class of molecules referred to as sterols, cholesterol possesses a 4-ringed steroidal structure (sterane) with a single alcohol group and an 8-carbon alkyl group. Dietary sources of cholesterol are limited to animal products. Non-animal foods are cholesterol free unless they are prepared with an animal product. Foods rich in cholesterol include meats and organ meats, seafood, egg yolk, and some dairy foods. Because cholesterol requirements can be met through biosynthesis, there is no dietary need for cholesterol.

Cholesterol is critical for normal body processes. It serves as an integral component of cellular membranes and steroid hormones, vitamin D, and bile acids are synthesized from cholesterol. The general public perceives cholesterol as a threat, however, due to the relationship between elevated serum cholesterol and risk for cardiovascular diseases.

B. Digestion and Absorption

After consumption, most dietary lipids require digestion prior to absorption. Humans are extremely efficient in digesting lipids from mixed meals. Fecal fat excretion is typically limited to approximately 4% of the dietary load.[134] The majority of lipid digestion occurs in the small intestine by the actions of pancreatic enzymes that enter the digestive system at the duodenum. Digestion cannot be accomplished without the emulsification of the dietary lipid components with the aqueous juices of the gastrointestinal tract, which occurs primarily due to the amphiphatic properties of bile acids. Bile acids are produced from cholesterol in the liver and stored and concentrated in the gallbladder. Upon consumption of a meal, particularly a fatty meal, the gallbladder contracts in response to the action of the hormone cholecystokinin, secreting bile into the duodenum via the common bile duct. Bile mixes with the aqueous chyme from the stomach and the digestive secretions of the pancreas, which allows the water-soluble pancreatic enzymes to interact with lipids in the chyme.

The enzyme primarily responsible for TG digestion is pancreatic lipase, which works in concert with colipase, which is also secreted from the pancreas. Colipase forms a complex between the emulsified lipid and lipase to allow digestion to occur. The function of pancreatic lipase is typically to hydrolyze the acyl groups from the glycerol backbone at the sn-1 and sn-3 positions, with greater specificity for cleavage at the sn-1 position. Typical products of TG digestion are monoglycerides and free fatty acids. Phospholipids must also be digested prior to absorption. This occurs through the function of the enzyme phospholipase A-2, which cleaves the acyl group at the sn-2 position, leaving a monoglyceride and lysophospholipid. A portion of dietary cholesterol is consumed as cholesterol esters in which a fatty acid is linked to cholesterol through an ester bond. The enzyme responsible for cholesterol ester digestion is cholesterol esterase. The activity of cholesterol esterase yields free cholesterol and a monoglyceride.

The products of digestion along with lipids not requiring digestion, by the action of bile acids, produce small lipid droplets referred to as micelles. The lipid components of micelles can be taken up by the epithelial cells of the small intestine. Short- and medium-chain fatty acids are then absorbed primarily into the mesenteric circulation for transport to the liver. Long-chain fatty acids and other products of digestion are transferred to the endoplasmic reticulum where TGs, phospholipids, and some cholesterol esters are reformed. The absorbed lipid components are ultimately packaged along with proteins (apoproteins) to form chylomicron lipoproteins. Chylomicrons are exported via lacteals of the intestinal villi to lymphatic vessels lining the small intestine. The content of these vessels are transported to the venous circulation via the left thoracic lymph duct; therefore, chylomicrons are delivered to the general circulation and peripheral tissues without first entering the liver.

C. Lipid Metabolism

1. General Metabolic Processes of Lipid Metabolism

Lipid metabolism encompasses an array of processes that relate to energy production, lipoprotein metabolism, fatty acid and TG production, synthesis of bioactive molecules, and numerous other processes related to the functions of various lipids.

Fatty acids serve as the major precursor for energy production from lipids. Initiation of the steps in energy production from fats depends on the source of the fatty acids. The primary sources of fatty acids catabolized for energy production are TGs. Triglycerides utilized for energy production reside primarily within the adipose tissue; however, TGs stored within muscle cells and those within both exogenous and endogenously produced lipoproteins, primarily chylomicrons and very low density lipoproteins (VLDL), respectively, are sources of energy as well.

When originating from adipose tissue TG, the first step in fat catabolism is mobilization of the fatty acids from the fat cell for export into the circulation. This is accomplished via the action of hormone sensitive lipase (HSL), which is responsive to an array of hormones. Hormones known to activate HSL include epinephrine, norepinephrine, glucagon, adrenocorticotropic hormone, thyroxine, thyroid stimulating hormone, and growth hormone. HSL hydrolyzes the fatty acids at the sn-1 and sn-3 positions, and monoacylglycerol lipase hydrolyzes the remaining fatty acid at the sn-2 position. As the fatty acids, usually described as free fatty acids (FFA), enter the circulation, they are bound to protein, principally albumin, for transport throughout the aqueous bloodstream. These fatty acids can be taken up by target tissues, particularly muscle tissue during exercise, where they can be catabolized for energy. During the postprandial state, insulin blocks the action of HSL, thereby decreasing fat mobilization.

Some TG is stored within the cells of the muscle tissue and is referred to as intramyocellular TG. These stores represent only a small fraction of the TG stored within the body, but can still play an important role in providing energy to working muscles. The fatty acids within this depot do not require mobilization for utilization. The TG within the muscle is broken down by the action of HSL present in the muscle cell.

Lipoprotein-bound TG is already in the circulatory system, particularly while in a postprandial state, and can also be taken up by target tissues after fatty acids are hydrolyzed by the action of lipoprotein lipase (LPL). LPL is a capillary bound TG hydrolase found in highest concentrations in muscle and adipose tissues. Upon hydrolyzing fatty acids from TG located primarily in VLDL or chylomicron particles, the FFA will predominantly enter the tissue in which it was cleaved, but a fraction will escape into the systemic circulation. The contributions of lipoproteins to the production of FFA available for energy catabolism is lower during fasting, because the concentrations of chylomicrons and VLDL are highest during the postprandial period. However, unlike adipose tissue, in which LPL expression is depressed during fasting, muscle LPL levels are maintained, which allows muscle-associated LPL to continue to hydrolyze lipoprotein-bound TG, particularly from VLDL, for ultimate oxidation within the muscle cell. During exercise, muscle LPL is increased, which enhances the ability of the muscle to obtain energy from lipoprotein-bound TGs.

Uptake of fatty acids by muscle cells occurs by processes that are not fully understood but may include a combination of diffusion and protein-mediated uptake particularly associated with fatty acid translocase, plasmalemmal-located fatty acid binding protein, and fatty acid transport protein.[135] Once inside the cell, fatty acids are linked to coenzyme A by fatty acyl CoA synthetase. Oxidation of fatty acids occurs in the mitochondria; however, long-chain fatty acids cannot diffuse into the mitochondria, so they must enter by an elaborate transport mechanism. Components of the transport mechanism include carnitine and the enzymes carnitine-acylcarnitine translocase, carnitine palmitoyltransferase-I (CPT-I) and carnitine palmitoyltransferase-II (CPT-II). CPT-I, associated with the outer mitochondrial membrane, allows the transfer of the acyl group from the cytosolic fatty acyl CoA to carnitine to transiently produce an acylcarnitine molecule. Carnitine-acylcarnitine translocase catalyzes the transport of the acylcarnitine molecule across the inner mitochondrial membrane, with subsequent reesterification of the acyl group to coenzyme A within the mitochondrial matrix through the action of CPT-II on the inner surface of the inner mitochondrial membrane.

Fatty acyl CoA molecules inside the mitochondria can be broken down through β-oxidation. The process of β-oxidation, which includes a series of reactions: an oxidation reaction followed by hydration, a second oxidation, and cleavage of acetyl CoA. β-oxidation is repeated on the remaining 2-carbon shorter fatty acyl Coenzyme-A (CoA) until the fatty acid is completely broken down. The process yields $FADH_2$ during the first oxidation step and NADH + H^+ in the second oxidation. Acetyl CoA molecules are obtained for every 2 carbons of the fatty acid oxidized. The resulting $FADH_2$ and NADH + H^+ can undergo oxidation with the production of energy via the electron transport chain as described for carbohydrate. The acetyl CoA molecules can also be further metabolized via Krebs cycle as previously described followed by further mitochondrial oxidation through the electron transport chain.

Under certain conditions, the use of fat for fuel is favored, while during others carbohydrate is the preferred substrate. For example, after a meal, insulin synthesis and secretion from the pancreas increases, which promotes the uptake of glucose, particularly in the muscles and adipose, by GLUT-4 as previously described. This enhanced uptake increases both glycogen storage and glucose oxidation. Insulin also inhibits lipolysis by decreasing hormone-sensitive lipase activity, which decreases efflux of fatty acids into the bloodstream. Furthermore, the increase in glucose uptake also promotes the production of malonyl CoA from acetyl CoA resulting from increased pyruvate dehydrogenase activity. Malonyl CoA inhibits CPT-I, which also decreases the utilization of fat for energy. The activity of adipose tissue lipoprotein lipase is also higher following a meal, which directs a greater proportion of circulating lipids to the adipose tissue. This state contrasts with the profile of fuel utilization during fasted conditions. During fasting, carbohydrate use by the muscle and adipose is suppressed, while fat utilization increases. Lipoprotein lipase activity in the muscle is enhanced, which promotes greater uptake of fatty acids from TG within circulating VLDL molecules. Lipolysis from the adipose tissue occurs at a greater rate, increasing the availability of FFA, which are taken up by the muscle for energy production. The increase in FFA uptake promotes β-oxidation, which yields acetyl CoA. This increase in acetyl CoA concentration decreases pyruvate utilization by lowering pyruvate dehydrogenase activity. Citrate concentrations are decreased by enhanced Krebs cycle activity, which suppresses glucose breakdown by inhibiting the activity of phosphofructokinase, the rate limiting enzyme in glycolysis. The rate of fatty acid utilization is proportional to the plasma FFA concentration; therefore, dietary strategies that produce elevations in plasma FFA concentration will typically increase fatty acid oxidation.

Exercise also increases fat utilization by increasing the use of ketone bodies produced primarily from fat and certain amino acids. In metabolism, ketones and ketoacids are produced from acetyl CoA. Acetone is a ketone and acetoacetate and beta-hydroxybutyrate are ketoacids. Ketone bodies can be utilized for energy by certain tissues, such as red blood cells and the central nervous system, that rely primarily on glucose as an energy substrate when glucose is less available. When their production increases to a rate greater than the rate of catabolism, a state of ketosis can occur. During exercise, ketone production and utilization are increased, providing athletes with an additional energy source. Little research is available to determine the impact of ketosis on athletic performance; however, many have speculated that it could be impaired due to a lack of available glucose for energy. Research has suggested that this is not always the case. For example, one study demonstrated that consumption of a diet extremely low in carbohydrate and high in fat for 1 month produced a state of ketosis that did not impair exercise performance.[136]

2. Lipid Metabolism during Exercise

Fat and carbohydrate are the key contributors to energy production at rest and during exercise, although amino acids produce energy to a lesser extent as well. While multiple factors influence energy production, the principal determinant of both total energy expenditure and the proportions of substrates utilized is exercise intensity. Because, under most conditions, amino acids serve as a minor contributor to energy production, the relative contributions of fat and carbohydrate are the key concern for this chapter. That proportion is most commonly determined by measurement of the respiratory exchange ratio (RER). RER, also know as respirator quotient (RQ), is assessed through determination of the volume of carbon dioxide produced divided by the volume of oxygen consumed as measured via expired gases. In general, as RER approaches 1.00, carbohydrate is providing a greater percentage of fuel for metabolism. Conversely, as RER approaches 0.70, fat is providing a larger percentage of fuel being utilized. The RER of protein is typically about 0.82; however, its impact in total fuel utilization is determined by urinary urea excretion and is usually not considered. As exercise intensity increases, carbohydrate utilization increases at an absolute rate and as a percentage of energy expenditure; thus, RER increases as well. While the proportion of oxidation of carbohydrate versus fat increases with greater exercise intensity, this is largely due to an increase in carbohydrate utilization rather than a decrease in fat consumption, although as intensity increased from 65% of aerobic capacity to 85%, a small decrease in fat utilization occurs as well.[137]

As described previously, the sources of fat and carbohydrate for energy production are varied. Fatty acids originating primarily from TGs are the major lipids utilized for energy during exercise and come principally from adipose tissue, intramuscular depots, and lipoproteins, as discussed. The relative contributions of these sources to energy production vary depending on numerous factors. A key factor that determines the proportion of energy production from these depots is exercise intensity. Research has demonstrated that, at lower intensities, the contribution of intramuscular TG is minor in comparison with FFA obtained from the plasma, and that as exercise intensity increases, the contributions of these sources for energy production tend to become more equal.[137] Furthermore, the duration of exercise participation influences fat source utilization. As duration continues during moderate steady state exercise, the plasma-borne FFAs make up a greater percentage of the fat utilized as intramuscular fat utilization decreases.[137]

D. Lipids and Exercise Performance

Strategies to modify fat intake as ways to improve athletic performance have not received the amount of attention that carbohydrate-related strategies have. This likely stems from the notion that acute consumption of fat produces less dramatic effects on metabolism and substrate utilization than alterations in acute carbohydrate intake. Much of the research related to lipids and performance has included (a) chronic adaptation to fat in general, (b) intake of particular types of lipids, or (c) dietary supplements that may alter fat metabolism in ways that could favorably affect performance.

1. Fat Loading

Fat loading derives its name from carbohydrate loading, the technique of consuming a very high carbohydrate diet in the days leading up to competition. Regimens of fat loading vary from carbohydrate loading in three major ways. One, as the name describes, is that the diet is very rich in fat instead of carbohydrate. Another is that the dietary modifications are often followed for longer periods of time to achieve the desired metabolic responses. A third difference is that carbohydrate loading is predicated on the notion of maximizing stores of carbohydrate energy within the body, while the goal of fat loading is to alter the body's metabolism in a way that will enhance fat utilization for energy production during competition. It is thought that this response would spare the utilization of stored carbohydrate for energetic processes, thereby promoting enhanced endurance.

Results of studies assessing the efficacy of fat loading for improving endurance performance have been equivocal. Furthermore, some of the research that has demonstrated enhancements in performance has been heavily criticized for design flaws. Because, as described previously, several studies have demonstrated that a carbohydrate-rich diet helps to maintain glycogen stores,[41] most believe it is counterintuitive to believe that fat loading could enhance performance. Empirically, however, some researchers examining the potential impact of fat loading have detected enhancements in performance[42,138,139] and fewer have actually detected adverse effects of a fat-rich diet.[140,141] Several other studies have yielded results suggesting that no difference in performance occurs in athletes adapted to a high fat versus a higher carbohydrate diet for up to several weeks, suggesting that consumption of a high fat diet at the expense of carbohydrate does not impair performance.[136,142–144] Overall, with equivocal data regarding fat loading as well as the risk of low muscle glycogen content while consuming a high fat diet, it is prudent to recommend that most endurance athletes consume a nutrient-dense lower fat diet until more conclusive data are available to suggest that fat loading is more effective.

As a method to maximize pre-event glycogen stores and to take advantage of the potential benefits of fat loading, several researchers have explored the potential of shifting to a carbohydrate-rich diet following fat adaptation in the days preceding the event. In one of the first such studies, Lambert et al.[145] demonstrated that adaptation to a diet rich in fats followed by short-term high carbohydrate intake in the days prior to competition enhanced cycling performance. Most other studies using a high fat adaptation followed by a short-term shift to a high carbohydrate intake have not observed similar improvements.[142,146,147] Most of those studies, however, used a shorter fat adaptation period followed by just a single day of high carbohydrate intake, both of which may have limited the opportunity for effective adaptation.

Many athletes and practitioners have expressed concern regarding the safety of such diets. Interestingly, as noted later in this chapter, the adverse blood lipid effects of a diet rich in fat, even primarily saturated fat, are blunted in athletes.[148] Because most other risk factors for chronic diseases have not been evaluated in athletes consuming a diet rich in saturated fatty acids; however, that research should not serve as a reason to consume excessive amounts of saturated fat. Because considerable data have demonstrated ergogenic benefits of a higher fat diet, athletes who do not have body weight control issues may wish to assess their exercise response to consuming a diet rich in "healthy" fats, particularly when followed by short-term carbohydrate loading, in comparison to a carbohydrate-rich diet regimen.

2. MCT Oil

Medium-chain triglyceride (MCT) oil is theorized to enhance endurance performance because medium-chain fatty acids are readily absorbed[149] and quickly metabolized independent of long-chain fatty acid transport mechanisms.[150] While long-chain fatty acids are absorbed into the cells of the gut, reesterified to glycerol, and packaged as part of chylomicrons for absorption via the lymphatic system, as previously described in this chapter, medium-chain fatty acids are predominantly absorbed directly into the portal circulation for transport to the liver. In the liver, these fatty acids are primarily converted to ketones and used for energy or secreted to the general circulation, where they can be taken up by peripheral tissues such as the muscle.[151] The ketones produced provide an alternative to endogenous carbohydrate as a fuel source, which may allow them to preserve muscle or liver glycogen during exercise.

The acute effects of feeding MCT before and during exercise on endurance performance have been assessed by several researchers. Significant muscle glycogen sparing, a purported mechanism by which some have suggested MCT could enhance performance, has not been observed in these acute feeding studies; however, Van Zyl et al.[152] did observe a significant improvement in endurance with acute feeding of carbohydrate plus MCT oil versus carbohydrate or MCT oil alone with cycling exercise. Because the energy content of the combination feeding was greater than in the trials of the separate components, these results have been subject to much criticism. Regardless, the addition of MCT oil to a carbohydrate feeding offers a potential additional energy source to the athlete that appears to translate to enhanced endurance, although that has not been demonstrated in similar studies.[153,154] Most studies assessing the potential ergogenic effects of acute MCT oil feedings versus isocaloric carbohydrate feedings provide no evidence of improved endurance.[155–157] In fact, Jeukendrup et al.[158] observed that intake of 85 g of MCT during exercise negatively affected performance. It is likely that the negative effect was associated with complaints of gastrointestinal distress rather than metabolic issues.

The influence of more chronic adaptation to MCT oil has been studied as well. Fushiki et al.[159] observed that chronic ingestion of MCT (17% total dietary kcal) for periods ranging from 2 to 6 weeks in duration by both trained and untrained mice caused glycogen sparing and produced significantly greater swimming endurance capacity. The authors suggested that upregulation of enzymes of lipid metabolism in response to MCT adaptation may play a part in glycogen sparing and improved endurance. Because long-term adaptation to MCT oil has been demonstrated to enhance lipid metabolism in mice, Misell et al.[160] conducted similar research in human subjects. Those researchers demonstrated that trained runners fed MCT oil versus corn oil for 2 weeks exhibited little differences in physiology and endurance performance than when tested following an overnight fast. Interestingly, chronic feeding led to a suppression in complaints of gastrointestinal discomfort, which would probably also eliminate the likelihood of adverse effects on performance. While these data fail to corroborate the results observed in animals, it is unclear whether the mice in the study by Fushiki et al.[159] were tested for endurance in a fasted or fed condition; therefore, it is possible that the combination of chronic MCT administration as well as an acute feeding to allow for adaptation as well as provision of an alternate fuel may prove useful. Thorburn et al.[161] recently tested that hypothesis by feeding a caprylate-based structured TG for 2 weeks along with an acute feeding during prolonged exercise. Adaptation to the MCT oil reduced gastrointestinal discomfort, but failed to enhance sprint performance at the end of the prolonged exercise bout. Future research is needed to examine the effects of a combination of chronic plus acute MCT oil ingestion on an endurance trial performance. While supplementation with MCT oil appears to be safe in most studies, negative effects of its consumption relative to corn oil on the resting blood lipid profile have been demonstrated in athletes.[162]

3. Conjugated Linoleic Acid

Conjugated linoleic acid (CLA) refers to isomers of linoleic acid containing conjugated diene units in which the two double bonds are separated by only 2 carbons rather than the typical 3 for linoleic acid. The predominantly consumed isomer in food presents the double bonds of the fatty acid in the *cis*-9 and *trans*-11 positions,[163] although *trans*-10, *cis*-12 isomers are typically used at equal levels to the *cis*-9 and *trans*-11 by most supplement manufacturers. Naturally occurring CLA is found primarily in meat and dairy products, and the average daily intake has been estimated to be approximately 150 mg for women and 200 mg for men.[164]

Little research has assessed the potential influence of CLA on endurance exercise performance. One study in young women initiating a training regimen demonstrated no improvement in endurance after consuming 3.6 grams of CLA per day for 6 weeks; however, improvements in body composition occurred with CLA intake and exercise training.[165] Research in mice, however, has demonstrated that CLA ingestion promotes fat oxidation and increases swimming endurance.[166] Early research in mice also demonstrated that CLA may stimulate norepinephrine-induced lipolysis.[167] Enhanced mobilization of FFAs from the adipose tissue to the blood stream elevates concentrations of plasma FFAs, which enhances fat oxidation and decreases utilization of carbohydrate for energy. Because these results have not been replicated in humans, this effect may be species specific; therefore, further research in humans assessing the influence of CLA in trained athletes is warranted.

More attention has been dedicated to the potential anabolic and fat-reducing effects of CLA during resistance training. Research has demonstrated no effect of 28 days of CLA supplementation on lean body mass or strength in resistance-trained men.[168] Another study indicated women ingesting 3 g/day of CLA for 64 days exhibited neither altered body composition nor changed energy expenditure or fat and carbohydrate utilization.[169] Furthermore, Zambell et al.[170] reported that 3.9 g CLA each day for 64 days failed to alter fatty acid or glycerol metabolism of adult women. More recently, Steck et al.[171] demonstrated that 12 weeks of CLA supplementation at 6.4 grams per day produced increased lean body mass, but that 3.2 grams per day failed to produce a similar effect in obese men and women who decreased their level of physical activity. This research suggests that a threshold above 3.2 grams of CLA per day may be needed before positive results can be detected. The need for a relatively high dose has been corroborated by other investigators as well.[172,173] The research by Pinkoski et al.[172] demonstrated that supplementation of 5 g of CLA per day for 7 weeks during resistance training increased lean mass and reduced fat mass more than resistance training alone, with some indication of enhanced strength, although less impressive results were obtained for a subgroup of participants that crossed over to the opposite treatment.

Although long-term human studies of safety per se have not been conducted, few, if any, adverse incidents or toxicity effects due to supplementation have been reported in the limited literature available. Overall, more research is needed before a solid recommendation for CLA supplementation in athletes can be made.

4. Omega-3 Fatty Acids

As described previously, omega-3 fatty acids are characterized by having the location of the first double from the methyl end of the hydrocarbon chain on the third carbon atom. Alpha-linolenic acid (ALA) is an essential fatty acid. Other important omega-3 fatty acids in the diet are eicosapentaenoic acid (EPA) and docosahexaenoic acid (DHA). Consuming EPA and DHA can reduce the daily requirement of ALA. Fish oils are particularly rich sources of EPA and DHA.

Eicosanoids are hormone-like compounds that are synthesized by cyclooxgenase and lipoxygenase enzyme systems from long-chain fatty acids including ALA, EPA, and DHA and non-omega-3 fatty acids. Classes of these compounds include thromboxanes, leukotrienes, and prostaglandins. The functions and potencies of eicosanoids depend upon their classes and the precursor fatty acids from which they are formed. A variety of functions including blood vessel or bronchiole dilation, platelet anti-aggregation, anti-inflammatory responses, and other roles are exhibited by various eicosanoids produced from omega-3 fatty acids, which has sparked an interest in the potential ergogenic as well as health benefits that might occur from consumption of these fatty acids.

Researchers have fed foods rich in omega-3 fatty acids and assessed potential benefits with no indication of an ergogenic effect. In one study, fish oil supplements containing 5.2 grams of total fat (1.60 g of EPA and 1.04 g of DHA) were fed to male soccer players each day for 10 weeks.[174] No improvements in maximal aerobic power, anaerobic power, or running performance were detected in comparison with corn oil supplementation. In similar research in trained cyclists, doses of 6 grams of fish oil per day failed to enhance endurance after 3 weeks of supplementation.[175] While oils rich in omega-3 fatty acids have significant metabolic effects that could theoretically influence exercise capacity, research has not established that such effects occur.

5. Carnitine and Choline

Carnitine and choline are both non-lipid compounds that play key roles in lipid metabolism. As described previously, the primary function of carnitine involves the transfer of long-chain fatty acids across the mitochondrial membrane from the cytoplasm. It has been hypothesized that supplementation of carnitine will increase fatty acid transport into the mitochondria, thus enhancing lipid oxidation at rest and during exercise.[176] Such an effect could reduce glycogen utilization and potentially prolong endurance. Carnitine is also involved in the conversion of acetyl-CoA into acetyl-L-carnitine and CoA. Enhancement of this process might favorably influence the citric acid cycle and decrease lactate accumulation during exercise.

Carnitine, a water-soluble vitamin-like compound synthesized in the body and present in relatively high concentrations in skeletal muscle and heart, is supplied from the diet as well. Key sources include animal products such as red meats, chicken, fish, eggs, and milk. Intake for non-vegetarian adults averages 100–300 mg per day.[176] When consumption is low, such as in vegan diets, the body compensates by increasing carnitine biosynthesis and decreasing renal carnitine clearance.[177] Within the body, carnitine is transported through the circulation and assimilated into the muscle, where it may impact both aerobic and anaerobic energy production during exercise.

Although carnitine functions to promote lipid oxidation, most research on carnitine supplementation does not support its use for ergogenic purposes. Although several researchers have demonstrated increases in plasma carnitine concentrations with the consumption of carnitine, fewer have reported improvements in muscle carnitine levels.[178] Most studies assessing muscle carnitine status have demonstrated no effect of carnitine supplementation on concentrations in that tissue.[179–182] Supplementation with choline, however, may enhance the incorporation of carnitine into the muscle cells,[183] which may ultimately prove to enhance the efficacy of carnitine supplementation.[184] Interestingly, some research has suggested that endurance training may increase endogenous carnitine synthesis,[185] which may lessen the likelihood that carnitine supplementation could be beneficial for athletes; however, other research has demonstrated lower status with exercise training.[178]

While research has relatively consistently yielded no improvement in exercise performance, a few studies have revealed some positive effects on physiological variables including increased fat utilization,[186] a decrease in respiratory exchange ratio,[185,187,188] and an increase in VO_{2max}.[187,189] This suggests that shifts in metabolism may occur that under some circumstances could prolong endurance. Several studies have demonstrated no difference in physiological variables such as heart rate, lactate, VO_{2max}, rate of perceived exertion (RPE), lipid metabolism, or exercise performance, with carnitine supplementation.[182,190–195] A rather small trial, however, did find that carnitine, especially when ingested with caffeine, significantly enhanced endurance performance.[196]

The dosing regimen that would be likely to maximize the potential for carnitine to enhance performance is unclear. Most researchers have provided 2–4 grams of carnitine for durations of between 1 and 12 weeks. Because these regimens typically have no effect on endurance performance and few physiological effects that could promote improved performance, some other dosing regimen is likely required if carnitine is ultimately determined to be effective. Carnitine supplements appear to be safe, because few adverse effects of carnitine supplementation occur with dosages ranging from 500 mg/day to 6 g/day for periods of 1–28 days.[176] In summary, because carnitine supplementation appears to have little effect on muscle carnitine status, the rate of fatty acid oxidation, or sport performance, its use in athletes is typically not recommended. If dosing regimens or interaction with other supplements such as choline or caffeine are demonstrated to consistently promote positive results, these recommendations should be revisited.

In addition to potentially enhancing cellular uptake of carnitine, choline and dietary components providing choline (i.e., lecithin, also known as phosphatidyl choline) have received some attention as being potentially ergogenic. Lecithin and choline have primarily been marketed for their ergogenic potential due to choline's role with acetylcholine and muscular contraction. While poor choline status will likely prevent optimal performance, evidence does not support claims that choline supplementation can provide an ergogenic effect.[197] Research has demonstrated that lecithin supplementation may prevent an exercise-induced decrease in choline status[198] however, which points to the need for a greater understanding of choline metabolism in athletes.

E. Influence of Exercise on Lipid Status

This chapter would not be complete without a brief description of research related to exercise and the blood lipid profile. Much research has examined the influence of physical activity on risk factors for heart disease, and many of these studies have been directed at the effects of exercise on blood lipid and lipoprotein metabolism. Lipoproteins, as described previously, are compound lipids deriving their name from their two primary components: lipids and proteins. The proteins that are constituents of lipoproteins are called apolipoproteins, sometimes shortened as apoproteins. Apoproteins serve a variety of roles including allowing transport of lipids within an aqueous environment, receptor recognition, and participating in a variety of biochemical reactions. Most lipids are transported as components of the various lipoproteins. The lipids producing the majority of mass in a lipoprotein include TGs, cholesterol, cholesterol esters, and phospholipids. Primary classes of lipoproteins include chylomicrons, VLDLs, low density lipoproteins (LDL), and high density lipoproteins (HDL). LDL particles are produced in the catabolism of VLDLs by the action of lipoprotein lipase. The cholesterol in LDL particles is referred to as LDL-cholesterol (LDL-C), and it is the fraction of cholesterol within LDL particles that is measured to determine a value for LDL-C. Because LDL can be deposited in the intima of arteries, high concentrations of LDL-C in the serum, particularly when LDL is oxidized, are associated with increased risk for heart disease. HDL particles are synthesized in the liver primarily but to a lesser degree in the cells of the gastrointestinal tract as well. The primary role of HDL particles is the removal of cholesterol from lower density lipoproteins and tissues along with its transportation to the liver via the reverse cholesterol transport system. This property is responsible for the negative association between elevelated HDL-cholesterol (HDL-C) and risk for heart disease.

As reviewed previously, exercisers typically exhibit lower serum cholesterol concentrations than non-exercisers[199] and are at lower risk for heart disease.[200] Many studies have also demonstrated that exercise training will produce a cholesterol-lowering response in previously untrained individuals.[199] Typically, total serum cholesterol concentration as well as LDL-C will be decreased by physical activity and the concentration of HDL-C will increase; therefore, exercise training, and in some studies just single bouts of exercise, produce decreases in the serum concentrations of LDL-C and increases in HDL-C.[199] Estimates by some scientists are that training that expends approximately 1000 kcals per week for at least 3 months is sufficient to provide elevations in HDL-C and thus protection against atherosclerosis.[199]

Research has demonstrated that both resistance training and aerobic exercise can have favorable effects on serum cholesterol concentrations; however, aerobic exercise appears to be the more effective of the two.[199] In aerobically trained athletes, several studies have even suggested that exercise may blunt the adverse effects of a diet rich in saturated fat on serum cholesterol concentrations.[148,201] While this is good news for the athlete, it should not send the message that athletes can eat any diet they wish with no risk of disease, because there are many other risk factors for heart disease and because research has not been conducted related to the adverse effects of a diet rich in saturated fat on risk factors for other diseases (e.g., cancer, etc.) in athlete-specific populations.

IV. CONCLUSIONS

The dietary and metabolic importance of both fat and carbohydrate for exercisers and athletes cannot be overstated. It is undeniable that dietary regimens and supplements that favorably alter the storage or utilization of these classes of nutrients can have significant impacts on performance as well as wellness. In the same way, as has been demonstrated with large doses of niacin,[202] it is likely that certain dietary choices could negatively impact carbohydrate or lipid metabolism and exercise performance, or risk factors for chronic diseases. As research on these issues continue, a clearer picture of those practices that are most beneficial will develop. From a health perspective, a food-first approach to eating is highly recommended. Many times it is impractical for athletes to meet all of their energy needs, particularly from carbohydrate, from natural food sources. However, as has been described in this chapter, whole foods can be used by athletes in a variety of conditions before, during, and after competition to help meet their macronutrient needs and promote less reliance on commercial sport foods that are often less palatable and lower in natural food constituents such as micronutrients and phytochemicals.

While extensive amounts of research have been published regarding the influences of carbohydrate and fats on exercise metabolism and performance, findings in many areas remain equivocal and much is yet to be learned. Research on dietary practices that optimally influence the health and exercise capacity of athletes is still needed. In most cases, combinations of various dietary regimens and supplements that alter carbohydrate or lipid metabolism have not been addressed. Furthermore, in some cases research has pointed to an influence of various dietary practices on physiological variables that could be related to performance without subsequent performance improvements. Additional research on these issues may demonstrate that performance can be enhanced for specific situations that have not yet been tested. As the base of research grows, athletes and practitioners will be better armed with tools that can be used to improve exercise performance.

REFERENCES

1. Jensen, C. D., Zaltas, E. S., and Whittam, J. H., Dietary intakes of male endurance cyclists during training and racing. *J. Am. Diet. Assoc.*, 92, 986–88, 1992.
2. Burke, L. M., Gollan, R. A., and Read, R. S. D., Dietary intakes and food use of groups of elite Australian male athletes. *Int. J. Sport Nutr.*, 1, 378–94, 1991.
3. Petersen, H. L., Peterson, C. T., Reddy, M. B., Hanson, K. B., Swain, J. H., Sharp, R. L., and Alekel, D. L., Body composition, dietary intake, and iron status of female collegiate swimmers and divers. *Int. J. Sport Nutr. Exerc. Metab.*, 16, 281–95, 2006.
4. Onywera, V. O., Kiplamai, F. K., Tuitoek, P. J., Boit, M. K., and Pitsiladis, Y. P., Food and macronutrient intake of elite Kenyan distance runners. *Int. J. Sport Nutr. Exerc. Metab.*, 14, 709–19, 2004.
5. Brooks, G., Fahey, T. D., White, T. and Baldwin, K., *Exercise Physiology: Human Bioenergetics and its Applications* (3rd ed.). New York: McGraw-Hill. 2000.
6. McArdle, W., Katch, F., and Katch, V., *Sports and Exercise Nutrition*. Lippincott, Williams and Wilkins. 1999.
7. Jeukendrup, A. E., Wagenmakers, A. J. M., Stegen, J. H. C. H., Gijsen, A. P., Brouns, F., and Saris, W. H. M. Carbohydrate ingestion can completely suppress endogenous glucose production during exercise. *Am. J. Physiol.* 276, E672–83, 1999.
8. Foster, C., Costill, D. L., and Fink, W. J., Effects of preexercise feedings on endurance performance. *Med. Sci. Sports.*, 11, 1, 1979.
9. Keller, K. and Schwarzkopf, R., Pre-exercise snacks may decrease exercise performance. *Phys. Sportsmed.*, 12, 89, 1984.
10. Davis, J. M., Alderson, N. L., and Welsh, R. S., Serotonin and central nervous system fatigue: Nutritional considerations. *Am. J. Clin. Nutr.* 72, 573S, 2000.
11. Jacobs, K. A. and Sherman, W. M., The efficacy of carbohydrate supplementation and chronic high carbohydrate diets for improving endurance performance. *Int. J. Sport Nutr.*, 1999;9:92–115.
12. Koivisto, V. A., Karvonen, S., and Nikkila, E. A., Carbohydrate ingestion before exercise: Comparison of glucose, fructose, and sweet placebo. *J. Appl. Physiol.* 51, 783–7, 1981.
13. Hargreaves, M., Costill, D. L., Fink, W. J., King, D. S., and Fielding, R. A., Effect of pre-exercise carbohydrate feedings on endurance cycling performance. *Med. Sci. Sports Exerc.* 19, 33–6, 1987.
14. Devlin, J. T., Calles-Escandon, J., and Horton, E. S., Effects of pre-exercise snack feeding on endurance cycle exercise. *J. Appl. Physiol.* 60, 980–5, 1986.
15. Palmer, G. S., Clancy, M. C., Hawley, J. A., Rodger, I. M., Burke, L. M., Noakes, T. D., Carbohydrate ingestion immediately before exercise does not improve 20 km time trial performance in well trained cyclists. *Int. J. Sports Med.* 19, 415–8, 1998.

16. Desbrow, B., Anderson, S., Barrett, J., Rao, E., and Hargreaves, M., Carbohydrate–electrolyte feedings and 1 h time trial cycling performance. *Int. J. Sport Nutr. Exerc. Metab.* 14, 541–9, 2004.
17. Burke, L. M., Wood, C., Pyne, D. B., Telford, R. T., and Saunders, P., Effect of carbohydrate intake on half-marathon performance of well-trained runners. *Int. J. Sport Nutr. Exerc. Metab.* 15, 573–89, 2005.
18. Van Nieuwenhoven, M. A., Brouns, F., and Kovacs, E. M. R., The effect of two sports drinks and water on GI complaints and performance during an 18-km run. *Int. J. Sports Med.* 26, 281–5, 2005.
19. Kovacs, E. M. R., Stegen, J. H. C. H., and Brouns, F., Effect of caffeinated drinks on substrate metabolism, caffeine excretion, and performance. *J. Appl. Physiol.* 85, 709–15, 1998.
20. Neufer, P. D., Costill, D. L., Flynn, M. G., Kirwan, J. P., Mitchell, J. B., and Houmard, J., Improvements in exercise performance: Effects of carbohydrate feedings and diet. *J. Appl. Physiol.* 62, 983–8, 1987.
21. Coggan, A. R., and Coyle, E. F., Reversal of fatigue during prolonged exercise by carbohydrate infusion or ingestion. *J. Appl. Physiol.* 63, 2388–95, 1987.
22. Wright, D. A., Sherman, W. M., Dernbach, A. R., Carbohydrate feedings before, during, or in combination improves cycling endurance performance. *J. Appl. Physiol.*, 71, 1082–8, 1991.
23. Anantaraman, R., Carmines, A. A., Gaesser, G. A., and Weltman, A., Effects of carbohydrate supplementation on performance during 1 hour of high-intensity exercise. *Int. J. Sports Med.* 16, 461–5, 1995.
24. Febbraio, M. A., Chiu, A., Angus, D. J., Arkinstall, M. J., and Hawley, J. A., Effects of carbohydrate ingestion before and during exercise on glucose kinetics and performance. *J. Appl. Physiol.* 89, 2220–6, 2000.
25. Below, P. R., Mora–Rodriguez, R., Gonzalez-Alonso, J., and Coyle, E. F., Fluid and carbohydrate ingestion independently improve performance during 1 hour of intense exercise. *Med. Sci. Sports Exerc.*, 27, 200–10, 1995.
26. Jeukendrup, A., Brouns, F., Wagenmakers, A. J., and Saris, W. H., Carbohydrate–electrolyte feedings improve 1 h time trial cycling performance. *Int. J. Sports Med.* 18, 125–9, 1997.
27. Vergauwen, L., Brouns, F., Hespel, P., Carbohydrate supplementation improves stroke performance in tennis. *Med. Sci. Sports Exerc.* 30, 1289–95, 1998.
28. Welsh, R. S., Davis, J. M., Burke, J. R., and Williams, H. G., Carbohydrates and physical/mental performance during intermittent exercise to fatigue. *Med. Sci. Sports Exerc.* 34, 723–31, 2002.
29. Winnick, J. J., Davis, J. M., Welsh, R. S., Carmichael, M. D., Murphy, E. A., and Blackmon, J. A., Carbohydrate feedings during team sport exercise preserve physical and CNS function. *Med. Sci. Sports Exerc.* 37, 306–15, 2005.
30. Dougherty, K. A., Baker, L. B., Chow, M., and Kenney, W. L., 2% dehydration impairs and 6% carbohydrate drink improves boys basketball skills. *Med. Sci. Sports Exerc.* 38, 1650–8, 2006.
31. Sherman, W. M., Brodowicz, G., Wright, D. A., Allen, W. K., Simonsen, J., Dernbach, A., Effects of 4 h preexercise carbohydrate feedings on cycling performance. *Med. Sci. Sports Exerc.*, 21, 598, 1989.
32. Sherman, W. M., Peden, M. C., Wright, D. A., Carbohydrte feedings 1 hour before exercise improves cycling performance. *Am. J. Clin. Nutr.*, 54, 866, 1991.
33. Coyle, E. F., Hagberg, J. M., Hurley, B. F., Martin, W. H., Ehsani, A. A., and Holloszy, J. O., Carbohydrate feeding during prolonged strenuous exercise can delay fatigue. *J. Appl. Physiol.*, 55, 230–5, 1983.

34. Niles, E. S., Lachowetz, T., Garfi, J., Sullivan, W., Smith, J. C., Leyh, B. P., and Headley S. A., Carbohydrate–protein drink improves time to exhaustion after recovery from endurance exercise. *J. Exerc. Physiol.* 4, 45–52, 2001.
35. Ivy, J. L., Res, P. T., Sprague, R. C., and Widzer, M. O., Effect of a carbohydrate–protein supplement on endurance performance during exercise of varying intensity. *Int. J. Sports Nutr. Exerc. Metab.*, 13, 382, 2003.
36. Ivy. J. L., Katz, A. L., Cutler, C. L., Sherman, W. M., and Coyle, E. F., Muscle glycogen synthesis after exercise: Effect of time of carbohydrate ingestion. *J. Appl. Physiol.*, 6, 1490, 1988.
37. Van Loon, L. J., Saris, W. H., and Kruijshoop, M., and Wagenmakers, J. M., Maximizing postexercise muscle glycogen synthesis: Carbohydrate supplementation and the application of amino acid or protein hydrolysate mixtures. *Am. J. Clin. Nutr.*, 72, 106, 2000.
38. Van Hall, G., Shirreffs, S., and Calbet, J., Muscle glycogen resynthesis during recovery from cycle exercise: No effect of additional protein ingestion. *J. Appl. Physiol.*, 88, 1631, 2000.
39. Rasmussen, B. B., Tipton, K. D., Miller, S. L., Wolf, S. E., and Wolfe, R. R., An oral essential amino acid–carbohydrate supplement enhances muscle protein anabolism after resistance exercise. *J. Appl. Physiol.*, 88, 386, 2000.
40. Karp, J. R., Johnston, J. D., Tecklenburg, S., Mickleborough, T. D., Fly, A. D., and Stager, J. M., Chocolate milk as a post-exercise recovery aid. *Int. J. Sport Nutr. Exerc. Metab.* 16, 78–91, 2006.
41. Sherman, W. M., Doyle, J. A., Lamb, D. R., and Strauss, R. H., Dietary carbohydrate, muscle glycogen, and exercise performance during 7 d of training. *Am. J. Clin. Nutr.*, 57, 27, 1993.
42. Lambert, E. V., Speechly, D. P., Dennis, S. C., and Noakes, T. D., Enhanced endurance in trained cyclists during moderate intensity exercise following 2 weeks adaptation to a high fat diet. *Eur. J. Appl. Physiol.*, 69, 287, 1994.
43. Williams, M. H., *Nutrition for Health, Fitness, & Sport*, 7th ed., McGraw-Hill, New York, NY, 2005, pp. 113–150.
44. Bussau, V. A., Fairchild, T. J., Rao, A., Steele, P. D., and Fournier, P. A., Carbohydrate loading in human muscle: an improved 1 day protocol. *Eur. J. Appl. Physiol.* 87, 290–5, 2002.
45. Williams, C. J., Brewer, J., and Walker, M., The effect of a high carbohydrate diet on running performance during a 30-km treadmill time trial. *Eur. J. Appl. Physiol.* 65, 18–24, 1992.
46. Tarnopolsky, M. A., Atkinson, S. A., Phillips, S. M., and MacDougall, J. D., Carbohydrate loading and metabolism during exercise in men and women. *J. Appl. Physiol.*, 78, 1360–8, 1995.
47. Pizza, F. X., Flynn, M. G., Duscha, B. D., Holden, J., Kubitz, E. R., A carbohydrate loading regimen improves high intensity, short duration exercise performance. *Int. J. Sport Nutr.* 5, 110–16, 1995.
48. Pitsiladis, Y. P., Duignan, C., and Maughan, R. J., Effects of alterations in dietary carbohydrate intake on running performance during a 10 km treadmill time trial. *Br. J. Sports Med.*, 30, 226–31, 1996.
49. Tarnopolsky, M. A., Zawada, C., Richmond, L. B., Carter, S., Shearer, J., Graham, T., and Phillips, S. M., Gender difference in carbohydrate loading are related to energy intake. *J. Appl. Physiol.* 91, 225–30, 2001.
50. Zehnder, M., Christ, E. R., Ith, M., J. Acheson, K. J., Pouteau, E., Kreis, R., et al., Intramyocellular lipid stores increase markedly in athletes after 1.5 days lipid supplementation and are utilized during exercise in proportion to their content. *Eur. J. Appl. Physiol.* 98, 341–54, 2006.

51. Larson-Meyer, D. E., Borkhsenious, O. N., Gullett, J. C., Russell, R. R., Devries, M. C., Smith, S. R., Ravussin, E., Effect of dietary fat on serum and intramyocellular lipids and running performance. *Med. Sci. Sports Exerc.* 40, 892–902, 2008.
52. Paddon-Jones, D. and Pearson, D. R. Cost-effectiveness of pre-exercise carbohydrate meals and their impact on endurance performance *J. Strength Cond. Res.* 12, 90–94, 1998.
53. Kern, M., Heslin, C. J., Rezende, R. S., Metabolic and performance effects of raisins versus sports gel as pre-exercise feedings in cyclists. *J. Strength Cond. Res.* 21, 1204–7, 2007.
54. Earnest CP, Lancaster SL, Rasmussen CJ, Kerksick CM, Lucia A, Greenwood MC, Almada AL, Cowan PA, Kreider RB. Low vs. high glycemic index carbohydrate gel ingestion during simulated 64–km cycling time trial performance. *J. Strength Cond. Res.* 2004 Aug;18(3):466–72.
55. DeMarco, H. M., Sucher, K. P., Cisar, C. J., and Butterfield, G. E., Pre-exercise carbohydrate meals: Application of glycemic index. *Med. Sci. Sports Exerc.*, 31, 164, 1999.
56. Kirwan, J. P., O'Gorman, D., and Evans, W. J., A moderate glycemic meal before endurance exercise can enhance performance, *J. Appl. Physiol.*, 84, 53, 1998.
57. Burns, J. H. and Berning, J. R., Sports beverages, in *Macroelements, Water, and Electrolytes in Sports Nutrition*, Driskell. J. A. and Wolinsky, I., Eds., CRC Press, Boca Raton, 1999.
58. Stricker, E. M., and Sved, A. F., Thirst, *Nutrition.* 16, 821, 2000.
59. Passe, D. H., Horn, M., and Murray, R., The effects of beverage carbonation on sensory responses and voluntary fluid intake following exercise. *Int. J. Sport Nutr.*, 7, 286, 1997.
60. Lamb, D. R. and Brodowicz, G. R., Optimal use of fluids of varying formulations to minimise exercise–induced disturbances in homeostasis. *Sports Med.*, 3, 247, 1986.
61. Currell, K., and Jeukendrup, A. E., Superior endurance performance with ingestion of multiple transportable carbohydrates. *Med. Sci. Sports Exerc.* 40, 275–81, 2008.
61. Murray, R., The effects of consuming carbohydrate–electrolyte beverages on gastric emptying and fluid absorption during and following exercise, *Sports Med.*, 4,322, 1987.
62. Wemple, R. D., Morocco, T. S., and Mack, G. S., Influence of sodium replacement on fluid ingestion following exercise-induced dehydration. *Int. J. Sports Med.*, 7, 104, 1997.
63. Rauch, H. G. L., Hawley, J. A., Woodey, M., Noakes, T. D., and Dennis, S. C., Effects of ingesting a sports bar versus glucose polymer on substrate utilisation and ultra-endurance performance. *Int. J. Sports Med.*, 20, 252, 1999.
64. Campbell, C., Prince, D., Braun, M., Applegate, E., and Casazza, G. A., Carbohydrate–supplement form and exercise performance. *Int. J. Sport Nutr. Exerc. Metab.* 18, 179–90, 2008.
65. Saunders, M. J., Luden, N. D., and Herrick, J. E., Consumption of an oral carbohydrate–protein gel improves cycling endurance and prevents postexercise muscle damage. *J. Strength Cond. Res.* 21, 678–84, 2007.
66. Burke, L. M., Collier, G. R., and Hargreaves, M., Glycemic index—a new tool in sport nutrition? *Int. J. Sport Nutr.*, 8, 401, 1998.
67. Coggan, A. R. and Coyle E. F., Carbohydrate ingestion during prolonged exercise: Effects on metabolism and performance. In *Exercise and Sports Science Reviews*, Vol. 19, Holloszy, J., Ed., Williams & Wilkins, Baltimore, 1991, 1.
68. Robergs, R. A., McMinn, S. B., Mermier, C., Leadbetter, G., Ruby, B., and Quinn, C., Blood glucose and glucoregulatory hormone response to solid and liquid carbohydrate ingestion during exercise. *Int. J. Sport Nutr.*, 8, 70, 1998.

69. Guezennec, C. Y., Oxidation rates, complex carbohydrates and exercise. *Sports Med.*, 19, 365, 1995.
70. Thomas, D. E., Brotherhood, J. R., and Brand, J. C., Carbohydrate feeding before exercise: Effect of glycemic index. *Int. J. Sports Med.*, 12, 180, 1991.
71. Thomas, D. E., Brotherhood, J. R., and Miller, J. B., Plasma glucose levels after prolonged strenuous exercise correlates inversely with glycemic response to food consumed before exercise. *Int. J. Sport Nutr.*, 4, 361, 1994.
72. Febbraio, M. A., Keenan, J., Angus, D. J., Campbell, S. E., and Garnham, A. P., Pre-exercise carbohydrate ingestion, glucose kinetics, and muscle glycogen use: Effect of the glycemic index. *J. Appl. Physiol.*, 89, 1845, 2000.
73. Febbraio, M. A. and Stewart, K. L., CHO feeding before prolonged exercise: Effect of glycemic index on muscle glycogenolysis and exercise performance. *J. Appl. Physiol.*, 81, 1115, 1996.
74. Sparks, M. J., Selig, S. S., and Febbraio, M. A., Pre-exercise carbohydrate ingestion: Effect of the glycemic index on endurance exercise performance. *Med. Sci. Sports Exerc.*, 30, 844, 1998.
75. Stannard, S. R., Constantini, N. W., and Miller J. C., The effect of glycemic index on plasma glucose and lactate levels during incremental exercise. *Int. J. Sport Nutr. Exerc. Metab.*, 10, 51, 2000.
76. Wee, S. L., Williams, C., Gray, S., and Horabin, J., Influence of high and low glycemic index meals on endurance running capacity. *Med. Sci. Sports Exerc.*, 31, 393, 1999.
77. Burke, L. M., Claasen, A., Hawley, J. A., and Noakes, T. D., Carbohydrate intake during prolonged cycling minimizes effect of glycemic index of preexercise meal. *J. Appl. Physiol.*, 85, 2220, 1998.
78. Jentjens, R. L., Achten, J., and Jeukendrup, A. E. High oxidation from combined carbohydrates ingested during exercise. *Med. Sci. Sports Exerc.* 36, 1551–8, 2004.
79. Jentjens, R. L., Moseley, L., Waring, R. H., Harding, L. K., and Jeukendrup, A. E. Oxidation of combined ingestion of glucose and fructose during exercise. *J. Appl. Physiol.* 96, 1277–84, 2004.
80. Jentjens, R. L., Shaw, C., Birtles, T., Waring, R. H., Harding, L. K., and Jeukendrup, A. E. Oxidation of combined ingestion of glucose and sucrose during exercise. *Metab.* 54, 610–8, 2005.
81. Wallis, G. A., Rowlands, D. S., Shaw, C., Jentjens, R. L., and Jeukendrup, A. E. Oxidation of combined ingestion of maltodextrins and fructose during exercise. *Med. Sci. Sports Exerc.* 37, 426–32, 2005.
82. Rowlands, D. S., Thorburn, M. S., Thorp, R. M., Broadbent, S., and Sh, X. Effect of graded fructose co-ingestion with maltodextrin on exogenous 14C-fructose and 13C-glucose oxidation efficiency and high-intensity cycling performance. *J. Appl. Physiol.* 104, 1709–19, 2008.
83. Carter, J. M., Jeukendrup, A. E., Jones, D. A., The effect of carbohydrate mouth rinse on 1-h cycle time trial performance. *Med. Sci. Sports Exerc.* 36, 2107–11, 2004.
84. Jozsi, A. C., Trappe, T. A., Starlling, R. D., Goodpaster, B., Trappe, S. W., Fink, W. J., and Costill, D. L. The influence of starch structure on glycogen resynthesis and subsequent cycling performance. *Int. J. Sports Med* 1996; 17: 373–378.
85. Leijssen, D. P., Saris, W. H., Jeukendrup, A. E., and Wagenmakers, A. J., Oxidation of exogenous [13C]galactose and [13C]glucose during exercise. *J. Appl. Physiol.*, 79(3),720–5, 1995.
86. Jentjens, R. L. and Jeukendrup A. E., Effects of pre-exercise ingestion of trehalose, galactose and glucose on subsequent metabolism and cycling performance. *Eur. J. Appl. Physiol.*, 88(4–5), 459–65, 2003.

87. Kerksick, C., Rasmussen, C., Bowden, R., Leutholtz, B., Harvey, T., Earnest, C., et al., Effects of ribose supplementation prior to and during intense exercise on anaerobic capacity and metabolic markers. *Int. J. Sport Nutr. Exerc. Metab.* 15, 653–64, 2005.
88. Hellsten, Y., Skadhauge, L., and Bangsbo J., Effect of ribose supplementation on resynthesis of adenine nucleotides after intense intermittent training in humans. *Am. J. Physiol. Reg. Integ. Comp. Physiol.*, 286, R182, 2004.
89. Op 't Eijnde, B., Van Leemputte, M., Brouns, F., Van Der Vusse, G. J., Labarque, V., Ramaekers, M., et al., No effects of oral ribose supplementation on repeated maximal exercise and de novo ATP resynthesis. *J. Appl. Physiol.*, 91, 2275, 2001.
90. Morrison, M. A, Spriet, L. L, and Dyck, D. J., Pyruvate ingestion for 7 days does not improve aerobic performance in well-trained individuals. *J. Appl. Physiol.*, 89, 549, 2000.
91. Stanko, R. T., Robertson, R. J., Galbreath, R. W., Reilly, J. J., Greenawalt, K. D., and Goss, F. L., Enhanced leg exercise endurance with a high-carbohydrate diet and dihydroxyacetone and pyruvate. *J. Appl. Physiol.*, 69, 1651, 1990a.
92. Stanko, R. T. Robertson, R. J., Spina, R. J., Reilly, J. J., Greenawalt, K. D., and Goss, F. L., Enhancement of arm exercise endurance capacity with dihydroxyacetone and pyruvate. *J. Appl. Physiol.*, 68, 119, 1990b.
93. Kalman, D., Colker, C. M., Wilets, I., Roufs, J. B., and Antonio, J., Effects of pyruvate supplementation on body composition and mood. *Curr. Ther. Res.*, 59, 793, 1998.
94. Vukovich, M. Fat reduction, In *Sports Supplements*, Antonio, J. and Stout, J. R., Eds., Lippincott Williams & Wilkins, Philadelphia, 2001, p. 101.
95. Brouns, F., Fogelholm, M., Van Hall, G., Wagenmakers, A., and Saris, W. H. M., Chronic oral lactate supplementation does not affect lactate disappearance from blood after exercise. *Int. J. Sport Nutr.*, 5, 117, 1995.
96. Bryner, R. W., Hornsby, W. G., Chetlin, R., Ullrich, I. H., and Yeater, R. A., Effect of lactate consumption on exercise performance. *J. Sports Med. Phys. Fitness*, 38, 116, 1998.
97. Swensen, T., Crater, G., Bassett, D. R., and Howley, E. T., Adding polylactate to a glucose polymer solution does not improve endurance. *Int. J. Sports Med.*, 15, 430, 1994.
98. Fahey, T. D., Larsen, J. D., Brooks, G. A., Colvin, W., Henderson, S., and Lary, D., The effects of ingesting polylactate or glucose polymer drinks during prolonged exercise. *Int. J. Sport Nutr.*, 1, 249, 1991.
99. Evans, G. W., The effect of chromium picolinate on insulin controlled parameters in humans. *Int. J. Biosoc. Med. Res.*, 11, 163, 1989.
100. Hasten, D. L., Rome, E. P., Franks, B. D., and Hegsted, M., Effects of chromium picolinate on beginning weight training students. *Int. J. Sports Nutr.*, 2, 343, 1992.
101. Antonio, J., and Stout, J. R., *Sports Supplements*, Lippincott Williams & Wilkins, Philadelphia, PA, 2001.
102. Trent, L. K., and Thieding-Cancel, D., Effects of chromium picolinate on body composition. *J. Sports Med. Phys. Fitness*, 35, 273, 1995.
103. Lukaski, H. C., Bolonchuk, W. W., Siders, W. A., and Milne, D. B., Chromium supplementation and resistance training: Effects on body composition, strength, and trace element status of men. *Am. J. Clin. Nutr.*, 63, 954, 1996.
104. Walker, L. S., Bemben, M. G., Bemben, D. A., and Knehans, A. W., Chromium picolinate effects on body composition and muscular performance in wrestlers. *Med. Sci. Sports Exerc.*, 30, 1730, 1998.
105. Lefavi, R. G., Anderson, R. A., Keith, R. E., Wilson, G. D., McMillan, J. L., and Stone, M. H., Efficacy of chromium supplementation in athletes: Emphasis on anabolism. *Int. J. Sports Nutr.*, 2, 111, 1992.

106. Hallmark, M. A., Reynolds, T. H., DeSouza, C. A., Dotson, C. O., Anderson, R. A., and Rogers, M. A., Effects of chromium and resistance training on muscle strength and body composition. *Med. Sci. Sports Exerc.*, 28, 139, 1996.
107. Campbell, W. W., Joseph, L. J. O., Davey, S. L., Cyr-Campbell, D., Anderson, R. A., and Evans, W. J., Effects of resistance training and chromium picolinate on body composition and skeletal muscle in older men. *J. Appl. Physiol.*, 86, 29, 1999.
108. Clancy, S. P., Clarkson, P. M., DeCheke, M. E., Nosaka, K., Freedson, P. S., Cunningham, J. J., and Valentine, B., Effects of chromium picolinate supplementation on body composition, strength, and urinary chromium loss in football players. *Int. J. Sports Nutr.*, 4, 142, 1994.
109. Grant, K. E., Chandler, R. M., Castle, A. L., and Ivy, J. L., Chromium and exercise training: Effect on obese women. *Med. Sci. Sports Exerc.*, 29, 992, 1994.
110. Miller, J. M., Coyle, E. F., Sherman, W. M., Hagberg, J. M., Costill, D. L., Fink, W. I., et al., Effect of glycerol feeding on endurance and metabolism during prolonged exercise in man. *Med. Sci. Sports Exerc.* 3, 237–42, 1983.
111. Latzka, W. A., Sawka, M. N., Montain, S. J., Skrinar, G. S., Fielding, R. A., Matott, R. P., and Pandolf, K. B., Hyperhydration: Tolerance and cardiovascular effects during uncompensable exercise–heat stress. *J. Appl. Physiol.*, 84, 1858, 1998.
112. Lyons, T., Riedesel, M. L., and Chick, T. W., Effects of glycerol-induced hyperhydration prior to exercise in the heat on sweating and core temperature. *Med. Sci. Sports Exerc.*, 22, 477, 1990.
113. Hitchins, S., Martin, D. T., Burke, L., Yates, K., Fallon, K., Hahn, A., and Dobson, G. P., Glycerol hyperhydration improves cycle time trial performance in hot humid conditions. *Eur. J. Appl. Physiol.*, 80, 494, 1999.
114. Scheet, T. P., Webster, M. J., and Wagoner, K. D., Effectiveness of glycerol as a rehydrating agent. *IInt. J. Sport Nutr. Exerc. Metab.*, 11, 63, 2001.
115. Montner, P., Stark, D. M., Riedesel, M. L., Murata, G., Robergs, R., Timms, M., and Chick, T. W., Pre-exercise glycerol hydration improves cycling endurance time. *Int. J. Sports Med.*, 17, 27, 1996.
116. Kavouras, S. A., Armstrong, L. E., Maresh, C. M., Casa, D. J., Herrera-Soto, J. A., Scheett, T. P., et al., Rehydration with glycerol: Endocrine, cardiovascular, and thermoregulatory responses during exercise in the heat. *J. Appl. Physiol.* 100, 442–50, 2006.
117. Inder, W. J., Swanney, M. P., Donald, R. A., Prickett, T. C. R., and Hellemans, J., The effect of glycerol and desmopressin on exercise performance and hydration in triathletes. *Med. Sci. Sports Exerc.* 30, 1263–9, 1998.
118. Marino, F. E., Kay, D., and Cannon, J., Glycerol hyperhydration fails to improve endurance performance and thermoregulation in humans in a warm humid environment. *Plugers Arch.* 446, 455–62, 2003.
119. Goulet, E. D., Robergs, R. A., Labrecque, S., Royer, D., and Dionne, I. J., Effect of glycerol-induced hyperhydration on thermoregulatory and cardiovascular functions and endurance performance during prolonged cycling in a 25 degrees C environment. *Appl. Physiol. Nutr. Metab.* 31, 101–9, 2006.
120. Goulet, E. D., Aubertin-Leheudre, M., Plante, G. E., and Dionne, I. J., A meta-analysis of the effects of glycerol-induced hyperhydration on fluid retention and endurance performance. *Int. J. Sport Nutr. Exerc. Metab.* 17, 391–410, 2007.
121. Goldberg, A. and Odessey, R., Oxidation of amino acid by diaphragms from fed and fasted rats. *Am. J. Physiol.*, 223, 1384, 1972.
122. White, T., and Brooks, G., [U-14C]glucose, -alanine, and -leucine oxidation in rats at rest and two intensities of running. *Am. J. Physiol.*, 240, E155, 1981.
123. Wolff, J., Kelts, D. G., Algert, S., Prodanos, C., and Nyhan, W. L., Alanine decreases the protein requirements of infants with inborn errors of amino acid metabolism. *J. Neurogenet.* 2: 41–9, 1985.

124. Bodamer, O. A. F., Halliday, D., and Leonard, J. V., The effects of L–alanine supplementation in late-onset glycogen storage disease type II. *Neurology*, 55, 710, 2000.
125. Kelts, D., Ney, D., Bay, C., Saudubray, J. M., and Nyhan, W. L., Studies on requirements for amino acids infants with disorders of amino acid metabolism: I. Effect of alanine. *Pediatr. Res.*, 19, 86, 1985.
126. Klein, J., Nyhan, W. L., and Kern, M. The effects of alanine supplementation on plasma amino acid concentrations, fuel substrates and endurance. *Amino Acids*, in press.
127. Kern, M., and Robinson, J. Metabolic and performance effects of alanine supplementation. *Med. Sci. Sports Exerc.*, 40, S166, 2008.
128. Ousley-Pahnke, L., Black, D. R., and Gretebeck, R. J., Dietary intake and energy expenditure of female collegiate swimmers during decreased training prior to competition. *J. Am. Diet. Assoc.* 101, 351–4, 2001.
129. Berning, J. R., Troup, J. P., Van Handel, P. J., Daniels, J., and Daniels, N. The nutritional habits of young adolescent swimmers. *Int. J. Sport Nutr.*, 1, 240–8, 1991.
130. Barr, S. I., Relationship of eating attitudes to anthropometric variables and dietary intakes of female collegiate swimmers. *J. Am. Diet. Assoc.* 91,976–7, 1991.
131. Barr, S. I., and Costill, D. L., Effect of increased training volume on nutrient intake of male collegiate simmers. *Int. J. Sports Med.* 13, 47–51, 1992.
132. Smith, M. P., Mendez, J., Druckenmiller, M., and Kris-Etherton, P. M., Exercise intensity, dietary intake and high-density lipoprotein cholesterol in young female competitive swimmers. *Am. J. Clin. Nutr.* 36, 251–5, 1982.
133. Grandjean, A. C., Macronutrient intake of U. S. athletes compared with the general population and recommendations made for athletes. *Am. J. Clin. Nutr.* 49, 1070–6, 1989.
134. Carey, M. C., Small, D. M., and Bliss, C. M., Lipid digestion and absorption. *Ann. Rev. Physiol.*, 45, 651–677, 1983.
135. Pelsers, M. M., Stellingwerff, T., and van Loon, J. J., The role of membrane fatty-acid transporters in regulating skeletal muscle substrate use during exercise. *Sports Med.*, 38, 387–99, 2008.
136. Phinney, S. D., Bistrian, B. R., Evans, W. J., Gervino, E., and Blackburn, G. L., The human metabolic response to chronic ketosis without caloric restriction: Preservation of submaximal exercise capability with reducted carbohydrate oxidation. *Metabolism*, 32, 769, 1983.
137. Romijn, J. A., Coyle, E. F., Sidossis, L. S., Gastaldelli, A., Horowitz, J. F., Endert, E., and Wolfe, R. R., Regulation of endogenous fat and carbohydrate metabolism in relation to exercise intensity and duration. *Am. J. Physiol.*, 265, E380–91, 1993.
138. Muoio, D. M., Leddy, J. J., Horvath, P. J., Aw, A. B., and Pendergrast, D. R., Effects of dietary fat on metabolic adjustments to maximal VO2 and endurance in runners. *Med. Sci Sports Exerc.*, 26, 81, 1994.
139. Horvath, P. J., Eagen, C. K., Fisher, N. M., Leddy, J. J., and Pendergrast, D. R., The effects of varying dietary fat on performance and metabolism in trained male and female runners. *J. Am. Coll. Nutr.*, 19, 52, 2000.
140. O'Keeffe, K. A., Keith, R. E., Wilson, G. D., and Blessing, D. L., Dietary carbohydrate intake and endurance exercise performance of trained female cyclists. *Nutr. Res.* 9, 819–30, 1989.
141. Helge, J. W., Richter, E. A., and Kiens, B., Interaction of training and diet on metabolism and endurance during exercise in man, *J. Physiol.*, 492, 293, 1996.
142. Rowlands, D. S., and Hopkins, W. G., Effects of high–fat and high–carbohydrate diets on metabolism and performance in cycling. *Metabolism*, 51, 678–90, 2002.
143. Goedecke, J. H., Christie, C., Wilson, G., Dennis, S. C., Noakes, T. D., Hopkins, W. G., and Lambert, E. V., Metabolic adaptations to a high-fat diet in endurance cyclists. *Metab.* 48, 1509–17, 1999.

144. Helge J. W., Wulff, B., and Kiens, B, Impact of a fat–rich diet on endurance in man: role of the dietary period. *Med. Sci. Sports Exerc.*, 30, 456, 1998.
145. Lambert,E. V., Goedecke, J. H., Van Zyl, C., Murphy, K., Hawley, J. A., Dennis, S. C., and Noakes, T. D., High–fat diet versus habitual diet prior to carbohydrate loading: Effects of exercise metabolism and cycling performance. *Int. J. Sport Nutr. Exerc. Metab.*, 11, 209, 2001.
146. Carey, A. L., Staudacher, H. M., Cummings, N. K., Stepto, N. K., Nikolopoulos, V., Burke, L. M., Hawley, J. A., Effects of fat adaptation and carbohydrate restoration on prolonged endurance exercise. *J. Appl. Physiol.* 91, 115–122, 2001.
147. Havemann, L. S., West, J. H., Goedecke, J. H., McDonald, I. A., St. Clair Gibson, A., Noakes, T. D., and Lambert, E. V., Fat adaptation followed by carbohydrate-loading compromises high-intensity sprint performance. *J. Appl. Physiol.* 100, 194–202, 2006.
148. Brown, R. C., and Cox, C. M., Effects of high fat versus high carbohydrate diets on plasma lipids and lipoproteins in endurance athletes. *Med. Sci. Sports Exerc.*, 30, 1677, 1998.
149. Beckers, E. J., Jeukendrup, A. E., Brouns, F., Wagenmakers, A. J., and Saris, W. H. M., Gastric emptying of carbohydrate-medium chain TG suspensions at rest. *Int. J. Sports Med.*, 13, 581, 1992.
150. Berning, J. R., The role of medium-chain TGs in exercise. *Int. J. Sports Nutr.*, 6, 121, 1996.
151. Bach, A. C. and Babayan, V. K., Medium-chain TGs: An update. *Am. J. Clin. Nutr.*, 36, 950, 1982.
152. Van Zyl, C. G., Lambert, E. V., Hawley, J. A., Noakes, T. D., and Dennis, S. C., Effects of medium-chain TG ingestion on fuel metabolism and cycling performance. *J. Appl. Physiol.*, 80, 2217, 1996.
153. Angus, D. J., Hargreaves, M., Dancey, J., and Febbraio, M. A., Effect of carbohydrate or carbohydrate plus medium–chain TG ingestion on cycling time trial performance. *J. Appl. Physiol.* 88, 113–9, 2000.
154. Vistisen, B. L., Nybo, L., Xuebing, X., Hoy, C. E., and Kiens, B., Minor amounts of plasma medium-chain fatty acids and no improved time trial performance after consuming lipids. *J. Appl. Physiol.* 94, 2434–43, 2003.
155. Goedecke, J. H., Elmer-English, R., Dennis, S. C., Schloss, I., Noakes, T. D., and Lambert, E. V., Effects of medium-chain triaclyglycerol ingested with carbohydrate on metabolism and exercise performance. *Int. J. Sport Nutr.*, 9, 35, 1999b.
156. Goedecke, J. H., Clark, V. R., Noakes, T. D., and Lambert, E. V., The effects of medium-chain triacylglycerol and carbohydrate ingestion on ultra-endurance performance. *Int. J. Sport Nutr. Exerc. Metab.* 15, 15–28, 2005.
157. Satabin, P., Portero, P, Defer, G., Bricout, J., and Guezennec, C. Y., Metabolic and hormonal responses to lipid and carbohydrate diets during exercise in man. *Med. Sci. Sports Exerc.*, 19, 218, 1987.
158. Jeukendrup, A. E., Thielen, J. J., Wagenmakers, A. J., Brouns, F., and Saris, W. H., Effects of medium-chain triacylglycerol and carbohydrate ingestion during exercise on substrate utilization and subsequent cycling performance. *Am. J. Clin. Nutr.*, 67, 397, 1998.
159. Fushiki, T. K., Matsumoto, K., Inoue, K., Kawada, T., and Sugimoto, E., Swimming capacity of mice is increased by chronic consumption of medium-chain TGs. *J. Nutr.*, 125, 531, 1995.
160. Misell, L. M., Lagomarcino, N. D., Schuster, V., and Kern, M., Chronic medium-chain triacylglycerol consumption and endurance performance in trained runners. *J. Sports Med. Phys. Fitness*, 41, 210, 2001.

161. Thorburn, M. S., Vistisen, B., Thorp, R. M., Rockell, M. J., Jeukendrup, A. E., Xu, X., and Rowlands, D. S., Attenuated gastric distress but no benefit to performance with adaptation to octanoate-rich esterified oils in well-trained male cyclists. *J. Appl. Physiol.* 101, 1733–1743, 2006.
162. Kern, M, Lagomarcino, N. D., Misell, L. M., and Schuster, V. The effect of medium-chain triacylglycerols on the blood lipid profile of male endurance runners. *J. Nutr. Biochem.*, 11, 288–93, 2000.
163. Pariza, M. W., Ha, Y. L., Benjamin, H., Sword, J. T., Gruter, A., Chin, S. F., et al., Formation and action of anticarcinogenic fatty acids. *Adv. Exp. Med. Biol.*, 289, 269, 1991.
164. Ritzenthaler, K. L., McGuire, M. K., Falen, R., Shultz, T. D., Dasgupta, N., and McGuire, M. A., Estimation of conjugated linoleic acid intake by written dietary assessment methodologies underestimates actual intake evaluated by food duplicate methodology. *J. Nutr.*, 131, 1548, 2001.
165. Colakoglu, S., Colakoglu, M., Taneli, F., Cetinoz, F., and Turkmen, M., Cumulative effects of conjugated linoleic acid and exercise on endurance development, body composition, serum leptin and insulin levels. *J. Sports Med. Phys. Fitness*, 46, 570–7, 2006.
166. Mizunoya, W., Haramizu, S., Shibakusa, T., Okabe, Y., and Fushiki, T., Dietary conjugated linoleic acid increases endurance capacity and fat oxidation in mice during exercise. *Lipids*. 40, 265–71, 2005.
167. Park, Y., Albright, K. J., Liu, W., Storkson, J. M., Cook, M. E., and Pariza, M. W., Effect of conjugated linoleic acid on body composition in mice. *Lipids.*, 32, 853, 1997.
168. Kreider, R. B., Ferreira, M. P., Greenwood, M., Wilson, M., and Almada, A. L., Effects of conjugated linoleic acid supplementation during resistance training on body composition, bone density, strength, and selected hematological markers. *J. Strength Cond. Res.*, 16, 325, 2002.
169. Zambell, K. L., Keim, N. L., Van Loan, M. D., Gale, B., Benito, P., Kelley, D. S., and Nelson, G. J., Conjugated linoleic acid supplementation in humans: Effects on body composition and energy expenditure. *Lipids*, 35, 777, 2000.
170. Zambell, K. L., Horn, W. F., and Keim, N. L., Conjugated linoleic acid supplementation in humans: Effects on fatty acid and glycerol kinetics. *Lipids*, 36, 767, 2001.
171. Steck, S. E., Chalecki, A. M., Miller, P., Conway, J., Austin, G. L., Hardin, J. W., et al. Conjugated linoleic acid supplementation for twelve weeks increases lean body mass in obese humans. *J. Nutr.* 137, 1188–93, 2007.
172. Pinkoski, C., Chilibeck, P. D., Candow, D. G., Esliger, D., Ewaschuk, J. B., Facci, M., et al. The effects of conjugated linoleic acid supplementation during resistance training. *Med. Sci. Sports. Exerc.* 38, 39–48. 2006.
173. Lowery, L. M., Appicelli, P. A., and Lemon, P. W. R., Conjugated linoleic acid enhances muscle size and strength gains in novice bodybuilders. *Med. Sci. Sports Exerc.* 30, S182, 1998.
174. Raastad, T., Hostmark, A. T., and Stromme, S. B., Omega-3 fatty acid supplementation does not improve maximal aerobic power, anaerobic threshold and running performance in well-trained soccer players. *Scand. J. Med. Sci. Sports*, 7, 25, 1997.
175. Oostenbrug, G. S., Mensink, R. P., Hardeman, M. R., DeVries, T., Brouns, F., and Hornstra, G., Exercise performance, red blood cell deformability, and lipid peroxidation: Effects of fish oil and vitamin E. *J. Appl. Physiol.*, 83, 746–52, 1997.
176. Kanter, M. M. and Williams, M. H., Antioxidants, carnitine, and choline as putative ergogenic aids. *Int. J. Sport Nutr.*, 5, S120, 1995.
177. Lombard, K. A., Olson, A. L, Nelson, S. E., and Rebouche, C. J., Carnitine status of lactoovovegetarians and strict vegetarian adults and children. *Am. J. Clin. Nutr.*, 50, 301–6, 1989.

178. Arenas, J., Ricoy, J. R., Encinas, A. R., Pola, P., D'Iddio, S., Zeviani, M., et al., Carnitine in muscle, serum, and urine of nonprofessional athletes: Effects of physical exercise, training, and L-carnitine administration. *Muscle Nerve*, 14, 598–604, 1991.
179. Barnett, C., Costill, D. L., Vukovich, M. D., Cole, K. J., Goodpaster, B. H., Trappe, S. W., and Fink, W. J., Effect of L-carnitine supplementation on muscle and blood carnitine content and lactate accumulation during high-intensity spring cycling. *Int. J. Sport Nutr.*, 4, 280–8, 1994.
180. Soop, M., Bjorkman, O., Cederblad, G., Hagenfeldt, L., and Wahren, J., Influence of supplementation on muscle substrate and carnitine metabolism during exercise. *J. Appl. Physiol.*, 64, 2394–9, 1988.
181. Vukovich, M., Costill, D., and Fink, W., Carnitine supplementation: Effect on muscle carnitine content and glycogen utilization during exercise. *Med. Sci. Sports Exerc.*, 26, 1122–29, 1994.
182. Wachter, S., Vogt, M., Kreis, R., Boesch, C., Bigler, P., Hoppeler, H., Krahenbuhl, S., Long-term administration of L-carnitine to humans: Effect on skeletal muscle carnitine content and physical performance. *Clin. Chim. Acta.*, 318, 51–61, 2002.
183. Daily, J. W. and Sachan, D. S., Choline supplementation alters carnitine homeostasis in humans and guinea pigs. *J. Nutr.*, 125, 1938, 1995.
184. Hongu, N. and Sachan, D. S., Carnitine and choline supplementation with exercise alter carnitine profiles, biochemical markers of fat metabolism and serum leptin concentration in healthy women. *J. Nutr.* 133, 84–9, 2003.
185. Gorostiaga E. M., Maurer, C. A., and Eclache, J. P., Decrease in respiratory quotient during exercise following L-carnitine supplementation. *Int. J. Sports Med.*, 10 169, 1989.
186. Natali, A., Santoro, D., Brandi, L. S., Faraggiana, D., Ciociaro, D., Pecori, N., et al., Effects of acute hypercarnitinemia during increased fatty substrate oxidation in man. *Metabolism*, 45, 594–600, 1993.
187. Vecchiet, L., Di Lisa, F., Pieralisi, G., Ripari, P., Menabo, R., Giamberardino, M. A., Siliprandi, N., Influence of L-carnitine administration on maximal physical exercise. *Eur. J. Appl. Physiol.* 61, 486–90, 1990.
188. Wyss, V., Ganzit, G. P., and Rienzi, A., Effects of L-carnitine administration on VO_{2max} and the aerobic–anaerobic threshold in normoxia and acute hypoxia. *Eur. J. Appl. Physiol.*, 60, 1–6, 1990.
189. Marconi, C., Sassi, G., Carpinelli, A., and Cerretelli, P., Effects of L-carnitine loading on the aerobic and anaerobic performance of endurance athletes. *Eur. J. Appl. Physiol.*, 54, 131–5, 1985.
190. Decombaz, J., Olivier, D., Acheson, K., Gmuender, B., and Jequier, E., Effect of L-carnitine on submaximal exercise metabolism after depletion of muscle glycogen. *Med. Sci. Sports Exerc.*, 25, 733–40, 1993.
191. Oyono-Enguelle, S., Freund, H., Ott, C., Gartner, M., Heitz, A., Marbach, J., et al., Prolonged submaximal exercise and L-carnitine in humans. *Eur. J. Appl. Physiol.*, 58, 53–61, 1988.
192. Greig, C., Finch, K. M., Jones, D. A., Cooper, M., Sargeant, A. J., and Forte, C. A., The effect of oral supplementation with L-carnitine on maximum and submaximum exercise capacity. *Eur. J. Appl. Physiol.*, 56, 457–60, 1985.
193. Colombani, P., Wenk, C., Kunz, I., Krahenbuhl, S., Kuhnt, M., Arnold, M., et al., Effects of L-carnitine supplementation on physical performance and energy metabolism of endurance-trained athletes: A double blind cross-over field study. *Eur. J. Appl. Phys.*, 73, 434–9, 1996.
194. Trappe, S. W., Costill, D. L., Goodpaster, B., Vukovich, M. D., and Fink, W. J., The effects of L-carnitine supplementation on performance during interval swimming. *Int. J. Sports Med.*, 15, 181–5, 1994.

195. Stuessi, C., Hofer, P., Meier, C., and Boutellier, U., L-Carnitine and the recovery from exhaustive endurance exercise: A randomised, double-blind, placebo-controlled trial. *Eur. J. Appl. Physiol.* 95, 431–5, 2005.
196. Cha, Y. S., Choi, S. K., Suh, H., Lee, S. N., Cho, D., and Li, K., Effects of carnitine coingested caffeine on carnitine metabolism and endurance capacity in athletes. *J. Nutr. Sci. Vitaminol.*, 47, 378–84, 2001.
197. Spector, S. A., Jackman, M. R., Sabounjian, L. A., Sakkas, C., Landers, D., and Willis, W. T., Effect of choline supplementation on fatigue in trained cyclists. *Med. Sci. Sports Exerc.* 27, 668–73, 1995.
198. Von Allworden, H. N., Horn, S., Kahl, J., and Feldheim, W., The influence of lecithin on plasma choline concentrations in triathletes and adolescent runners during exercise. *Eur. J. Appl. Physiol.* 67, 87–91, 1993.
199. Durstine, J. L. and Haskell, W. L., Effects of exercise training on plasma lipids and lipoproteins. *Exerc. Sports Sci. Rev.*, 22, 477, 1994.
200. Paffenbarger, R. S., Hyde, R. T., Wing, A. L., Lee, I. M., Jung, D. L., and Kampert, J. B., The association of changes in physical activity level and other lifestyle characteristics with mortality among men. *New Eng. J. Med.*, 328, 538, 1993.
201. Leddy, J., Horvath, P., Rowland, J., and Pendergrast, D., Effect of a high or a low fat diet on cardiovascular risk factors in male and female runners. *Med. Sci. Sports Exerc.*, 29, 17, 1997.
202. Pernow, B., and Saltin, B., Availability of substrates and capacity for prolonged heavy exercise. *J. Appl. Physiol.* 31, 416–22, 1971.

3 Proteins

Tom J. Hazell and Peter W. R. Lemon

CONTENTS

I. INTRODUCTION

Interest in determining the protein need for physically active individuals from a scientific standpoint has waxed and waned over the years, yet from the point of view of athletes it has remained consistently high. Although the placebo effect is often significant, this discrepancy in thinking is reason enough to investigate why opinions differ so much on what would seem to be a very straightforward question. Likely the controversy stems from the fact that scientists have focused on requirements using laboratory methodology primarily while athletes have always been most interested in performance, i.e., whether they can run faster or jump higher, etc. Consequently, it could be that there is some truth to both viewpoints.

Although energy intake is of course critical for many types of athletic performance, recent data indicate that the focus on requirements, at least from a protein standpoint, is quite possibly misdirected. Rather, other factors such as timing of protein intake, type of dietary protein or more specifically amino acid (AA) intake may be critical. For those unfamiliar with the history of the protein-exercise studies, a number of comprehensive reviews dating back almost 30 years are available.[1–6] The focus of this chapter is on the timing of protein ingestion relative to exercise and whether certain AA might act as important signals controlling protein metabolism.

II. HISTORICAL PERSPECTIVE

During the 1800s, protein was considered the major fuel for exercise[7] so it is easy to understand why it held such a significant place relative to exercise metabolism at that time. However, during the early part of the 20th century, this idea was largely discounted[8] and the emphasis switched to carbohydrate (CHO) and fat metabolism where it has remained for the most part ever since. This body of work, using the needle biopsy technique initially and, more recently, the utilization of both isotope and magnetic resonance spectroscopy methodologies, has established clearly the major role of CHO and fat in exercise metabolism. Interestingly, from time to time and especially in the 1980s and 90s, some published data have indicated that protein should not be overlooked so quickly and, as a result, more investigators returned to this all but abandoned topic. This work, summarized elsewhere,[1,3] suggests a small but important increased protein need for athletes undergoing most types of vigorous training. However, in contrast to earlier understanding, this has little to do with providing exercise fuel because, in reality, protein contributes very little energy under most exercise circumstances (generally less than 5% and rarely more than 10% of exercise energy expenditure). Clearly, dietary CHO and fat are the predominant exercise fuels. However, protein, and more specifically some of its component parts, especially the indispensable AA (or essential AA [EAA]), may play a significant role in exercise performance via their role as a signal for protein metabolism.

III. CONTROVERSY

Although the age-old debate has focused on dietary protein requirements, it has become clear in recent years that most athletes can maintain positive nitrogen status (dietary requirement is the protein intake when nitrogen excretion = nitrogen intake) during vigorous training with daily protein intakes around 1.4–1.8 g/kg.[9] This is ~75–100% above the dietary recommendations of most countries,[10] but this dietary protein need, unlike CHO, can be attained quite easily by most athletes, even vegetarians, without any special dietary supplementation. This is because most athletes, at least male athletes, increase energy intake substantially with training and, assuming one's diet comes from a variety of food sources, protein intake increases proportionately.

Importantly, anyone who restricts energy intake is at greater risk of a deficiency because protein fuel use increases as total energy intake decreases and this is especially true during periods of growth because the component parts of protein, AA, are key building blocks. Also, an important gender difference exists, as many female athletes left to their own choice will under-eat relative to their daily expenditure resulting in a slowing of metabolic rate to compensate. This phenomenon, especially when combined with less than average protein intakes (common in women who avoid dietary animal protein), could cause insufficient protein intake for optimum performance.

Unfortunately, protein metabolism studies are labor intensive and both complicated and expensive from a technique standpoint. Together with the relatively small number of investigators working in this area, the result is that far fewer definitive data are available versus that of CHO and fat metabolism. Consequently, the controversy continues. Regardless, protein deficiency is uncommon among athletes in the developed countries, and the more critical factors are likely timing of protein ingestion relative to training or competition and perhaps even the type of dietary protein or AA. Discussion of these topics will form the focus of this review.

IV. CRITICAL FACTORS FOR PROTEIN METABOLISM

A. Background

Typically, exercise, especially heavy resistance (strength) exercise, increases muscle protein synthesis (MPS).[11–18] Specifically, it appears that strength exercise stimulates the molecular signalling pathways that promote these increases in MPS.[13] However, exercise also increases muscle protein breakdown (MPB).[11,14,16] Of course, for muscle growth (hypertrophy) to result, the sum total of these two processes (net muscle protein balance) must be positive, either through greater increases in MPS or smaller decreases in MPB (or some combination of both).

Although hypertrophy can occur with exercise and inadequate dietary intake,[19] exercise alone is not sufficiently anabolic to result in optimal net positive muscle protein balance due to the magnitude of the associated increase in MPB. The ingestion of nutrients (especially protein or AA) is also anabolic in nature even without exercise due to an increase in MPS.[20–24] Apparently, from a dietary standpoint, the EAA (or indispensable AA) are the major stimulators of MPS,[25,26] and the branched chain amino acid leucine may be particularly effective.[27] Fujita et al.[22] demonstrated that even without exercise of any kind, ingesting EAA and CHO together causes a significant anabolic response by increasing the AA availability (especially leucine), which stimulates MPS. Carbohydrate ingestion can also result in increases in MPS as long as there is a sufficient amount of AA available,[28] due, at least in part, to the resulting increase in circulating insulin.[29] Some research also suggests that, although the effect of insulin post exercise on MPS may be minimal, it can cause a decrease in MPB,[30] resulting in an even greater net protein balance.

Unfortunately, as mentioned, apparently the singular effects of either exercise or the ingestion of nutrients alone result in a suboptimal net protein balance. As a result, considerable recent research has focused on the combined effects of nutrient ingestion and exercise (particularly strength exercise) in an attempt to maximize muscle anabolism.

B. Nutrient Ingestion Timing

1. Following Exercise

The majority of attempts to enhance net muscle protein balance have focused on the ingestion of nutrients following an exercise bout. The effects of post-exercise feeding on net muscle protein balance appear to be important, as both the ingestion[26,31] or infusion[20] of AA increase MPS further versus ingestion or infusion alone, i.e., without exercise. Muscle protein synthesis increases ($P < 0.05$) during the hour following ingestion and 4 hour totals are similar when ingestion is 1 or 3 hours post exercise, especially when consideration is given for the fact that measures were collected for

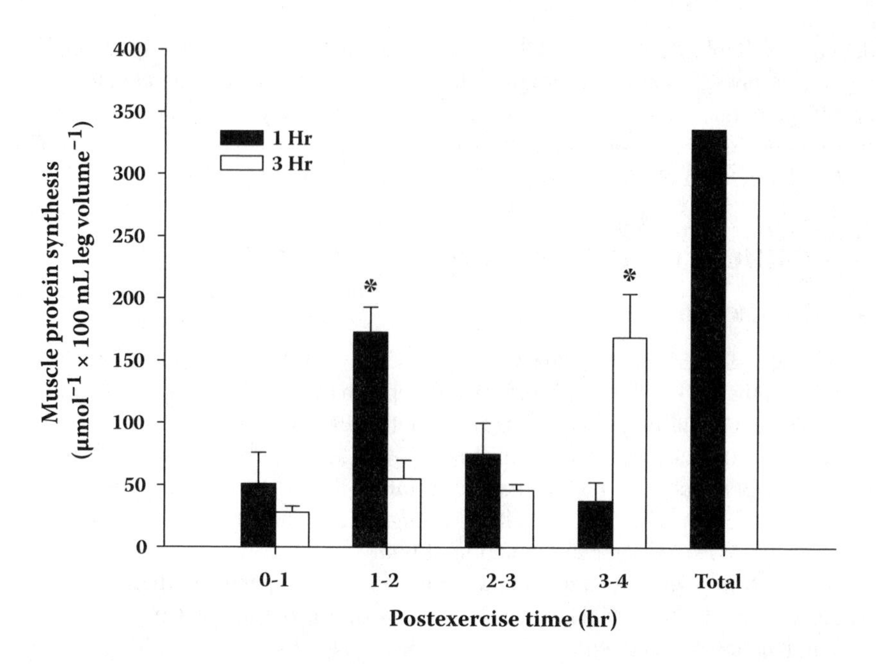

FIGURE 3.1 Muscle protein synthesis increases following the ingestion of an essential amino acid (EAA)–carbohydrate (CHO) drink (6 g EAA + 35 g CHO) ingested either 1 hour (black) or 3 hours (open) post exercise. Values are means ± SEM. *Significantly different from placebo and pre-drink values, $P < 0.05$. (Adapted from Rasmussen, B.B., Tipton, K.D., Miller, S.L., Wolf, S.E., and Wolfe, R.R. An oral essential amino acid–carbohydrate supplement enhances muscle protein anabolism after resistance exercise, *J. Appl. Physiol.* 88, 386–392, 2000.)

3 hours post ingestion for the 1 hour post group and only 2 hours for the 3 hour post group (Figure 3.1).[26] These data suggest any window of time for accelerated muscle protein anabolism post exercise is at least 3 hours. However, Esmarck et al.[32] observed muscle hypertrophy and greater ($P < 0.05$) strength gains in 74+-year-old men undertaking 12 weeks of strength training when ingesting a 409-kJ snack (10 g milk and soy protein, 7 g CHO, and 3.3 g fat) immediately post training versus 2 hours later. Consequently, age may affect the timing of this post-exercise anabolic window.

Interestingly, a similar effect of early post exercise CHO intake on muscle glycogen synthesis exists, but its duration is < 2 hours.[33] Apparently, the effects of exercise lingering into the immediate post-exercise period promote both protein and glycogen synthesis in comparison with other times. Use of this information is critical if optimal recovery from exercise is to occur.

Considerable research suggests that eating and exercise have a cumulative effect, i.e., eating increases MPS ~94–150%[20,22] and exercise increases MPS ~41–100%,[20,21] while their combined effects result in a much larger increase in MPS ~145–200+%.[20,21] The ingestion of protein results in an increased AA availability post exercise, which increases MPS likely due to its stimulation of the molecular cell-signaling pathways involving rapamycin (mTOR) and messenger ribonucleic acid (mRNA) translation initiation and elongation.[21,22] However, it's not just the ingestion of AAs that promote an anabolic state in muscle because CHO ingestion as well as the co-ingestion of protein and CHO also do so.

The ingestion of CHO with the aim of increasing circulating insulin post exercise has been shown to result in a decrease in MPB.[26,28,30,34–36] Consequently, the co-ingestion of protein or AAs, and CHO post exercise could increase the anabolic effect further by increasing MPS with the AAs and decreasing MPB because of the insulin. The ingestion of protein with CHO may even increase AA uptake by the muscle.[37–39] Miller and colleagues[36] reported that CHO and protein co-ingestion post exercise produces additive effects, and several subsequent research studies have corroborated this.[21,22,35,40,41] However, at least one paper suggests that MPS is not increased further with the co-ingestion of CHO and protein as long as there is a sufficient amount of protein ingested.[42] Regardless of any CHO effect on MPS, CHO ingestion is likely anabolic via its effect on blunting the exercise-induced increase in MPB[26,28,30,34–36,43] and, of course, needs to be included in post-exercise supplementation whenever glycogen use has been significant, or subsequent performance, whether a training bout or competition, will be adversely affected due to impaired glycogen resynthesis.

Taken together, these data indicate that eating immediately post exercise is anabolic and the co-ingestion of CHO and protein or AA results in the most anabolic response compared with neither (fasting) or either alone. Unfortunately, as of yet, there is uncertainty as to what quantities of these nutrients are optimal, but likely quite small quantities suffice.

The early research on post-exercise ingestion or infusion used relatively large amounts (~40g) of AA (infusion[20]; ingestion[31]). But Rasmussen and colleagues[26] demonstrated that only a small amount of EAA (6 g) with CHO (35 g) is effective and, although some data indicate a shorter post-exercise window of increased protein anabolism,[44] timing may not be critical (except possibly in older individuals) as long as the nutrient ingestion occurs within 3 hours post exercise. Apparently, large amounts of CHO are not required, because only small increases in insulin have a permissive effect on both MPS and MPB.[42,45] The presence of insulin simply allows the AA ingested to be used for MPS. Recently, Tang and colleagues[46] demonstrated that even smaller amounts of AA (4.2g) and CHO (21g) are effective.

Besides CHO, some other nutrients have significant effects on insulin release, especially the branched chain amino acids.[47] As insulin is a potent anabolic hormone, this response could be critical relative to protein metabolism, although this may be by insulin's effect on inhibition of MPB primarily rather than via its stimulation of MPS.[48] Further, changes in insulin sensitivity could be important (see below).

Some of the current research focus has even shifted to the co-ingestion of protein with the free EAA leucine and CHO. These data suggest that the addition of leucine results in a further decrease in MPB.[40] Moreover, leucine appears to be a potent stimulator of the MPS pathway.[21,27]

The majority of post-exercise ingestion data would suggest that as long as protein and CHO are ingested within 2–3 hours post exercise there will be a significant increase in MPS and a decrease in MPB. Essential amino acids are important, especially leucine, and only small quantities are needed to influence both MPS and MPB.

The result is a positive net muscle protein balance relative to fasting. Therefore, this strategy is recommended for both optimal muscle growth and exercise recovery.

2. Before Exercise

With all of the data demonstrating that eating post exercise is anabolic, it has been suggested that eating before exercise may also be anabolic, possibly even more so, and several very intriguing studies have attempted to shed light on this issue. Tipton et al.[49] first examined the effects of ingesting EAA and CHO before compared with after strength exercise and demonstrated that eating before was more anabolic, perhaps due to a greater total AA uptake in the group eating before exercise compared with the group eating post exercise (Figure 3.2). They hypothesized that providing AA before exercise combined with the increased blood flow during exercise increased MPS further as a result of an enhanced AA availability.[49] Later, Tipton and colleagues[39] retested this hypothesis with the ingestion of intact protein (20 g) and found no advantage to the pre-exercise feeding, i.e., eating whole protein before or after exercise resulted in similar increases in MPS. However, in this second study, there was no CHO ingested with the whole protein, which might have been important, especially as the concentration of AA in the blood increased only 30%, whereas in their previous study there was a 100% increase.[49]

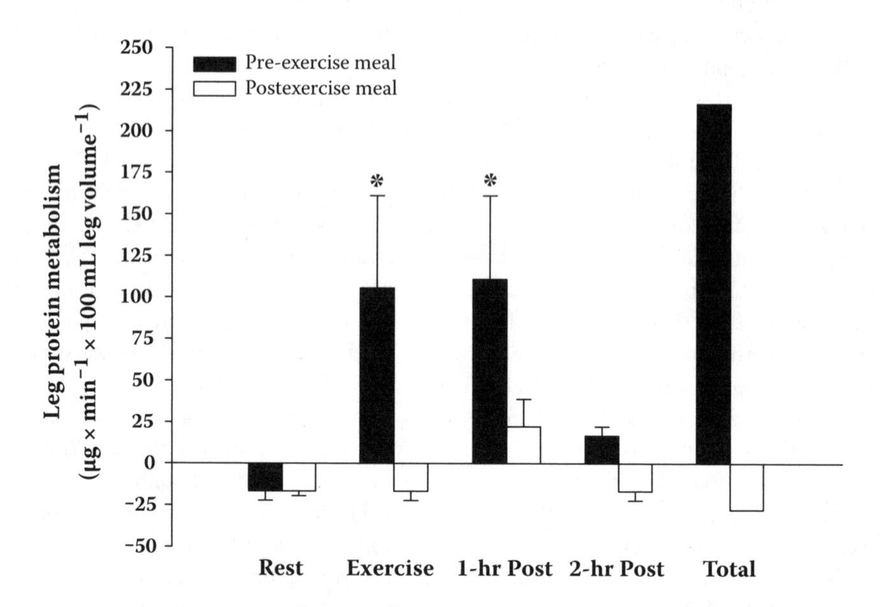

FIGURE 3.2 Muscle net phenylalanine balance following the ingestion of an essential amino acid (EAA)–carbohydrate (CHO) drink (6 g EAA + 35 g CHO) either immediately before (black) or immediately after (open) strength exercise. Values are means ± SEM. *Significantly different from resting values, $P<0.05$. (Adapted from Tipton, K.D., Rasmussen, B.B., Miller, S.L., Wolf, S.E., Owens-Stovall, S.K., Petrini, B.E., and Wolfe, R.R. Timing of amino acid–carbohydrate ingestion alters anabolic response of muscle to resistance exercise, *Am. J. Physiol. Endocrinol. Metab.* 281, E197–206, 2001.)

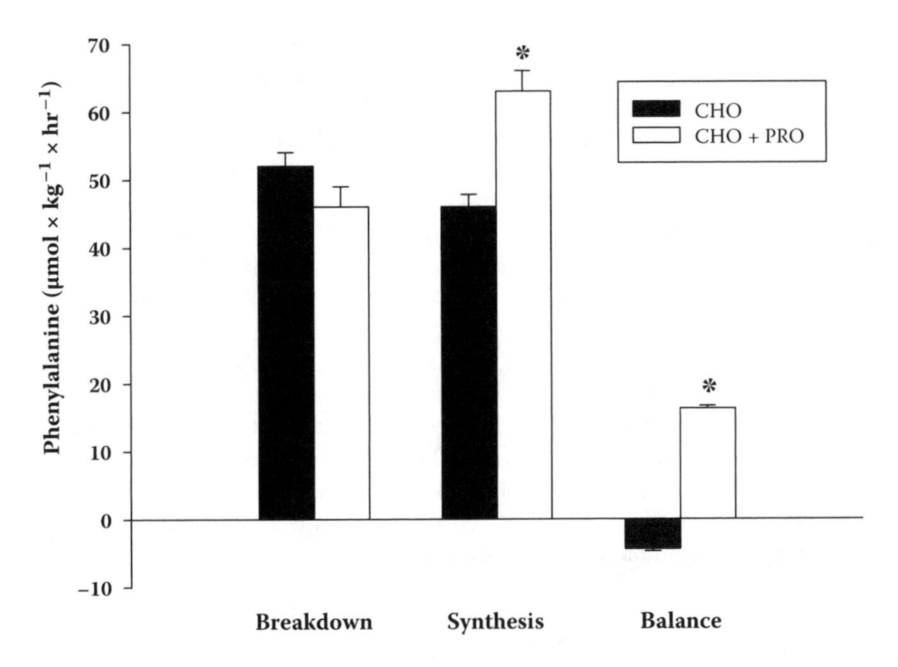

FIGURE 3.3 Whole body protein breakdown, synthesis, and net protein balance rates when ingesting carbohydrate and protein (CHO + PRO, open bars) or carbohydrate alone (CHO, black) both before and during strength exercise. Values are means ± SEM. *Significantly different from CHO, $P < 0.05$. (Adapted from Beelen, M., Koopman, R., Gijsen, A.P., Vandereyt, H., Kies, A.K., Kuipers, H., et al. Protein co-ingestion stimulates muscle protein synthesis during resistance type exercise, *Am. J. Physiol. Endocrinol. Metab.* 295, E70–77, 2008.)

More recently, Beelen et al.[50] examined the co-ingestion of protein and CHO during strength exercise conducted in the evening for subjects who had eaten a standardized diet during the day. Their results demonstrated that, for subjects in the fed state, the co-ingestion of protein and CHO during exercise increased MPS versus CHO alone (Figure 3.3). They hypothesized that nutrient ingestion (in this case EAA and CHO) during exercise in fed subjects may have provided additional time for an elevated MPS, resulting in a positive anabolic state. Bird et al.[51] observed a reduced index of muscle breakdown (urinary 3-methlyhistidine excretion on a meat-free diet) when subjects consumed a liquid CHO-EAA mixture during a strength training session in comparison with CHO, EAA, or placebo conditions. Although these latter data are indirect, they are consistent with the observation that during exercise CHO–EAA ingestion has important effects on MPB. Berardi et al.[52] observed increased ($P < 0.05$) glycogen resynthesis and enhanced ($P < 0.05$) endurance cycling time trial performance[53] 6 hours following a 1-hour time trial with pre- and immediate post-exercise feeding of small meals (7 kcal/kg; 1.2 g/kg CHO, 0.3 g/kg protein, 0.1 g/kg fat) indicating that pre- and immediate post feedings can enhance recovery and subsequent same day endurance performance. Together, these data suggest that ingesting nutrients (CHO and EAA, especially leucine) immediately before, during, and following exercise can be beneficial for both strength and endurance exercise. Consequently, ingestion before, during, and following may be optimal for protein anabolism.

However a recent study by Fujita et al.[54] clouds this issue. This particular study examined the ingestion of CHO and EAA with additional leucine 1 hour before strength exercise and hypothesized that this pre-exercise ingestion would prevent the exercise-induced decrease in MPS as well as promote a greater MPS stimulus during early post-exercise recovery. In contrast, their data demonstrate that eating before or not eating at all resulted in similar increases in MPS during exercise and at both 1 and 2 hours post, suggesting that eating before exercise may be of little benefit. Such conflicting data are confusing; however, nutrient ingestion in the Fujita et al.[54] study was 1 hour prior to exercise and this might be important because for the others the nutrient intake was immediately before[49] or immediately before and during exercise.[50] Moreover, at several measured time points in the Fujita and colleagues'[54] experiment, the EAA plus CHO condition resulted in a nonsignificantly greater effect and, when all data collected are summed, the overall MPS appeared to be greater in the EAA plus CHO condition (Figure 3.4). Finally, and perhaps importantly, eating 1 hour pre-exercise did not prevent the exercise-induced increase

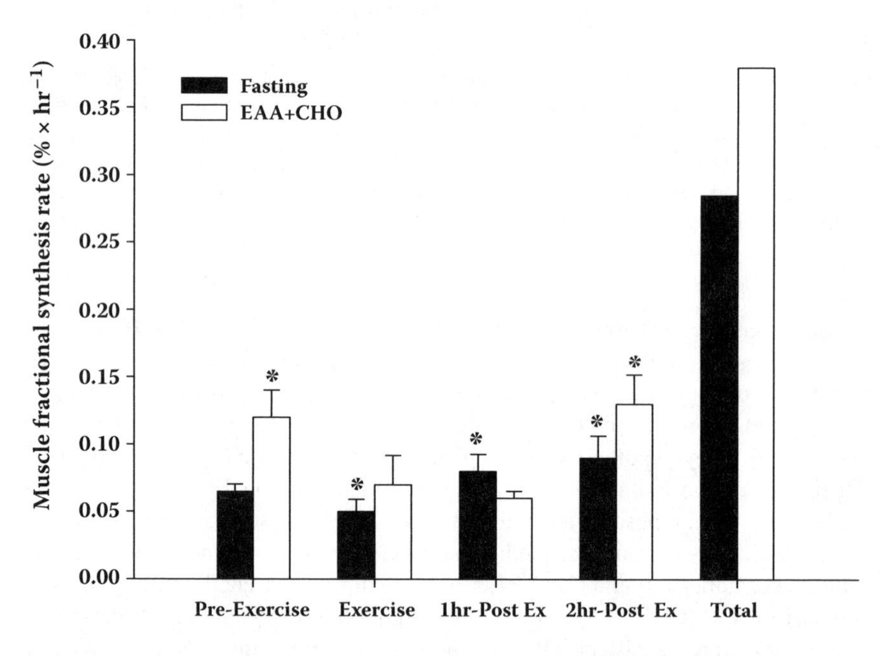

FIGURE 3.4 Muscle protein synthesis following ingestion of an essential amino acid (EAA)–carbohydrate (CHO) drink (17.5 g EAA + 25 g CHO) ingested 1 hour prior to exercise (open) versus no nutrient ingestion (black). Values are means ± SEM. *Significantly different from fasting pre-exercise fasting values, $P < 0.05$. EAA + CHO was greater pre-exercise but there were no between-condition differences during exercise or at either 1 or 2 hours post exercise (Adapted from Fujita, S., Dreyer, H.C., Drummond, M.J., Glynn, E.L., Volpi, E., and Rasmussen, B.B. Essential amino acid and carbohydrate ingestion prior to resistance exercise does not enhance post–exercise muscle protein synthesis, *J. Appl. Physiol.* in press.)

in MPB. As both post- and during-exercise feeding do decrease any MPB typically, nutrient ingestion 1 hour pre-exercise may not be the best approach.

At this time a definitive solution to explain these conflicting data is not possible, so we must await future studies. For now, the majority of evidence indicates that early post exercise intake of small quantities of EAA, especially leucine and CHO, is beneficial for both muscle growth and performance. The value of pre- and during-exercise nutrient intake on these parameters is much less clear but certainly worth pursuing as research topics.

C. Protein Type

Although AA or EAA ingestion in the immediate post-exercise period is clearly beneficial for exercise recovery, other research has demonstrated that intact protein ingestion post exercise can also result in a significant increase in MPS.[37–40,42,55–57] Interestingly, different types of intact protein have been shown to have different effects on MPS. For example, whey protein results in a large and rapid increase with a short duration, whereas casein protein causes a more moderate increase with a much longer duration.[58,59] However, significantly, casein appears to have greater effects on chronic protein deposition, perhaps because it inhibits MPB more than whey. This mechanism could explain the observed greater gains in lean mass and strength during 12 weeks of strength training in men when the dietary protein source was primarily casein versus whey.[60]

Interestingly, differences in circulating insulin are likely not responsible because insulin concentrations were similar in the experiments of Boirie and colleagues.[58,59] However, it is possible that changes in insulin sensitivity are important. Some protein sources, especially deep-ocean fish, have powerful effects on insulin sensitivity due to their omega-3 fatty acid content, but others, such as cod, which have a low omega-3 content, have significant positive effects on insulin sensitivity, presumably due to their AA profile.[61,62] This appears to be the result of normalizing insulin activation of the phosphatidylinositol 3-kinase/Akt and by selectively improving GLUT 4 translocation to the T-tubules in skeletal muscle.[63] Such differing effects of protein type could be critical to the resulting protein anabolic effect and need to be investigated more fully.

In addition, the post-exercise ingestion of milk as a source of protein can result in acute increases in MPS[37,57] and more chronic increases in lean body mass versus soy protein.[55] Cow's milk contains about 4.8% CHO, 3.4% protein (of this 2.8% is casein and 0.6 is whey), 3.7% fat, 0.8% minerals (of this 0.3% is sodium and potassium), and 87.3% water.[64] Of course, for skim milk, the fat is removed during the skimming process so the percentages of everything else increase proportionately. Essentially then, milk is a CHO-protein-electrolyte fluid whose composition is quite appropriate as a post-exercise nutritional supplement to enhance protein balance. Others have noted post-exercise ingestion of chocolate milk (immediately and at 2 hours post) can enhance recovery following exhaustive endurance exercise bouts.[65] This should not be surprising because, although the CHO content of chocolate milk varies (typically, it is approximately double that of regular milk), the additional CHO content means that glycogen resynthesis would also be enhanced. Hence, it would appear that chocolate milk is a very effective post-exercise drink.

Other potential explanations for the observed effects of pre-, during-, or post-exercise protein ingestion on protein metabolism could involve physical or chemical differences that exist among dietary protein sources, as these affect digestion or absorption rates and, therefore, AA availability to muscle. For example, it is well known that whey protein is absorbed much more quickly than casein[58,66] and this, not the specific AA content, is likely responsible for the differing effects on protein metabolism. Support for this hypothesis can be found from experiments where repeated intakes of small quantities of whey protein at regular intervals result in effects on protein metabolism essentially like casein (which is absorbed relatively slowly).[59] Moreover, intake of a free AA mixture mimicking the composition of casein has effects on protein metabolism more like whey (which is absorbed quickly) (Figure 3.5). Consequently, AA availability to muscle overtime appears to be an important determinant of protein balance.

Vegetarian diets are now very popular to reduce saturated fat intake for health reasons but this approach may not be optimal relative to protein balance because

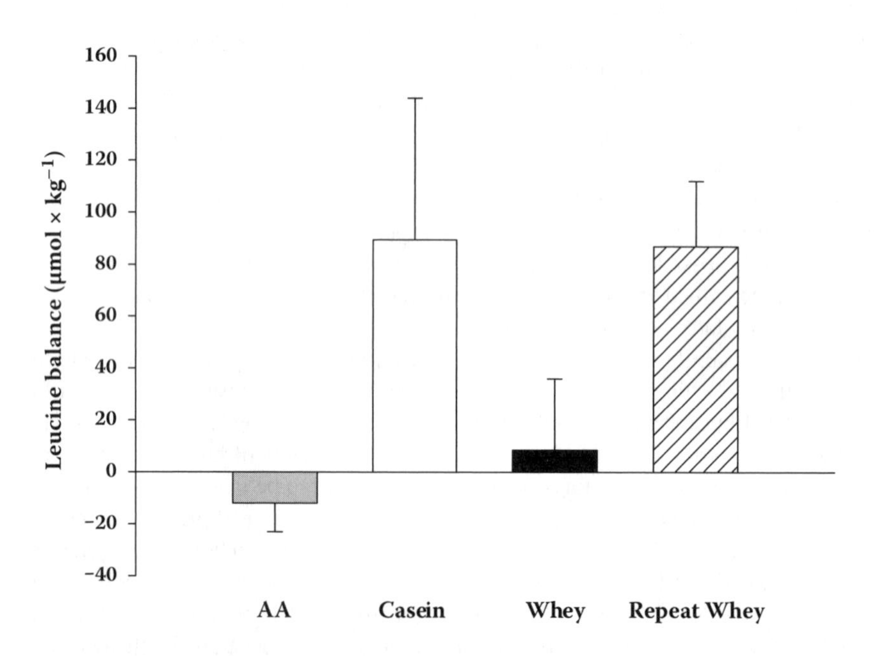

FIGURE 3.5 Leucine balance over 7 hours after ingestion of 30 g of a free amino acid composition mimicking casein AA (gray), casein (open), whey (black), or repeated, smaller ingestions of whey (repeat whey, hatched) where 13 small ingestions (~2.3 g) took place at 20-minute intervals over 4 hours. Values are means ± SEM. No significance is shown as the data are combined from two studies but clearly the effects are dramatic. (Adapted from Boirie, Y., Dandin, M., Gachon, P., Vasson, M-P., Maubois, J-L., Beaufrère, B. Slow and fast dietary protein differently modulate postprandial protein accretion, *Proc. Nat. Acad. Sci.* 94, 14930–14935, 1997; Dangin, M., Boirie, Y., Garcia-Rodenas, C., Gachon, P., Fauquant, J., Callier, P., et al. The digestion rate of protein is an independent regulating factor of postprandial protein retention, *Am. J. Physiol. Endocrinol. Metab.* 280, E340–348, 2001.)

51- to 69-year-old men who consumed a vegetarian diet over a 12-week strength study obtained lower ($P < 0.05$) gains in body density, fat-free mass, and creatinine excretion, as well as nonsignificant and less than 50% increase in fast twitch muscle fiber area than their counterparts who followed an identical training program but ate meat.[67] Several possibilities could explain these observations, including the lower amino score, the lower digestibility, or the catabolic effects of post-ingestion increases in circulating cortisol associated with the consumption of vegetarian diets.[68–71]

V. RESEARCH NEEDS

Switching emphasis from investigations on dietary protein requirements for physically active individuals to detailed study of the intake timing of specific nutrients, especially CHO, EAA, and leucine is now needed to advance our understanding of how to optimize protein metabolism. Clearly, post-exercise feedings of EAA, leucine, and CHO can enhance both protein and glycogen resynthesis. Details of the precise post-exercise timing and quantities for optimal responses need to be worked out as well as whether pre- and during-exercise feedings may also be important. Finally, which AA or intact proteins are best could form the basis of many future studies. When understood fully, this information will be most valuable not only for athletes attempting to maximize their performance or to recover more quickly from training sessions or competitions, but also for a host of others who need to increase or retain muscle mass (seniors, dieters, astronauts, those with a variety of degenerative diseases associated with aging, etc). This latter point is especially critical as it becomes increasingly clear that decreases in muscle mass (sarcopenia) are responsible for a variety of health problems prevalent today.[72,73]

VI. CONCLUSIONS

Protein requirements of exercising individuals have been debated for hundreds of years. It now appears that protein needs are increased by perhaps 75–100% for athletes engaged in serious exercise training but, importantly, these intakes can be obtained quite easily, assuming a balanced diet with adequate energy intake. Consequently, from this perspective, protein supplementation is not necessary under normal circumstances. Exceptions might include women who under-eat relative to their exercise training expenditure or those who are restricting energy intake for some other reason.

On the other hand, recent data indicate clearly that protein and CHO ingestion immediately post exercise (and perhaps also during or shortly before exercise) definitely can enhance acute exercise performance as well as training adaptations by activating both protein and glycogen metabolic pathways. The timing of this nutrient intake may be critical, but the duration of time that any post- or pre-exercise window exists is not yet clear (but closer to the exercise bout is likely best). Moreover, much more study is needed to elucidate the possible benefits of pre- or during-exercise nutrient intake. Specific amino acids (EAA, especially leucine) and CHO appear to be important and only very small amounts are necessary.

REFERENCES

1. Lemon, P.W.R. and Nagle, F.J. Effects of exercise on protein and amino acid metabolism, *Med. Sci. Sports Exerc.* 13,141–149, 1981.
2. Lemon, P.W.R. Effects of exercise on dietary protein requirements, *Int. J. Sport Nutr.* 8, 426–447, 1998.
3. Rennie, M.J. Physical exertion, amino acid and protein metabolism, and protein requirements, in *The Role of Protein and Amino Acids in Sustaining and Enhancing Performance,* Institute of Medicine, National Academy Press, Washington, 1999, 243–253.
4. Lemon, P.W.R., Berardi, J.M., and Noreen, E.E. The role of protein and amino acid supplementation in the athlete's diet: Does type or timing of ingestion matter? *Curr. Sport Med. Rep.* 4, 214–221, 2002.
5. Tipton, K.D. and Wolfe, R.R. Protein and amino acids for athletes, *J. Sport. Sci.* 22, 65–79, 2004.
6. Gibala, M.J. Protein metabolism and endurance exercise, *Sports Med.* 37, 337–340, 2007.
7. von Liebig, J. *Animal Chemistry of Organic Chemistry in Its Application to Physiology,* Gregory, G. (Translator), Taylor & Walton, London, 1842.
8. Cathcart, E.P., and Burnett, W.A. Influence of muscle work on metabolism in varying conditions of diet, *Proc. Roy. Soc. London [Biology]* 99, 405–426, 1926.
9. American College of Sports Medicine; American Dietetic Association; Dieticians of Canada. Joint Position Statement: Nutrition and athletic performance, *Med. Sci. Sports. Exerc.* 32, 2130–2145, 2000.
10. Institute of Medicine, *Dietary Reference Intakes for Energy, Carbohydrate, Fiber, Fat, Fatty Acids, Cholesterol, Protein, and Amino Acids.* Food and Nutrition Board, Washington, 2002.
11. Biolo, G., Maggi, S.P., Williams, B.D., Tipton, K.D., and Wolfe, R.R. Increased rates of muscle protein turnover and amino acid transport after resistance exercise in humans, *Am. J. Physiol.* 268, E514–520, 1995b.
12. Kim, P.L., Staron, R.S., and Phillips, S.M. Fasted-state skeletal muscle protein synthesis after resistance exercise is altered with training, *J. Physiol.* 568, 283–290, 2005.
13. Koopman, R., Zorenc, A.H., Gransier, R.J., Cameron-Smith, D., and van Loon, L.J. Increase in S6K1 phosphorylation in human skeletal muscle following resistance exercise occurs mainly in type II muscle fibers, *Am. J. Physiol. Endocrinol. Metab.* 290, E1245–1252, 2006.
14. Phillips, S.M., Tipton, K.D., Aarsland, A., Wolf, S.E., and Wolfe, R.R. Mixed muscle protein synthesis and breakdown after resistance exercise in humans, *Am. J. Physiol.* 273, E99–107, 1997.
15. Phillips, S.M., Parise, G., Roy, B.D., Tipton, K.D., Wolfe, R.R., and Tarnopolsky, M.A. Resistance-training-induced adaptations in skeletal muscle protein turnover in the fed state, *Can. J. Physiol. Pharmacol.* 80, 1045–1053, 2002.
16. Sheffield-Moore, M., Yeckel, C.W., Volpi, E., Wolf, S.E., Morio, B., Chinkes, D.L., et al. Post exercise protein metabolism in older and younger men following moderate-intensity aerobic exercise, *Am. J. Physiol. Endocrinol. Metab.* 287, E513–522, 2004.
17. Tipton, K.D., Ferrando, A.A., Williams, B.D., and Wolfe, R.R. Muscle protein metabolism in female swimmers after a combination of resistance and endurance exercise, *J. Appl. Physiol.* 81, 2034–2038, 1996.
18. Wilkinson, S.B., Phillips, S.M., Atherton, P.J., Patel, R., Yarasheski, K.E., Tarnopolsky, M.A., Rennie, M.J. Differential effects of resistance and endurance exercise in the fed state on signalling molecule phosphorylation and protein synthesis in human muscle, *J. Physiol.* 586, 3701–3717, 2008.

19. Goldberg, A.L., Etlinger, J.D., Goldspink, D.F., and Jablecki, C. Mechanism of work-induced hypertrophy of skeletal muscle, *Med. Sci. Sports.* 7, 248–261, 1975.
20. Biolo, G., Tipton, K.D., Klein, S., and Wolfe, R.R. An abundant supply of amino acids enhances the metabolic effect of exercise on muscle protein, *Am. J. Physiol.* 273, E122–129, 1997.
21. Dreyer, H.C., Drummond, M.J., Pennings, B., Fujita, S., Glynn, E.L., Chinkes, D.L., et al. Leucine-enriched essential amino acid and carbohydrate ingestion following resistance exercise enhances mTOR signaling and protein synthesis in human muscle, *Am. J. Physiol. Endocrinol. Metab.* 294, E392–400, 2008.
22. Fujita, S., Dreyer, H.C., Drummond, M.J., Cadenas, J.G., Yoshizawa, F., Volpi, E., and Rasmussen, B.B. Nutrient signalling in the regulation of human muscle protein synthesis, *J. Physiol.* 582, 813–823, 2007.
23. Paddon-Jones, D., Sheffield-Moore, M., Zhang, X.J., Volpi, E., Wolf, S.E., Aarsland, A., et al. Amino acid ingestion improves muscle protein synthesis in the young and elderly, *Am. J. Physiol. Endocrinol. Metab.* 286, E321–328, 2004.
24. Wolfe, R.R. Regulation of muscle protein by amino acids, *J. Nutr.* 132, 3219S–3224S, 2002.
25. Tipton, K.D., Gurkin, B.E., Matin, S., and Wolfe, R.R. Nonessential amino acids are not necessary to stimulate net muscle protein synthesis in healthy volunteers, *J. Nutr. Biochem.* 10, 89–95, 1999.
26. Rasmussen, B.B., Tipton, K.D., Miller, S.L., Wolf, S.E., and Wolfe, R.R. An oral essential amino acid–carbohydrate supplement enhances muscle protein anabolism after resistance exercise, *J. Appl. Physiol.* 88, 386–392, 2000.
27. Layman, D.K. Role of leucine in protein metabolism during exercise and recovery, *Can. J. Appl. Physiol.* 27, 646–663, 2002.
28. Bell, J.A., Fujita, S., Volpi, E., Cadenas, J.G., and Rasmussen, B.B. Short-term insulin and nutritional energy provision do not stimulate muscle protein synthesis if blood amino acid availability decreases, *Am. J. Physiol. Endocrinol. Metab.* 289, E999–1006, 2005.
29. Biolo, G., Fleming, R.Y., and Wolfe, R.R. Physiologic hyperinsulinemia stimulates protein synthesis and enhances transport of selected amino acids in human skeletal muscle, *J. Clin. Invest.* 95, 811–819, 1995.
30. Biolo, G., Williams, B.D., Fleming, R.Y., and Wolfe, R.R. Insulin action on muscle protein kinetics and amino acid transport during recovery after resistance exercise, *Diabetes* 48, 949–957, 1999.
31. Tipton, K.D., Ferrando, A.A., Phillips, S.M., Doyle, D., Jr, and Wolfe, R.R. Post exercise net protein synthesis in human muscle from orally administered amino acids, *Am. J. Physiol.* 276, E628–634, 1999.
32. Esmarck, B., Andersen, J.L., Olsen, S., Richter, E.A., Mizuno, M., and Kjaer, M. Timing of postexercise protein intake is important for muscle hypertrophy with resistance training in elderly humans, *J. Physiol.* 535, 301–311, 2001.
33. Ivy, J.L., Katz, A.L., Culter, C.L., Sherman, W.M., and Coyle, E.F. Muscle glycogen synthesis after exercise: Effect of time of carbohydrate ingestion, *J. Appl. Physiol.* 64, 1480–1485, 1988.
34. Borsheim, E., Tipton, K.D., Wolf, S.E., and Wolfe, R.R. Essential amino acids and muscle protein recovery from resistance exercise, *Am. J. Physiol. Endocrinol. Metab.* 283, E648–657, 2002.
35. Borsheim, E., Cree, M.G., Tipton, K.D., Elliott, T.A., Aarsland, A., and Wolfe, R.R. Effect of carbohydrate intake on net muscle protein synthesis during recovery from resistance exercise, *J. Appl. Physiol.* 96, 674–678, 2004.

36. Miller, S.L., Tipton, K.D., Chinkes, D.L., Wolf, S.E., and Wolfe, R.R. Independent and combined effects of amino acids and glucose after resistance exercise, *Med. Sci. Sports Exerc.* 35, 449–455, 2003.
37. Elliot, T.A., Cree, M.G., Sanford, A.P., Wolfe, R.R. and Tipton, K.D. Milk ingestion stimulates net muscle protein synthesis following resistance exercise, *Med. Sci. Sports. Exerc.* 38, 667–674, 2006.
38. Tipton, K.D., Elliott, T.A., Cree, M.G., Wolf, S.E., Sanford, A.P., and Wolfe, R.R. Ingestion of casein and whey proteins result in muscle anabolism after resistance exercise, *Med. Sci. Sports Exerc.* 36, 2073–2081, 2004.
39. Tipton, K.D., Elliott, T.A., Cree, M.G., Aarsland, A.A., Sanford, A.P., and Wolfe, R.R. Stimulation of net muscle protein synthesis by whey protein ingestion before and after exercise, *Am. J. Physiol. Endocrinol. Metab.* 292, E71–76, 2007.
40. Koopman, R., Wagenmakers, A.J., Manders, R.J., Zorenc, A.H., Senden, J.M., Gorselink, M., Keizer, H.A., and van Loon, L.J. Combined ingestion of protein and free leucine with carbohydrate increases postexercise muscle protein synthesis in vivo in male subjects, *Am. J. Physiol. Endocrinol. Metab.* 288, E645–653, 2005.
41. Koopman, R., Verdijk, L., Manders, R.J., Gijsen, A.P., Gorselink, M., Pijpers, E., Wagenmakers, A.J., and van Loon, L.J. Co–ingestion of protein and leucine stimulates muscle protein synthesis rates to the same extent in young and elderly lean men, *Am. J. Clin. Nutr.* 84, 623–632, 2006.
42. Koopman, R., Beelen, M., Stellingwerff, T., Pennings, B., Saris, W.H., Kies, A.K., Kuipers, H., and van Loon, L.J. Coingestion of carbohydrate with protein does not further augment postexercise muscle protein synthesis, *Am. J. Physiol. Endocrinol. Metab.* 293, E833–842, 2007.
43. Roy, B.D., Tarnopolsky, M.A., MacDougall, J.D., Fowles, J., and Yarasheski, K.E. Effect of glucose supplement timing on protein metabolism after resistance training, *J. Appl. Physiol.* 82, 1882–1888, 1997.
44. Levenhagen, D.K., Gresham, J.D., Carlson, M.G., Maron, D.J., Borel, M.J., Flakoll, P.J. Postexercise nutrient intake timing in humans is critical to recovery of leg glucose and protein homeostasis, *Am. J. Physiol. Endorcrinol. Metab.* 280, E982–993, 2001.
45. Rennie, M.J., Bohé, J., Smith, K., Wackerhage, W., and Greenhaff, P. Branched-chain amino acids as fuels and anabolic signals in human muscle, *J. Nutr.* 136 (Supplement 1), 264S–268S, 2006.
46. Tang, J.E., Manolakos, J.J., Kujbida, G.W., Lysecki, P.J., Moore, D.R., and Phillips, S.M. Minimal whey protein with carbohydrate stimulates muscle protein synthesis following resistance exercise in trained young men, *Appl. Physiol. Nutr. Metab.* 32, 1132–1138, 2007.
47. Sener, A., and Malaisse, W.J. The stimulus-secretion coupling of amino acid-induced insulin release: Insulinotropic action of branched-chain amino acids at physiological concentrations of glucose and glutamine, *Eur. J .Clin. Invest.* 11, 455–460, 2008.
48. Gelfand, R.A., and Barrett, E.J. Effect of physiologic hyperinsulinemia on skeletal muscle protein synthesis and breakdown in man, *J. Clin. Invest.* 80, 1–6, 1987.
49. Tipton, K.D., Rasmussen, B.B., Miller, S.L., Wolf, S.E., Owens-Stovall, S.K., Petrini, B.E., and Wolfe, R.R. Timing of amino acid–carbohydrate ingestion alters anabolic response of muscle to resistance exercise, *Am. J. Physiol. Endocrinol. Metab.* 281, E197–206, 2001.
50. Beelen, M., Koopman, R., Gijsen, A.P., Vandereyt, H., Kies, A.K., Kuipers, H., et al. Protein co-ingestion stimulates muscle protein synthesis during resistance type exercise, *Am. J. Physiol. Endocrinol. Metab.* 295, E70–77, 2008.
51. Bird, S.P., Tarpenning, K.M., and Marino, F.E. Liquid carbohydrate/essential amino acid ingestion during a short term bout of resistance exercise suppresses myofibrillar protein degradation, *Metab. Clin. Exp.* 55, 570–577, 2006.

52. Berardi, J.M., Price, T.B., Noreen, E.E., and Lemon, P.W.R. Postexercise muscle glycogen recovery enhanced with a carbohydrate–protein supplement, *Med. Sci. Sports Exerc.* 38, 1106–1113, 2006.
53. Berardi, J.M., Noreen, E.E., and Lemon, P.W.R. Recovery from a cycling time trial is enhanced with carbohydrate–protein supplementation versus isoenergetic carbohydrate supplementation, *J. Int. Soc. Sport Nutr.* 5, 24, 2008.
54. Fujita, S., Dreyer, H.C., Drummond, M.J., Glynn, E.L., Volpi, E., and Rasmussen, B.B. Essential amino acid and carbohydrate ingestion prior to resistance exercise does not enhance post–exercise muscle protein synthesis, *J. Appl. Physiol.* in press.
55. Hartman, J.W., Tang, J.E., Wilkinson, S.B., Tarnopolsky, M.A., Lawrence, R.L., Fullerton, A.V., and Phillips, S.M. Consumption of fat-free fluid milk after resistance exercise promotes greater lean mass accretion than does consumption of soy or carbohydrate in young, novice, male weightlifters, *Am. J. Clin. Nutr.* 86, 373–381, 2007.
56. Koopman, R., Pennings, B., Zorenc, A.H., and van Loon, L.J. Protein ingestion further augments S6K1 phosphorylation in skeletal muscle following resistance type exercise in males, *J. Nutr.* 137, 1880–1886, 2007.
57. Wilkinson, S.B., Tarnopolsky, M.A., Macdonald, M.J., Macdonald, J.R., Armstrong, D., Phillips, S.M. Consumption of fluid skim milk promotes greater muscle protein accretion after resistance exercise than does consumption of an isonitrogenous and isoenergetic soy-protein beverage, *Am. J. Clin. Nutr.* 85, 1031–1040, 2007.
58. Boirie, Y., Dandin, M., Gachon, P., Vasson, M-P., Maubois, J-L., Beaufrère, B. Slow and fast dietary protein differently modulate postprandial protein accretion, *Proc. Nat. Acad. Sci.* 94, 14930–14935, 1997.
59. Dangin, M., Boirie, Y., Garcia-Rodenas, C., Gachon, P., Fauquant, J., Callier, P., et al. The digestion rate of protein is an independent regulating factor of postprandial protein retention, *Am. J. Physiol. Endocrinol. Metab.* 280, E340–348, 2001.
60. Demling, R.H., and DeSanti, L. Effect of a hypocaloric diet, increased protein intake and resistance training on lean mass gains and fat mass loss in overweight police officers, *Ann. Nutr. Metab.* 44, 21–29, 2000.
61. Lavigne, C., Marette, A., and Jacques, H. Cod and soy proteins compared with casein improve glucose tolerance and insulin sensitivity in rats, *Am. J. Physiol. Endocrinol. Metab.* 278, E491–500, 2000.
62. Lavigne, C., Tremblay, F., Asselin, G., Jacques, H., and Marette, A. Prevention of skeletal muscle insulin resistance by dietary cod protein in high fat-fed rats. *Am. J. Physiol. Endocrinol. Metab.* 281, E62–71, 2001.
63. Tremblay, F., Lavigne, C., Jacques, H., and Marette, A. Dietary cod protein restores insulin-induced activation of phosphatidylinositol 3-kinase/Akt and GLUT 4 translocation to the t-tubules in skeletal muscle of high-fat-fed obese rats, *Diabetes* 52, 29–37, 2003.
64. Hoogenkamp, H.W. bv: BA Veghel, *Milk Protein*. DMV Campina, The Netherlands, 1989, p 2.
65. Karp, J.R., Johnston, J.D., Tecklenburg, S., Mickleborough, T.D., Fly, A.D., and Stager, J.M. Chocolate milk as a post-exercise recovery aid, *Int J. Sport Nutr. Exerc. Metab.* 16, 78–91, 2006.
66. Mahe, S., Roos, N., Benamouzig, R., Davin, L., Luengo, C., Gagnon, L., Gaussergès, N., Rautureau, J., Tomé, D. Gastrojejunal kinetics and the digestion of [^{15}N] beta-lactoglobulin and casein in humans: the influence of the nature and quantity of the protein, *Am. J. Clin. Nutr.* 63, 546–552, 1996.
67. Campbell, W.W., Barton, M.L. Jr, Cyr–Campbell, D., Davey, S.L., Beard, J.L., Parise, G. et al. Effects of an omnivorous diet compared with a lactoovovegetarian diet on resistance–training–induced changes in body composition and skeletal muscle in older men, *Am. J. Clin. Nutr.* 170, 1032–1039, 1999.

68. Baglieri, A., Mahe, S., Benamouzig, R., Savoie, L., and Tomé, D. Digestion patterns of endogenous and different exogenous proteins affect the composition of intestinal effluents in humans, *J. Nutr.* 125, 1894–1903, 1995.
69. Food and Agricultural Organization World Health Organization and United Nations University, *Energy and protein requirements.* World Health Organization, Geneva, 1985.
70. Henley, E.C., and Kuster, J.M. Protein quality evaluation by protein digestibility-corrected amino acid scoring, *Food Technol.* 48, 74–77, 1994.
71. Lohrke, B., Saggau, E., Schadereit, R., Beyer, M., Bellmann, O., Kuhla, S., Hagemeister, H. Activation of skeletal muscle protein breakdown following consumption of soyabean protein in pigs, *Br. J. Nutr.* 85, 447–457, 2001.
72. Booth, F. and Roberts, C.K. Linking performance and chronic disease risk: Indices of physical performance are surrogates for health, *Br. J. Sports Med.* 42, 950–952, 2008.
73. Johnson, A.P., De Lisio, M., and Parise, G. Resistance training, sarcopenia, and the mitochondrial theory of aging, *Appl. Physiol. Nutr. Metab.* 33,191–199, 2008.

4 Vitamins

Young-Nam Kim and Judy A. Driskell

CONTENTS

I. INTRODUCTION

Vitamins are a group of complex organic compounds that are essential to normal functioning and metabolic reactions in the body. They are divided into two categories: fat-soluble or water-soluble. The fat-soluble vitamins are vitamins A, D, E, and K. The water-soluble vitamins include vitamin C, the B-complex vitamins (thiamin, riboflavin, niacin, vitamin B_6, folate, vitamin B_{12}, pantothenic acid, and biotin), and perhaps choline. The B-complex vitamins are required for the energy-producing pathways and the synthesis or repair of cells in the body. Other vitamins function in maintaining immune function, protecting the body tissues from oxidative damages, and maintaining bone health. Therefore, vitamin deficiencies may influence physiological processes important to exercise or sport performance.

TABLE 4.1
Definitions of the Categories of Dietary Reference Intakes (DRIs)

DRI	Definition
Recommended Dietary Allowance (RDA)	The average daily dietary intake level that is sufficient to meet the nutrient requirement of nearly all (97 to 98%) healthy individuals in a particular life stage and gender group.
Adequate Intake (AI)	A recommended daily intake value based on observed or experimentally determined approximations of nutrient intake by a group (or groups) of healthy people that are assumed to be adequate—used when an RDA cannot be determined.
Tolerable Upper Intake Level (UL)	The highest level of daily nutrient intake that is likely to pose no risk of adverse health effects to almost all individuals in the general population. As intake increases above the UL, the risk of adverse effects increases.
Estimated Average Requirement (EAR)	A daily nutrient intake value that is estimated to meet the requirement of half the healthy individuals in a group.

Adapted from: Otten, J.J., Hellwig, J.P., and Meyers, L.D., Eds., *Dietary Reference Intakes: The Essential Guide to Nutrient Requirements*, National Academy Press, Washington, DC, 2006, pp. 8.[1]

TABLE 4.2
Fat-Soluble Vitamin Recommendations for 19+-Year-Old Adults: Recommended Dietary Allowances (RDAs)/Adequate Intakes (AIs),[a] Daily Values (DVs),[b] and Tolerable Upper Intake Levels (ULs)[a]

	RDA/AI		DV	UL
Vitamin	Men	Women	4+ Years	All Adults[c]
Vitamin A (μg/d)[d]	900	700	5,000 IU	3,000
Vitamin D (μg/d)[e]	5/10[f]	5/10	400 IU	50
Vitamin E (mg/d)[g]	15	15	30 IU	1,000[h]
Vitamin K (μg/d)	120	90	80	ND[i]

[a] DRI publications.[5,12,16,30]

[b] DVs are used on food and supplement labels.[2]

[c] 19+ year-old adults.

[d] As retinol activity equivalents (RAE). 1 RAE = 1 μg retinol, 12 μg β-carotene, 24 μg α-carotene, or 24 μg β-cryptoxanthin. 1 μg retinol = 3.33 IU vitamin A.

[e] As cholecalciferol. 1 μg cholecalciferol = 40 IU vitamin D.

[f] Recommendations for 19–50 y/51+ y.

[g] As α-tocopherol. 1 IU = 1 mg *all rac*-α-tocopheryl acetate, 0.67 mg *RRR*-α-tocopherol, or 0.74 mg *RRR*-α-tocopheryl acetate.

[h] The ULs apply to synthetic forms obtained from supplements, fortified foods, or a combination of the two.

[i] Not determinable.

The U.S. Institute of Medicine (IOM), National Academy of Sciences,[1] has established Dietary Reference Intakes (DRIs) including Estimated Average Requirements (EARs), Recommended Dietary Allowances (RDAs), Adequate Intakes (AIs), and Tolerable Upper Intake Levels (ULs) for vitamins that healthy people should consume. The definitions of the various categories of DRIs are provided in Table 4.1. EARs are the average nutrient intakes estimated to meet the requirement of half the individuals in a group. EARs are utilized in evaluating the prevalence of inadequate intakes within a group. RDAs were established to meet the needs of nearly all (97 to 98 %) individuals in a group. AIs were set when sufficient data were not available to calculate RDAs. RDAs and AIs can both be used as goals for individual intake. Because some vitamins can be toxic, ULs for some of the vitamins were established that are likely to pose no risk of adverse health effects to almost all individuals in the general population.[1] The Daily Value (DV), established by the U.S. Food and Drug Administration, is a nutrient reference value used on food and supplement labels.[2] The RDAs/AIs and ULs of 19+-year-old adults and the DVs of 4+-year-old individuals for fat-soluble and water-soluble vitamins are given in Table 4.2 and Table 4.3,

TABLE 4.3
Water-Soluble Vitamin Recommendations for 19+-Year-Old Adults: Recommended Dietary Allowances (RDAs)/Adequate Intakes (AIs),[a] Daily Values (DVs),[b] and Tolerable Upper Intake Levels (ULs)[a]

	RDA/AI		DV	UL
Vitamin	**Men**	**Women**	**4+ Years**	**All Adults[c]**
Vitamin C (mg/d)	90	75	60	2,000
Thiamin (mg/d)	1.2	1.1	1.5	ND[d]
Riboflavin (mg/d)	1.3	1.1	1.7	ND
Niacin (mg/d)[e]	16	14	20	35[f]
Vitamin B_6 (mg/d)	1.3/1.7[g]	1.3/1.5	2.0	100
Folate (μg/d)[h]	400	400[i]	400	1,000[f]
Vitamin B_{12} (μg/d)	2.4	2.4	6.0	ND
Pantothenic Acid (mg/d)	5	5	10	ND
Biotin (μg/d)	30	30	300	ND
Choline (mg/d)	550	425	ND	3,500

[a] DRI publications.[33,42,54,62,80,92,97,103,105]
[b] DVs are used in food and supplement labels.[2]
[c] 19+ year-old adults.
[d] Not determinable.
[e] As niacin equivalents (NE). 1 mg of niacin = 60 g of tryptophan.
[f] The ULs apply to synthetic forms obtained from supplements, fortified foods, or a combination of the two.
[g] Recommendations for 19–50 y/51+ y.
[h] As dietary folate equivalents (DFE). 1 DFE = 1 μg food folate = 0.6 μg of folic acid from fortified food or as a supplements consumed with food = 0.5 μg of a supplements taken on an empty stomach.
[i] All women capable of becoming pregnant should consume 400 μg from supplements or fortified foods in addition to intake from a varied diet.

respectively. Various methods have been used for the measurement of status of most of the individual nutrients. These methods have been reviewed by Sauberlich.[3]

II. FAT-SOLUBLE VITAMINS

Vitamins A, D, E, and K are classified as fat-soluble vitamins due to their solubility in fat. Fat-soluble vitamins are absorbed and transported along with fats in the body. They are primarily stored in the liver and adipose tissues, and can accumulate in these tissues and cause harmful effects to the body. Recommendations for the fat-soluble vitamins, including RDAs/AIs, ULs, and DVs, are provided in Table 4.2.

A. Vitamin A

Fat-soluble vitamin A includes retinoids and provitamin A carotenoids. The term retinoids refers to retinol, its metabolites (retinal, retinoic acid, and retinyl esters), and synthetic analogues that are structurally similar to retinol. The retinoids are often referred to as preformed vitamin A. Carotenoids are long-chained hydrocarbon compounds, of which more than 600 forms exist. Of the many carotenoids in nature, about 50 forms have provitamin A activity. The most prevalent provitamin A carotenoids in diets include α-carotene, β-carotene, and β-cryptoxanthin.[4]

Vitamin A is known for its role in the visual system. The 11-cis retinal in the retina of the eye functions as a coenzyme with the protein opsin to form rhodopsin. After exposure to light, 11-cis retinal isomerizes to trans-retinal, releasing opsin. The release of opsin initiates an impulse along the optic nerve to send visual images to the brain. Another critical function of vitamin A is its requirement for cellular differentiation. Retinoic acid, a vitamin A metabolite, regulates the various gene expressions that encode for structural proteins, enzymes, extracellular matrix proteins, growth factors, and receptors. Retinoids play a role in normal reproduction, fetal development, and growth. In addition, retinoic acid is involved in normal immune function, maintaining adequate levels of natural killer cells.[5] Carotenoids have been shown to possibly have antioxidant activity, and to be associated with the following health effects: decreased risk of macular degeneration and cataracts, decreased risk of some cancers, and decreased risk of some cardiovascular diseases. However, in humans, the only clear function of carotenoids is vitamin A activity.[4]

Vitamin A deficiency occurs when there is an inadequate vitamin A intake, requirements are increased, or intestinal absorption, transport, or metabolism are impaired as a result of conditions such as diarrhea.[6] Night blindness is one of the first signs of vitamin A deficiency. A more severe deficiency contributes to xerophthalmia (dry eye) and if untreated, permanent blindness. Other signs and symptoms of vitamin A deficiency include anorexia, immune deficiencies, follicular hyperkeratosis, and growth difficulties.[7] Vitamin A deficiency is uncommon in the most developed countries.[8] However, vitamin A deficiency in the United States is most often associated with strict dietary restrictions and excessive alcohol intake.[9]

The conversion factors for provitamin A activity of carotenoids were recently changed to reflect the findings of studies on carotenoid bioavailability. Previously, the biological activity of vitamin A was quantified by conversion of retinol and

TABLE 4.4
Interconversion of Vitamin A and Carotenoid Units

Retinol Activity Equivalent (μg RAE)	International Unit (IU)
1 μg RAE	1 IU
= 1 μg of all-trans-retinol	= 0.3 μg retinol
= 2 μg of supplemental all-trans-β-carotene	= 0.6 μg supplemental β-carotene
= 12 μg of dietary all-trans-β-carotene	= 3.6 μg dietary β-carotene
= 24 μg of other dietary provitamin A carotenoids	

Adapted from: Institute of Medicine, *Dietary Reference Intakes for Vitamin A, Vitamin K, Arsenic, Boron, Chromium, Copper, Iodine, Iron, Manganese, Molybdenum, Nickel, Silicon, Vanadium, and Zinc*, National Academy Press, Washington, DC, 2001, chap. 4.[5]

provitamin A carotenoids to retinol equivalents (REs). One RE was defined as 1 μg of retinol, 6 μg of β-carotene, or 12 μg of other provitamin A carotenoids. However, in 2001, IOM introduced a new term, retinol activity equivalent (RAE) to express the vitamin A activity of carotenoids[5] based on very low vitamin A activity of plant-derived foods in combating vitamin A deficiency despite high provitamin A carotenoid content.[10] One RAE is equivalent to 1 μg of retinol, which is nutritionally equivalent to 12 μg of β-carotene or 24 μg of other provitamin A carotenoids. Currently, International Units (IUs) of vitamin A (1 IU = 0.3 μg retinol or 0.6 μg supplemental β-carotene) are utilized on food and supplement labels in the United States. Interconversions of currently used vitamin A units, RAE and IU, are given in Table 4.4.

The recommendations for vitamin A intakes for the United States and Canada are given in μg RAE. The RDAs for men and women are 900 and 700 μg RAE/d, respectively. Preformed vitamin A is found in animal-derived foods, particularly organ meats, egg yolks, and fortified food products. Nonfat and low-fat milk products are frequently fortified with retinoids. Provitamin A carotenoids are abundant in dark green leafy vegetables and yellowish-orange fruits and vegetables.

Vitamin A toxicity symptoms are variable and nonspecific. The symptoms may include nausea, vomiting, headaches, increased cerebrospinal fluid pressure, vertigo, blurred vision, muscular incoordination, and bulging fontanel in infants. Chronic hypervitaminosis A may include central nervous system effects, liver abnormalities, and bone and skin changes.[5] Carotenoids are relatively nontoxic. Carotenodermia has been reported only from the large consumption of carotenoids in foods. Carotenodermia is harmless and results in a yellowish discoloration of the skin due to the elevation of carotene concentrations. The UL of vitamin A for adults is set at 3,000 μg/d. Currently, DRIs including ULs for carotenoids are not available.

Physical exercise may raise oxygen consumption and increase free radical production, leading to lipid peroxidation or possible tissue damage.[10] Although vitamin A is a weak antioxidant, vitamin A is probably needed for tissue repair, and an increased metabolism of the vitamin would be expected during strenuous exercise. Adult athletes reportedly are well-nourished with respect to the total vitamin A.

Some athletes reportedly have excessive vitamin A intakes, which can be harmful and potentially toxic. Studies indicate that supplementation has no beneficial effect on physical activity. Because vitamin supplements usually contain 100% of the RDA in one dose, it is easy to exceed the UL for vitamin A by taking multiple doses along with a diet rich in animal products.[10] Carotenoids have been shown to possess antioxidant properties. Thus, carotenoids may influence exercise-induced lipid peroxidation or muscle damage. β-carotene has been most investigated for its antioxidant activity to reduce exercise-induced lipid peroxidation in combination with other antioxidant nutrients such as vitamins E and C. Clear evidence of beneficial roles of carotenoids in exercise-induced lipid peroxidation and in the abilities of carotenoids to improve physical performance has not yet been reported.[11] Currently, no specific recommendations for either vitamin A or carotenoids have been set for athletes.

B. Vitamin D

Vitamin D is a fat-soluble vitamin found in foods and also synthesized in the body after exposure to ultraviolet rays from the sun. Several forms of vitamin D have been described, but the two major physiologically relevant ones are vitamin D_2 and vitamin D_3.[12] Vitamin D_2 (ergocalciferol) is a synthetic form of vitamin D that is produced by irradiation of plant steroid ergosterol in plants. Vitamin D_3 (cholecalciferol) is the naturally occurring form of vitamin D produced from 7-dehydrocholesterol when the skin of animals and humans is exposed to sunlight. Both forms are used in supplements.

The main function of vitamin D is in maintaining calcium and phosphorus homeostasis by its influence on the intestines, kidneys, and bones. Other physiologic functions of vitamin D in the brain, heart, pancreas, mononuclear cells, activated lymphocytes, and skin are still unknown, but its biologic function has been identified as a potent antiproliferative and prodifferentiation hormone.[12]

In children, vitamin D deficiency results in a bone disease called rickets, which is characterized by failure to properly mineralize bone tissue. The physical symptoms of rickets include bowed legs, knock knees, curvature of the spine, and thoracic and pelvic deformities. In adults, vitamin D deficiency leads to demineralization of the skeleton causing osteomalacia. Vitamin D deficiency causes a decreased in calcium concentrations in blood, which increases the production and secretion of parathyroid hormone (PTH).[12] Elevated PTH concentrations lead to a normal bone matrix turnover, resulting in a mineralization defect. Vitamin D deficiency may be caused by poor dietary intake or limited exposure to sunlight. Vitamin D interacts with iron; therefore, iron deficiency can induce a concomitant decrease in vitamin D absorption.[13]

The recommendations for vitamin D, as AIs, for 19–50 year-old and 51+-year-old adults are 5 and 10 μg/d, respectively. Vitamin D contents of food and dietary supplement labels are expressed as IU. The biological activity of 1 μg vitamin D is equal to 40 IU. Natural sources of vitamin D in foods are few. Fish and fish oils are the richest sources. Almost all of the vitamin D intake in the United States comes from fortified milk products and other fortified foods such as breakfast cereals.[12]

Vitamin D toxicity may occur with chronic intake of large doses of vitamin D supplements or fish oils, but overexposure to sunlight does not cause vitamin D toxicity. The symptoms of vitamin D toxicity include nausea, vomiting, poor appetite, constipation, weakness, and weight loss.[15] Consequences of severe hypervitaminosis D can lead to hypercalcemia, hypercalcinuria, and possible calcification of soft tissues such as the kidneys.[12] The UL for vitamin D established by IOM is 50 μg/d for all children and adults.

There is little evidence that the deficiency or supplementation of vitamin D influences exercise performance. Vitamin D deficiency was indicated in one-third of female gymnasts aged 10–17 years (n = 18).[14] Because vitamin D does help maintain bone strength and mineralization through regulation of calcium and phosphate homeostasis, monitoring of vitamin D status may be needed in some groups of athletes, such as gymnasts and possibly other indoor athletes.[14] However, intake of large doses may result in vitamin D toxicity.

C. Vitamin E

Natural vitamin E exists in eight different forms, four tocopherols (α-, β-, γ-, and δ-) and four tocotrienols (α-, β-, γ-, and δ-). Alpha-tocopherol is considered the only form of vitamin E that is biologically active in the human body.[16]

The main function of vitamin E is its role as an antioxidant. Free radicals are produced in the body during normal metabolism and exposure to various environmental factors. As a peroxyl radical scavenger, it protects unsaturated lipid components in cells and plasma from free-radical attack by itself becoming oxidized. The antioxidant capacity of vitamin E is lost by oxidation with free radicals, but vitamin E can be reduced by other antioxidants such as vitamin C, regenerating the antioxidant capacity of vitamin E.[16] Besides its antioxidant activity, vitamin E has been shown to have anti-atherogenic and anti-inflammatory effects through its modulation of some molecular signaling pathways.[17]

Although vitamin E deficiency is rare in humans, it has been observed in individuals with genetic abnormalities in α-tocopherol transfer protein, fat malabsorption syndromes, or protein-energy malnutrition.[16] Newborn babies may be at risk of vitamin E deficiency because the vitamin does not cross the placenta. Symptoms of vitamin E deficiency include degeneration of the sensory nerves (peripheral neuropathy), impaired balance and coordination (ataxia), muscle weakness (myopathy), and damage to the retina of the eye (pigmented retinopathy).[16]

Previously, vitamin E activity in foods and dietary recommendations were reported as α-tocopherol equivalents (α-TE) based on the biological activity of tocopherols and tocotrienols in rats.[18] However, it is now known that α-tocopherol is biologically active in humans because only α-tocopherol is repackaged into lipoproteins by the hepatic α-tocopherol transfer protein.[19] DRIs for vitamin E published by the IOM in 2000 were expressed as mg α-tocopherol, and the U.S. Department of Agriculture has updated its nutrient database for vitamin E expressing content in mg α-tocopherol.[20] Alpha-tocopherol in natural foods is in the form of the isomer *RRR*-α-tocopherol (formally *d*-α-tocopherol). The synthetic form of vitamin E is *all-rac*-α-tocopherol, formally *dl*-α-tocopherol, containing all eight isomers of α-tocopherol (*RRR*-, *RSR*-, *RRS*-, *RSS*, *SRR*-, *SSR*-, *SRS*-, and *SSS*-α-tocopherol) in the mixture. Both natural and synthetic forms are used for vitamin E supplementation of foods and supplements,

TABLE 4.5
Vitamin E Content (mg α-tocopherol) of Selected Foods

Food	mg α-tocopherol/100g	mg α-tocopherol/Serving
Olive oil	14.35	1.94 (1 tbsp)[a]
Safflower oil	34.10	4.64 (1 tbsp)
Sunflower oil	41.08	5.59 (1 tbsp)
Mayonnaise	6.43	0.90 (1 tbsp)
Almonds	26.22	7.43 (1 oz)
Peanuts, dry-roasted	7.80	2.21 (1 oz)
Peanut butter	8.99	2.88 (2 tbsp)
Sunflower seeds, dry-roasted	26.10	7.40 (1 oz)
Asparagus, raw	1.13	0.76 (1/2 cup)
Spinach, raw	2.03	0.61 (1 cup)
Turnip greens, raw	2.86	1.57 (1 cup)
Apples, raw	0.18	0.33 (1 medium)
Bananas, raw	0.10	0.12 (1 medium)
Oranges, raw	0.18	0.24 (1 medium)
Eggs	0.97	0.48 (1 large)
Whole milk	0.06	0.15 (1 cup)
Bread, whole-wheat	0.51	0.14 (1 slice)

[a] Serving size.

Adapted from: U.S. Department of Agriculture, Agricultural Research Service, USDA National Nutrient Database for Standard Reference, Release 20.[20]

and typically sold either as acetate esters or succinate esters.[21] Currently, the IU is used in labeling fortified foods and dietary supplements for vitamin E content. One IU of vitamin E activity was defined as 1 mg of *all rac*-α-tocopherol acetate, 0.67 mg *RRR*-α-tocopherol, or 0.74 mg *RRR*-α-tocopheryl acetate by the U.S. Pharmacopeia.[22]

The RDA for adults is 15 mg α-tocopherol/d. Alpha-tocopherol includes *RRR*-α-tocopherol in natural foods and the 2*R*-stereoisomeric forms of α-tocopherol (*RRR*-, *RSR*-, *RRS*-, and *RRS*-α-tocopherol) in fortified foods and dietary supplements. Other isometric forms of α-tocopherol also found in fortified foods and supplements are not usable by the body according to IOM.[16] Major dietary sources of α-tocopherol are vegetable oils (olive, sunflower, and safflower oils), nuts, whole grains, and green leafy vegetables. The vitamin E content of selected foods is found in Table 4.5.

There is no evidence of toxicity from the consumption of vitamin E naturally occurring in foods. The IOM established an UL for vitamin E at 1,000 mg/d for any form of supplementary α-tocopherol, which is based on the prevention of hemorrhage. Vitamin E can act as an anticoagulant, thus high amounts of vitamin E supplementation may increase the risk of bleeding problems.

The greatly increased oxygen consumption indicated during exercise results in the generation of free radicals and lipid peroxidation. Strenuous exercise may induce oxidative damage and result in muscle injury.[23] Vitamin E, the major antioxidant in cellular membranes, may lower the oxidative stress associated with exercise. In vitamin E-deficient rats, exercise increased susceptibility to free radical damage and declined exercise endurance capacity.[24]

Supplementation of vitamin E alone or in combination with other antioxidants such as vitamin C and carotenoids has been shown to result in inconclusive results varying from reduced lipid peroxidation to no effects for protecting against exercise-induced lipid peroxidation.[17] Several studies have reported that vitamin E supplementation has an effect in attenuating exercise-induced lipid peroxidation in aerobic or endurance exercise,[25–27] but not strength training,[28] by decreasing lipid peroxidation markers such as malondiadehyde, F_2-isoprostanes, or breath pentane. However, the vitamin E effects in antioxidant combinations on exercise-induced oxidative stress have been shown to produce inconsistent results.[17]

Athletes often use vitamin E supplementation to prevent exercise-induced muscular damages and fatigue.[29] Damage to skeletal muscle cell membranes by exercise-induced oxidative stress can impair cell viability, resulting in necrosis and an acute-phase inflammatory response.[17] However, the evidence of antioxidant protection provided by vitamin E supplementation on membrane damage following exercise and recovery is limited; thus, further research is needed in this area.

Many studies have been conducted to investigate the effects of vitamin E supplementation as an ergogenic aid. Most studies have shown no improvement in exercise performance of humans with vitamin E supplementation.[17]

The current RDAs for vitamin E meet the needs of normal healthy people, but no specific recommendations have been set for athletes. Vitamin E may be of some benefit in endurance exercise to decrease exercise-induced oxidative stress, although vitamin E supplementation seems to have no effect on exercise performance, muscle damage, or recovery. Athletes who consume low intakes of antioxidants including vitamin E may be at risk for the harmful effects of oxygen radicals, and endurance athletes may need more than the recommendation of vitamin E.

D. Vitamin K

Vitamin K is a fat-soluble vitamin. There are three biologically active forms: vitamin K_1 (phylloquinone), vitamin K_2 (menaquinone), and vitamin K_3 (menadione). Vitamin K_1 is synthesized by plants and is the predominant form of vitamin K in U.S. diets.[30] Vitamin K_2 is produced by bacteria in the intestinal microflora and absorbed by the human body. Vitamin K_3 is a synthetic form of vitamin K, utilized clinically as a coagulant.

Vitamin K functions as a coenzyme in the synthesis of the active form of proteins involved in blood coagulation and bone metabolism.[30] It is required to catalyze the post-translational γ-carboxylation of glutamic acid residues for the normal coagulation of the blood. Carboxylated proteins include plasma prothrombin (coagulation factor II) and the plasma procoagulants, factors VII, IX, and X. Another vitamin K-dependent protein, osteocalcin, which is localized in the bone matrix, may have a role in the calcification of bone.[13]

A symptom of vitamin K deficiency is an increase in prothrombin time, which increases risk of spontaneous hemorrhage. Although vitamin K deficiencies are rare, individuals with fat malabsorption, liver diseases, or chronic antibiotic therapy are at risk of vitamin K deficiency. Newborn infants may be at risk of abnormal vitamin K status due to poor placental transfer of vitamin K and a lack of intestinal microflora to produce vitamin K_2.

Because of the lack of data to estimate an average requirement for vitamin K, AIs have been established based on dietary intake data from healthy individuals.[30] The AIs of vitamin K for adult men and women are 120 and 90 μg/d, respectively. Vitamin K_1 is the major dietary form of vitamin K. Green leafy vegetables and plant oils are major sources of dietary vitamin K. Also, vitamin K_1 is the form of the vitamin generally utilized in dietary supplements.

No evidence of toxicity has been associated with large intakes of either vitamin K_1 or vitamin K_2. However, high doses of the synthetic form, vitamin K_3, may cause liver damage.[30] No UL has been established for vitamin K.

There is no clear association between vitamin K and exercise; thus, research has not been conducted with regard to vitamin K and exercise performance. The vitamin K-dependent protein, osteocalcin, is involved in bone formation in the body. An improvement of bone metabolism was reported in female athletes after vitamin K supplementation.[31] Therefore, adequate dietary intakes of vitamin K may be of importance with regard to the skeletal growth for young athletes.

III. WATER-SOLUBLE VITAMINS

Water-soluble vitamins consist of the B-complex vitamins and vitamin C. These vitamins are generally excreted in urine with little storage, thus regular consumption is needed. Recommendations of water-soluble vitamins including RDAs/AIs, ULs, and DVs are provided in Table 4.3.

A. Thiamin

Thiamin, also known as vitamin B_1, is one of the B-complex vitamins. Thiamin exists in the human body as free thiamin and as interconvertible phosphorylated form: thiamin monophosphate, thiamin triphosphate, and thiamin pyrophosphate (TPP). The active form of thiamin as a coenzyme is TPP.

Thiamin, as TPP, is a coenzyme for two types of enzymes, α-keto acid dehydrogenases and transketolases. These TPP-dependent enzymes require a divalent cation, commonly Mg^{2+}. TPP is needed for the oxidative decarboxylation of pyruvate, α-ketoglutarate, and branched-chain amino acids in the citric acid cycle. TPP is involved as a coenzyme for transketolase reaction, which functions for the hexose monophosphate shunt (also called pentose phosphate shunt). The hexose monophosphate shunt is a pathway for the synthesis of pentoses and generating NADPH for the synthesis of fatty acids. Thus, thiamin is needed for the metabolism of carbohydrates, fats, and proteins. Thiamin also has a role in electrical generative cells such as nerves, brain, and muscles.[32]

Thiamin deficiency is known as beriberi. Its symptoms include anorexia, weight loss, muscle weakness, cardiovascular effects, and mental changes such as short-term memory loss, confusion, and irritability. Dry beriberi includes muscle wasting.

In wet beriberi, edema occurs.[33] Thiamin deficiency occurs from inadequate thiamin intake or consumption of excessive alcohol. Wernicke-Korsakoff Syndrome is a neurological condition associated with thiamin deficiency among alcoholics. Thiaminase, an enzyme found in raw fish, break down thiamin in food. Individuals who habitually consume raw fish may have a risk of thiamin deficiency. Thiamin deficiencies are rare in the United States except with severe alcoholism.

The RDA for adults ages 19 years and older is 1.2 mg/d for men and 1.1 mg/d for women. Dietary sources of thiamin include pork, beef, organ meats, yeast, whole grains, and legumes. Most thiamin is lost in the production of polished rice and white flour; therefore, thiamin-enriched grain products such as white rice, bread, and pasta are widely available in the United States.

The amounts of thiamin consumed in excess of needs are excreted in the urine. Because there are not sufficient data regarding adverse effects from the consumption of excess thiamin in food or through long-term oral supplementation, the IOM did not establish an UL for thiamin.[33]

Thiamin functions in the metabolism of both carbohydrate and branched-chain amino acids; thus, thiamin has an important role in producing energy during exercise. Consequently, it has been assumed that individuals with thiamin deficiency reduce their abilities to perform physical activity, because thiamin deficient status could result in impaired carbohydrate metabolism and accumulation of lactic acid.[34] However, the prevalence of deficiency appears to be low in active individuals.[35]

Several studies have been conducted to determine the effects of thiamin supplementations on exercise performance.[36–39] Suzuki and Itokawa reported that a high dose of thiamin (100 mg/d) significantly decreased the number of complaints shortly after exercise in a fatigue assessment.[36] The improvement of neurological and motor movement control was indicated in target shooting after thiamin supplementation.[37] However, supplementation with a thiamin derivative did not improve high-intensity exercise performance when thiamin status was adequate.[37] Supplementation with thiamin along with pantothenic acid did not enhance performance in knee extension and flexion exercises.[39] Thus, thiamin supplementation may not impact exercise performance or influence energy production when athletes have an adequate status of thiamin, while the supplementation may help to achieve optimal neurological activity.

Currently, there are no specific thiamin recommendations for athletes. Athletes who are engaged in physically demanding occupations or who spend much time training for active sports may have a higher requirement for thiamin.[33] Individuals consuming excessive amounts of dietary carbohydrates in a diet are recommended increased thiamin intakes.[40]

B. Riboflavin

Riboflavin is a water-soluble B vitamin that is also known as vitamin B_2. In the body, riboflavin acts as an integral component of two coenzymes: flavin adenine dinucleotide (FAD) and flavin mononucleotide (FMN); these coenzymes are called flavoproteins.

Riboflavin is essential for the metabolism of glucose, fatty acids, glycerol, and amino acids for energy formation.[41] Riboflavin, as FAD and FMN, functions as a catalyst for redox reactions in numerous metabolic pathways and in energy production.[42] The redox reactions include flavoprotein-catalyzed dehydrogenations that are both pyridine nucleotide dependent and independent, reactions with sulfur-containing compounds, hydroxylations, oxidative decarboxylations, dioxygenations, and reduction of oxygen to hydrogen peroxide. Riboflavin has a role in the formation of some vitamins and their coenzymes.[42]

Riboflavin deficiency (ariboflavinosis) can be associated with sore throat, redness, and swelling of the lining of the mouth and throat, cheilosis, angular stomatitis, tongue swelling (glossitis), seborrheic dermatitis, and normocytic anemia. Riboflavin deficiencies are rare in developed countries, except in chronic alcoholics. Riboflavin deficiency is rarely found in isolation; it occurs frequently in combination with deficiencies of other water-soluble vitamins.

The recommendations for riboflavin intake, as RDAs, for adults ages 19 years and older are 1.3 mg/d for men and 1.1 mg/d for women. Riboflavin is widely distributed in foods. Dietary sources include organ meats, dairy products, enriched cereals and breads, and green leafy vegetables.

The IOM did not establish an UL for riboflavin because no toxic or adverse effects of high riboflavin consumption from food or supplements have been reported. Although no adverse effects have been associated with excess riboflavin intake, this does not mean there is no potential for adverse effects from high intakes. Data on adverse effects are limited. Thus, caution may be warranted.[42]

Because riboflavin functions in the many metabolic reactions including energy production in the body, several studies[43–48] have been conducted to investigate the effects of riboflavin supplementation on physical performance. The results of these studies indicated that riboflavin supplementation did not improve exercise performance in children,[43,44] adolescents,[45] elderly,[46] and athletes,[47,48] which seems that there is no advantage to riboflavin supplementation on physical performance. However, it is possible that the requirement of the vitamin is increased for individuals who are ordinarily very active physically, but data are not available to adjust their riboflavin requirements.[42]

The current RDAs for riboflavin meet the needs of normal healthy people. There are no specific riboflavin recommendations for athletes. However, physical activity would be expected to increase riboflavin requirements due to increased energy expenditure or increased incorporation of riboflavin into new muscle tissue.[49] According to the research regarding riboflavin requirements as influenced by physical activity,[46,49,50] some of the indices of riboflavin status seem to be altered by exercise in sedentary or non-athletic women. In these studies, it was indicated that exercise, dieting, and dieting along with exercise may increase the requirements of riboflavin above previous RDA for riboflavin published in 1989.[51] Therefore, riboflavin requirements may be increased for those who are ordinarily very active physically.[42] However, athletes can maintain adequate riboflavin status when adequate energy is consumed.[52]

C. Niacin

Niacin is one of the water-soluble B-vitamins and is also known as vitamin B_3. The term niacin is the generic descriptor for nicotinic acid and nicotinamide, which are essential for formation of the coenzymes nicotinamide adenine dinucleotide (NAD) and nicotinamide adenine dinucleotide phosphate (NADP).

Approximately 200 enzymes, primarily dehydrogenases, are dependent on the coenzymes NAD and NADP, which both serve as a hydrogen donor or electron acceptor.[53] NAD functions as a coenzyme with enzymes involved in the oxidation of fuel molecules such as glyceraldehyde 3-phosphate, lactate, alcohol, 3-hydroxybutyrate, and α-ketoglutarate. NADP functions as a hydrogen donor in reductive biosynthesis such as in fatty acid and steroid syntheses, and is involved in the pentose phosphate pathways.[54] In addition, NAD acts as donor of adenosine diphosphate ribose (ADP-ribose) for the post-translational modification of proteins and for the formation of cyclic ADP-ribose. Two enzymes, mono ADP-ribosyl transferase and poly ADP-ribose polymerase, function to transfer ADP-ribose from NAD to an acceptor proteins including histone and histone proteins. These proteins seem to function in DNA replication and repair and in cell differentiation.[54]

The niacin deficiency disease is known as pellagra, whose symptons include pigmented rash developed by sunlight exposure, changes in the digestive tract causing vomiting, constipation or diarrhea, a bright red tongue, and neurological symptoms including apathy, depression, fatigue, headache, and loss of memory.[54] The symptoms of pellagra are often referred to as the four D's: dermatitis, dementia, diarrhea, and death. Niacin deficiency is rare in industrialized countires except in malnourished alcoholics and in individuals having disorders of tryptophan pathways.

In that trypophan can be converted to niacin, niacin contents in foods and dietary recommendations are commonly expressed as mg of niacin equivalents (NE). Sixty milligrams of dietary tryptophan is considered equivalent to 1 mg of niacin. Thus, 1 mg NE is equal to 1 mg of niacin or 60 mg of dietary tryptophan. The recommendations for niacin intake as RDAs for adults are 16 mg NE/d for men and 14 mg NE/d for women. Niacin is widely distributed in both animal foods and plant-derived foods. The dietary sources of niacin are yeasts, meats, poultry, fish, nuts, and enriched products such as cereals and grains. The dietary sources of the amino acid tryptophan include lean meats, fish, poultry, and nuts. In supplements and in food fortification, niacin is generally found as nicotinamide, while nicotinic acid is often used as a cholesterol-lowering agent.[53]

Large doses of nicotinic acid are used in the treatment of hypercholesterolemia. The pharmacological doses have been shown to significantly lower total serum cholesterol and low-density lipoproteins and increase high-density lipoproteins.[55] Despite the therapeutic effect of nicotinic acid, side effects are associated with these large doses. The side effects are flushing of the skin with a concomitant itching and feeling of heat, liver cell damage (hepatotoxicity) including elevated liver enzymes and jaundice, and gastrointestinal problems such as heartburn, nausea, and vomiting. Because flushing is the first observed adverse effects after large doses of nicotinic acid, as this symptom is observed at lower doses than other adverse effects, the IOM selected flushing as the most appropriate endpoint on which to base a UL. Nicotinamide is generally better tolerated than nicotinic acid, and does not generally cause flushing. However, a UL for niacin is considered protective against potential adverse effects of nicotinamide.[54] The UL for niacin is 35 mg NE/d for adults, and is limited to niacin that is obtained from supplements or fortified foods. There is no evidence of adverse effects from naturally occurring niacin from foods.

Niacin functions in energy metabolism like other B vitamins; therefore, exercise performance could be affected by niacin status. However, there is no evidence of inadequate niacin status in athletes or physically active individuals. Large doses of nicotinic acid have been reported to decrease mobilization of free fatty acids (FFAs) during exercise,[56–59] which could affect exercise performance because circulating FFAs provide energy in the muscle during exercise.[55] A decrease in FFA availability with large doses of niacin as nicotinic acid does not impact physical performance unless carbohydrate sources are limited.[55] Although experimental data are lacking, the IOM has recommended at least 10% increase in the niacin requirement to allow for increased energy utilization and the physical size of individuals who exercise vigorously.[54]

D. Vitamin B_6

Vitamin B_6 is a water-soluble vitamin that consists of derivatives of 3-hydroxy-2-methylpyridine, i.e., pyridoxal (PL), pyridoxine (PN), pyridoxamine (PM), and their respective 5′-phosphates, (PLP, PNP, and PMP). PLP is a metabolically active B_6 vitamer.

The active form of vitamin B_6, PLP, plays an important role in its function as a coenzyme for enzymes involved in amino acid metabolism. Vitamin B_6 is required for transamination, racemization, deamination, or desulfhydration of amino acids. The vitamin has a role in the conversion of glycogen to glucose (gluconeogenesis). PLP functions in the synthesis of heme from porphyrin precursors as a cofactor for δ-aminolevulinic acid synthase.[60] In the brain, the vitamin functions in the synthesis of serotonin from the amino acid tryptophan. Other neurotransmitters, such as γ-aminobutyric acid, dopamine, epinephrine, and norepinephrine, are also synthesized using PLP-dependent enzymes.[61] Vitamin B_6 is also involved in the synthesis of the sphingolipids for the myelin sheath, the synthesis of nucleic acids, and the synthesis of niacin from tryptophan.

The signs of vitamin B_6 deficiency include weakness, sleeplessness, cheilosis, glossitis, stomatitis, and impaired cell-mediated immunity.[60] Other symptoms noted in vitamin B_6 deficiency are microcytic anemia, epileptiform convulsions, depression, and confusion.[62] Vitamin B_6 deficiency is rare in the United States, but it is found in alcoholics and those taking certain drugs including isoniazid, penicillamine, corticosteroid, and anticonvulsants.

The RDA for vitamin B_6 is 1.3 mg/d for 19–50 years old adults. The RDAs for adults ages 51 years and older are 1.7 mg/d for men and 1.5 mg/d for women. Dietary sources of vitamin B_6 in commonly consumed foods include meats, whole-grain products, vegetables, some fruits (e.g., banana), nuts, and fortified cereals. Vitamin B_6 in supplements is generally found as pyridoxine hydrochloride. PLP is also available as a dietary supplement.

No adverse effects have been reported for high vitamin B_6 intakes from food sources. However, when taken in high levels of supplemental vitamin B_6 intakes (200 mg or more per day) as pyridoxine hydrochloride, vitamin B_6 can cause neurological disorders such as loss of sensation in legs and imbalance. To prevent sensory neuropathy, the IOM set a UL for vitamin B_6 of 100 mg/d for adults 19 years or older.

Vitamin B_6 is involved in the metabolic pathways required for exercise, principally amino acid metabolism and glycogen breakdown. Therefore, adequate vitamin B_6 status is important for athletes because they typically have higher protein consumption and vitamin B_6, as PLP, is required to break down muscle glycogen for energy during exercise. Adequate vitamin B_6 intakes have been reported for most male athletes,[63–65] while several studies indicated vitamin B_6 intake of female athletes are lower than recommended.[66–68] Inadequate intakes of vitamin B_6 in athletes are often related to low energy intake for maintaining bodyweight or to poor food choices.[69] Inadequate biochemical status of vitamin B_6 in male and female athletes was indicated in some studies.[41,70,71] Telford et al.[70] found that 60% of male and female athletes ($n = 86$) had poor baseline vitamin B_6 status while consuming their typical diets.

Researchers have reported that exercise may increase the turnover and loss of vitamin B_6 in the body.[13] Increasing plasma concentrations of PLP was indicated during exercise, which in turn increases the probability that PLP will be metabolized to 4-pyridoxic acid (4-PA) and lost in the urine during exercise.[69] Active individuals had higher 4-PA losses compared to sedentary controls or periods of inactivity.[72,73] Higher 4-PA acid losses were reported after strenuous physical activity.[74] However, no study has reported decreased plasma PLP concentrations by exercise-induced 4-PA losses. And, the amount of vitamin B_6 loss is small and could be easily met through appropriate food choices.[69]

Because vitamin B_6 has a role in energy production during exercise, inadequate status of vitamin B_6 may compromise exercise performance. The effect of vitamin B_6 deficiency on exercise performance has been determined in several studies[45,75,76] that indicated that inadequate status of vitamin B_6 due to poor dietary intakes may decrease the ability to do work, especially maximal work and exercise.[69] However, it was reported that, during exercise, supplemental vitamin B_6 has not enough beneficial effect to alter performance.[77,78] Although vitamin B_6 supplementation did not result in the improvements of exercise performance, athletes may increase their vitamin B_6 intakes as they consume higher protein diets because vitamin B_6 is required for enzymes in protein metabolism.[79] However, there are currently no specific vitamin B_6 recommendations for athletes.

E. Folate

Folate, a generic term for one of the water-soluble vitamins, includes naturally occurring food folates and folic acid found in dietary supplements and used in food fortification. Folate can vary in structure by reduction of the pteridine moiety to dihydrofolic acid and tetrahydrofolic acid (THF). Folate exists predominately as polyglutamyl forms of THF, which are biologically active folate coenzymes in the body.

Folate functions in the body as a coenzyme to accept one-carbon units typically generated from amino acid metabolism. Folate is involved in DNA synthesis, purine synthesis, generation of formate into the formate pool, and amino acid metabolism.[80] Folate is needed for synthesis of methionine from homocysteine, which helps maintain normal levels of homocysteine in the body. Folate is also required for the synthesis of normal red blood cells and prevention of macrocytic anemia.

Folate deficiency can cause megaloblastic anemia characterized by enlarged immature red blood cells and neutrophil hypersegmentation. Megaloblastic anemia also occurs in vitamin B_{12} deficiency. Weakness, fatigue, difficulty concentrating, irritability, headache, palpitations, and shortness of breath can occur at an advanced stage of anemia.[80] Pregnant women with folate deficiency are at greater risk of having infants with low birth weight, premature birth, or neural tube defects. Atrophic glossitis may occur in folate-deficient people. Folate deficiency is commonly caused by insufficient dietary intake. Also, it has been observed in people with excessive alcohol ingestion, those with malabsorption disorders such as inflammatory bowel disease, and in individuals taking anticonvulsants, oral contraceptives, methotrexate (used for rheumatoid arthritis), sulfasalazine (used to treat inflammatory bowel disease), and cholestyramine (used to treat high cholesterol concentrations).[81]

The DRIs for folate are expressed in a term called the Dietary Folate Equivalents (DFEs), which reflects the higher bioavailablity of synthetic folic acid used in supplements than that of naturally occurring food folates. Folic acid taken with food is 85% bioavailable, but folate *in* food is about 50% bioavailable; thus, folic acid taken with food is 1.7 times more available. Only half as much folic acid taken on an empty stomach is comparable to food folate. Table 4.6 shows this explanation as presented by the IOM.[80]

The recommendations for folate intakes for the United States and Canada are given in μg DFEs. The RDA for adults is 400 μg DFEs/d. All women capable of becoming pregnant should consume 400 μg from supplements or fortified foods in addition to intake from a varied diet. Green leafy vegetables, orange juice, and dried beans and peas are all natural rich sources of folate. In 1996, the Food and Drug Administration published regulations requiring fortification with folic acid to enriched breads, cereals, flours, pastas, rice, and other grain products.[82] Thus, cereals, breads, and other grain products have become the primary sources of folate in the United States.

No adverse effects have been associated with the consumption of the amounts of folate in foods, and the risk of toxicity from folic acid is low. Megaloblastic anemia with vitamin B_{12} deficiency is indistinguishable from that associated with folate deficiency. Large doses of folic acid may relieve this, but the irreversible neurological

TABLE 4.6
Dietary Folate Equivalents (DFEs)

1 μg of DFEs
= 1 μg of food folate
= 0.5 μg of folic acid taken on an empty stomach
= 0.6 μg of folic acid with meals

Adapted from: Institute of Medicine, *Dietary Reference Intakes for Thiamin, Riboflavin, Niacin, Vitamin B_6, Folate, Vitamin B_{12}, Pantothenic Acid, Biotin, and Choline,* National Academy Press, Washington, DC, 1998, chap. 8.[80]

damage in vitamin B_{12}-deficient individuals continues. Hence, the UL for adults is set at 1000 μg/d of folate from fortified food or supplements, exclusive of naturally occurring food folate.[80]

Folate is required for synthesis of new cells and for the repair of damaged cells and tissues. Thus, folate status might be of importance to athletes. Generally, active men have adequate folate intakes due to high energy intakes.[83] However, low folate intakes have been observed in athletic women in several studies[84–86] that were conducted prior to the FDA mandatory fortification of folic acid in 1996. Beshgetoor and Nichols in 2003[87] reported that female cyclists and runners had mean folate intakes greater than the RDA, whereas a study reported in 2002[88] found that more than 80% of elite female adolescent volleyball players had folate intakes less than the RDA. In Brazil, 89% of adolescent athletes consumed folate less than the EAR.[89] Research examining the biochemical status of folate in athletes is limited, although several studies have been conducted.[90,91] Matter et al.[90] reported that 33% of non-supplemented female marathon runners (n = 85) had less than normal serum folate concentrations. Ziegler et al.[91] found that 20% of female figure skaters (n = 18) had lower serum folate concentrations than normal.

Supplementation with folate has been shown to have no effects on exercise performance. Exercise performance on a treadmill of female marathon runners having folate deficiency were not changed by folate supplementation (5 mg/d folic acid) although hematological parameters for folate status improved.[90] In a study of multivitamin and mineral supplementation including folate, there was no measurable difference in exercise performance as a result of vitamin and mineral supplementation in male runners.[47] There are no specific folate recommendations for athletes. Although folate supplementation did not result in the improvement of exercise performance, athletes, especially females, may need to increase their folate intakes to prevent megaloblastic anemia caused by folate deficiency. Any type of anemia could have an effect on the exercise performance of athletes.

F. Vitamin B_{12}

Vitamin B_{12} is a group of compounds called cobalamins which contain cyanocobalamin, hydroxocobalamin, and the two coenzymes forms 5′-deoxyadenosylcobalamin (adenosylcobalamin) and methylcobalamin. Cyanocobalamin and hydroxocobalamin are the forms of vitamin B_{12} used in most dietary supplements, and are converted to adenosylcobalamin and methylcobalamin in the body.

Methylcobalamin and adenosylcobalamin are required for the functioning of the enzymes methionine synthase and L-methylmalonyl-CoA mutase, respectively. Methionine synthase requires methylcobalamin as a cofactor for methyl group transfer from methyltetrahydrofolate to homocysteine to form methionine and tetrahydrofolate. Adenosylcobalamin is needed for methylmalonyl-CoA mutase, which converts L-methylmalonyl-CoA to succinyl-CoA. This reaction plays an important role in energy production from fats and proteins.

Deficiency of vitamin B_{12}, like that of folate, can lead to megaloblastic anemia, which is characterized by large red blood cells. Symptoms of this vitamin deficiency include skin pallor, fatigue, shortness of breath, palpitations, tingling and numbness (paresthesia) in extremities, abnormal gait, disorientation, swelling of myelinated fibers, memory loss, and possible dementia. Neurological complications are observed in 75–90% of deficient individuals.[92] Megaloblastic anemia of vitamin B_{12} deficiency is indistinguishable from that of folate deficiency. If vitamin B_{12} deficiency is not corrected, it can cause demyelination of nerves so that nerve damage may occur.[93] Therefore, folate supplementation can resolve the anemia, but not correct the demyelination of vitamin B_{12} deficiency, if vitamin B_{12} deficiency is the cause. Most vitamin B_{12} deficiencies result from inadequate absorption, rather than poor intakes. However, strict vegetarians can have deficiencies of the vitamin. Malabsorption of the vitamin is due to a lack or insufficiency of intrinsic factor or hydrochloric acid. An autoimmune condition (pernicious anemia), atrophic gastritis, or gastrectomy are the causes of decreasing intrinsic factor production, thereby impairing absorption of the vitamin. Hydrochloric acid is required to release the vitamin from dietary proteins. Thus, reduced hydrochloric acid production decreases the release of the vitamin bound to food, causing malabsorption of the vitamin.

The RDA for vitamin B_{12} is 2.4 μg/d for adults ages 19 years and older. For those older than 50 years, it is advisable for most of this amount to be consumed in foods fortified with vitamin B_{12} or a vitamin B_{12}-containing supplement because 10 to 30% of older people may not be able to absorb naturally occurring vitamin B_{12}.[92] Dietary sources of vitamin B_{12} include meats, poultry, fish, shellfish, eggs, fermented foods, milk, and milk products. Because vitamin B_{12} is present in animal products, athletes who eat no animal products (strict vegetarians or vegans) need to include food sources fortified with vitamin B_{12} such as breakfast cereals and may take supplements containing vitamin B_{12} to meet their requirements.

No adverse effects have been associated with large doses of vitamin B_{12} from food or supplements in healthy individuals.[92] No UL for vitamin B_{12} has been set by IOM because there is not sufficient scientific evidence to set the UL.

Those athletes who are on energy-restricted diets or who are on strict vegetarian diets without vitamin B_{12} supplementation or fortification may have inadequate intakes of vitamin B_{12}. Steen et al.[67] indicated that 80% of female collegiate heavyweight rowers consumed over the RDA for vitamin B_{12}. However, in the study of male and female participants in a triathlon, 45% of females and 30% of the males had vitamin B_{12} intakes lower than the RDA although 40% of the participants supplemented.[84] Keith et al.[86] reported that over 33% of trained female cyclists (n = 23) consumed less than the recommended intake of vitamin B_{12}; however, only one subject had a lower serum vitamin B_{12} concentrations than the normal range. Generally, highly trained endurance athletes do not show vitamin B_{12}-deficient status according to their blood vitamin B_{12} levels, and short-term rigorous exercise has no effect on the plasma vitamin B_{12} concentrations in trained athletes.[93]

Most of studies examining the effects of vitamin B_{12} on exercise performance have been conducted in conjunction with the intake of the B vitamins. Existing evidence shows that vitamin B_{12} supplementation has no effect on performance.[94–96] There are no specific vitamin B_{12} recommendations for athletes, and there appears to be no need to recommend an increased requirement of vitamin B_{12} for athletes as compared with the general population.[93] Vitamin B_{12} supplementation may be needed for elderly athletes and athletes who are strict vegetarians to prevent hematopoietic defects caused by vitamin B_{12} inadequacy.

G. Pantothenic Acid

Pantothenic acid, also known as vitamin B_5, consists of β-alanine and pantoic acid. Pantothenic acid is a component of coenzyme A (CoA) and acyl-carrier protein. CoA is required for chemical reactions that generate energy from carbohydrate, fat, and protein. CoA also functions in the synthesis of sterols, membrane phospholipids, choline, acetylcholine, and porphyrin rings found in hemoglobin and myoglobin. Acyl-carrier protein is a component of the fatty acid synthase complex. The acyl-carrier protein requires pantothenic acid in the form of 4′-phosphopanthetheine for its activity in the synthesis of fatty acids.[97]

Pantothenic acid deficiency is very rare and has been observed in individuals having severe malnutrition or who have taken the pantothenic acid antagonist ω-methyl pantothenic acid. Pantothenic acid deficiency was reported to cause the "burning foot syndrome," characterized by abnormal skin sensations of the feet and lower legs. Other symptoms of the deficiency include vomiting, fatigue, weakness, irritability, numbness, and tingling.

Because of the lack of data to estimate an average requirement for pantothenic acid, AIs have been established based on dietary intake data from healthy individuals.[97] The AI for pantothenic acid is 5 mg/d for adult men and women. Pantothenic acid is widely distributed in all plant and animal foods. Dietary sources include meats, egg yolks, whole grains, potatoes, broccoli, mushrooms, and avocadoes. About a third of the vitamin present in foods is lost during ordinary cooking.[98]

The adverse effects of oral pantothenic acid have not been reported in humans or animals. Intakes of up to 20 g/d may be associated with mild intestinal distress and diarrhea.[99] Due to the lack of the evidence of adverse effects, the IOM did not establish a UL for pantothenic acid in 1998.

There is no conclusive evidence for beneficial effects of pharmacological doses of pantothenic acid on exercise, and there are no specific recommendations for athletes. Pantothenic acid plays a key role in energy metabolism, thus several researchers have indicated that it may affect exercise performance.[100,101] However, Webster[39] found that supplementation with pantothenic acid derivatives had no effect on exercise metabolism or exercise performance in highly trained cyclists. Rokitzki et al.[102] indicated that more than 30% of high-performance athletes ($n = 96$) had blood values of pantothenic acid lower than a normal range. And, pantothenic acid might have some effects on glycogen homeostasis and physical performance.[98] Therefore, more research is needed to understand pantothenic acid status and metabolism in athletes.

H. Biotin

Biotin is a water-soluble B-vitamin that contains sulfur. The biotin molecule contains three asymmetric carbon atoms, and therefore eight different isomers are possible. Of these isomers, only the dextrorotatory (+) *d*-biotin possesses biotin activity as a coenzyme.

Biotin functions as a coenzyme for four carboxylases acetyl-CoA carboxylase, pyruvate carboxylase, propionyl-CoA carboxylase, and β-methylcrotonyl-CoA carboxylase.[103] Acetyl-CoA carboxylase forms malonyl-CoA from acetyl-CoA in the initiation of fatty acid synthesis. Pyruvate carboxylase is an essential enzyme in gluconeogenesis, the formation of glucose from amino acids and fats. Propionyl-CoA carboxylase is involved in the metabolism of the amino acids isoleucine, threonine, methionine, valine, and odd-chain fatty acids. β-Methylcrotonyl-CoA carboxylase functions in the catabolism of the amino acid leucine. Thus, biotin is required for the synthesis and degradation of fatty acids and gluconeogenesis as well as protein degradation.

Biotin deficiency is rare in humans, but the deficiency occurs in two different situations: the consumption of large amounts of raw egg whites over long periods and total parenteral nutrition without biotin supplementation. Egg whites contain the protein avidin, which binds biotin and prevents its absorption. Avidin is denatured by cooking. Gastrointestinal disorders such as inflammatory bowel disease and achlorhydria may result in impaired biotin absorption.[104] The symptoms of biotin deficiency include lethargy, depression, hallucinations, muscle pain, paresthesia in extremities, anorexia, nausea, hair loss, and scaly red dermatitis.

The IOM has established recommendations for biotin as AIs because sufficient scientific evidence is not available for estimating an average requirement for biotin.[103] The AI for biotin is 30 μg/d for men and women aged 19 years and older. Biotin is widely distributed in foods. Liver, egg yolks, soybeans, and bakers and brewer's yeasts are relatively rich sources.

Toxicity of biotin has not been reported. Large doses of biotin (up to 200 mg/d) have been given daily to individuals with inherited disorders of biotin metabolism without side effects.[103] Due to the lack of the evidence of adverse effects, ULs for intake of biotin have not been set by the IOM.

Biotin is involved in energy metabolism; thus, biotin might have some effects on physical activity. Research has not been conducted regarding biotin status in athletes and effects of biotin supplementation on exercise performance. There are no specific biotin recommendations for athletes.

I. Choline

Choline is an essential nutrient for humans, providing the structural integrity of cell membranes, methyl metabolism, cholinergic neurotransmission, transmembrane signaling, and lipid and cholesterol transport and metabolism.[105] Humans can synthesize choline in small amounts from ethanolamine and a methyl group donor such as methionine, folate, or vitamin B_{12}, but synthesis rates are not adequate to meet the demand for choline in the body. Thus, choline was classified as an essential nutrient by IOM in 1998.

Choline provides structure to cell membranes and facilitating transmembrane signaling as well as synthesis and release of acetylcholine. Choline functions as a component of phosphatidylcholine for intracellular signaling and hepatic export of very low-density lipoproteins and sphingomyelin for structural and signaling functions.[105] It is a precursor for the synthesis of acetylcholine, which is an important neurotransmitter involved in memory, muscle control, and many other functions.

Choline functions as a precursor for the methyl group donor betaine, used as an organic osmolyte to adapt to osmotic stress by renal glomerular cells.[105]

Choline is required for the transport of fat from the liver; thus, symptoms of choline deficiency may include fat accumulation in the liver, "fatty liver", and liver damage. Decreased choline stores and liver damage were indicated in healthy men fed choline-deficient diets containing adequate amounts of methionine, folate, and vitamin B_{12}.[106] In adults, choline-deficient diets for 42 days induced DNA damage and apoptosis in peripheral lymphocytes.[107]

For a recommendation of choline intake, AIs have been established based on dietary intake data from healthy individuals.[105] The AIs for adult men and women are 550 and 425 mg/d, respectively. All natural fats contain some choline; thus, choline is found in a wide variety of foods. Dietary sources of choline include meats, whole grains, egg yolks, peanuts, and legumes. The vitamin occurs mostly in the form of phosphatidylcholine, also known as lecithin. Phosphatidylcholine is frequently added to foods as an emulsifier during processing by the food industry.

Large quantities of choline have been associated with several adverse effects including a fishy body odor, nausea, vomiting, diarrhea, salivation, and increased sweating. The fish body odor results from the increased presence of a breakdown product of choline called trimethylamine. Doses of choline in the 5–10 g/d range[105] have been reported to reduce blood pressure (hypotension), which could result in faintness or dizziness. In 1998, the IOM established the UL for choline at 3.5 g/d for generally healthy adults, based on primarily preventing decreased blood pressure and secondarily preventing the fishy body odor.

Decreased plasma choline concentrations have been reported after prolonged exercise[108–110]; however, the mechanism that might account for a decrease in plasma choline is unknown.[111] There are no conclusive results for beneficial effects of choline supplementation on exercise performance.[111] Because choline is required for the synthesis of acetylcholine involved in muscle control during physical activity, choline deficiency or supplementation might have some effects on exercise performance. Therefore, more research is needed to investigate choline status of athletes and roles in physical activity.

J. Vitamin C

Vitamin C, also known as ascorbic acid, is a water-soluble vitamin. It is essential, as humans do not have the ability to biosynthesize vitamin C in the body or only in very low, inadequate amounts. Ascorbic acid is reversibly oxidized to dehydroascorbic acid (DHA). Because both forms exhibit anti-scorbutic activity, the term vitamin C refers to ascorbic acid and DHA.[112]

Vitamin C is a strong water-soluble antioxidant protecting cells and cellular components from free radicals by donating electrons. Vitamin C seems to regenerate other antioxidants such as vitamin E.[113] Because of its reducing power, the vitamin functions primarily as a cofactor for reactions requiring a reduced iron or copper metalloenzyme.[112] Vitamin C also has a role in the transport of non-heme iron. Vitamin C is necessary for the synthesis of collagen, which is a structural component of cartilage, ligaments, tendons, and other connective tissue. The vitamin is required for the synthesis of neurotransmitters, norepinephrine, and epinephrine and for the synthesis of carnitine, which is essential for the transport of fatty acids into the mitochondria for conversion to energy. Vitamin C functions in the conversion of cholesterol to bile acids and probably in the reduction of folic acid intermediates and the proper metabolism of the stress hormone cortisol.[113]

The vitamin C deficiency disease is scurvy, characterized by symptoms related to connective tissue defects.[112] Symptoms of scurvy include follicular hyperkeratosis, swollen or bleeding gums, perifollicular hemorrhages, joint effusions, arthralgia, fatigue, depression, and impaired wound healing. Scurvy is rare in developed countries, but does appear in children and the elderly on restricted diets and in alcoholics.

The RDA for adults is 90 mg/d for men and 75 mg/d for women. For smokers, intakes of 35 mg vitamin C higher than for nonsmokers are recommended daily as smokers generally have lower blood vitamin C concentrations and are under increased oxidative stress from the toxins in cigarette smoke.[112] The vitamin C content of selected fruits and vegetables is found in Table 4.7. Dietary sources of vitamin C include fruits and vegetables. Some foods such as breakfast cereals, sports drinks, and various nutrition bars, are fortified with vitamin C. Vitamin C in supplements is typically free ascorbic acid, calcium ascorbate, sodium ascorbate, and ascorbyl palmitate.[114]

TABLE 4.7
Vitamin C Content of Selected Foods

Food	Vitamin C mg/100g	Vitamin C mg/Serving
Asparagus, raw	5.6	7.5 (1 cup)[a]
Banana, raw	8.7	10.3 (1 medium)
Broccoli, raw	89.2	81.2 (1 cup)
Brussels sprouts, raw	85.0	74.8 (1 cup)
Cantaloupe, raw	36.7	58.7 (1cup)
Cauliflower, raw	46.4	46.4 (1 cup)
Grapefruit, raw	34.4	44.0 (1 fruit)
Kale, raw	120.0	80.4 (1 cup)
Kiwi fruits, raw	92.7	70.5 (1 medium)
Lemons, raw	53.0	30.7 (1 medium)
Lettuce, green leaf, raw	18.0	6.5 (1 cup)
Oranges, raw	53.2	69.7 (1 medium)
Orange juice	50.0	124.0 (1 cup)
Papayas, raw	61.8	86.5 (1 cup)
Peaches, raw	6.6	9.9 (1 medium)
Peppers, sweet, green, raw	80.4	74.0 (1 cup)
Strawberries, raw	58.8	84.7 (1 cup)
Tomatoes, red, raw	12.7	22.9 (1 cup)

[a] Serving size.

Adapted from: U.S. Department of Agriculture, Agricultural Research Service, USDA National Nutrient Database for Standard Reference, Release 20.[20]

Adverse effects from vitamin C intakes have been reported primarily with large doses (> 3000 mg/d), which may include diarrhea and other gastrointestinal disturbances.[112] Possible adverse effects include increased oxalate excretion and kidney stone formation, increased uric acid excretion, pro-oxidant effects, systemic conditioning, increased iron absorption leading to iron overload, reduced vitamin B_{12} and copper status, increase oxygen demand, and erosion of dental enamel; however, the relationship between these effects and excess vitamin C intakes have not been clearly confirmed.[112] Therefore, the UL for vitamin C established by IOM is 2000 mg/d for adults to prevent diarrhea and gastrointestinal disturbances.

Vitamin C has certain biological functions that can influence physical performance. It is needed for synthesis of collagen for ligament and tendon formation, synthesis of carnitine to use fatty acids as an energy source during exercise, synthesis of neurotransmitters for metabolic responses to exercise, and iron metabolism related to anemia and fatigue with consequential decreases in aerobic performance.[113] Thus, adequate status of vitamin C is of importance for athletes. Physically active adults generally have been reported to have adequate amounts of vitamin C intakes and plasma vitamin C concentrations in the range of normal values.[113] However, suboptimal intakes of vitamin C were determined in some athletic groups, such as male wrestlers[115] and female basketball player and gymnasts.[116] Approximately 12% of a group of athletes had lower levels of plasma vitamin C concentrations than the normal range.[70] Because physical activity can increase plasma vitamin C concentrations for up to 24 hours,[117,118] caution should be taken when interpreting plasma ascorbic acid values of athletes.

Improved performance is to be expected in vitamin C-deficient individuals administered the vitamin. After administrations of 100 mg to 500 mg vitamin C daily, individuals initially having low blood concentrations of vitamin C were reported to improve VO_{2max} with normalized plasma vitamin C concentrations,[119] work efficiency[120] and to decrease fatigue and normalize plasma vitamin C concentrations.[121]

Vitamin C may indirectly have a benefit on physical performance by enhancing physiologic functions. Supplemental vitamin C of 100 mg to 1500 mg daily has shown increased adaptation in the heat,[122] reduction of upper respiratory tract infections in marathon runners,[123] reduction of plasma cortisol concentrations responding to physiological and psychological stress,[13] and muscle soreness markers following exercises.[124,125] However, additional studies are needed to define the mechanisms of these effects by vitamin C supplementation.

Several studies indicate that vitamin C has an ergogenic effect, while an equal number of studies report no effect on physical performance. In other studies, supplemental vitamin C at 200–1000 mg seemed to show no ergogenic effects regarding a variety performance measures in individuals having initially adequate vitamin C status.[113] Currently, no specific recommendations for vitamin C have been set for athletes. Inadequate status of vitamin C can cause decreased physical performance, and exercise is another physiologic stressor that may increase vitamin C needs. The recommendations for adults may not be sufficient for individuals engaged in strenuous prolonged exercise. Appropriate vitamin C intakes for these individuals may range from 100 mg to 1000 mg daily.[113] This level can easily be obtained by a consumption of diets that include fruits and vegetables. Vitamin C was indicated to be the most ingested supplement by athletes.[126] Because the intakes of large doses may results in vitamin C toxicity, vitamin C intakes including supplements should not exceed the UL for this vitamin. Some athletes may not have adequate intakes, so their health would be improved by dietary changes or modest supplementation.

IV. CONCLUSIONS AND FUTURE RESEARCH NEEDS

Vitamins play many roles in maintaining the health of active individuals and assuring that energy can be produced for physical activity. Inadequate or marginal nutritional status may result in adverse effects on physical performance. The effects of vitamin supplementation are different in individuals deficient in the nutrient from those with adequate status. Individuals with vitamin deficiency or deficiencies may benefit from supplementation of the limiting vitamins. In general, most studies do not suggest an effect of vitamins on physical activity, exercise, and sport if individuals consume adequate amounts of these nutrients; however, additional well designed studies are needed on vitamins, including supplementation, related to physical performance. The efficacy of certain vitamin supplementation might vary by different forms of physical activity and measurements. Some age and gender differences might exist.

Generally, adequate vitamin intakes have been observed in athletes. However, some groups of athletes, such as gymnasts, long-distance runners, and wrestlers, may not consume adequate amounts of vitamins by restricting energy intakes or eliminating food groups from a diet for esthetic requirement or competition. Long periods of deficient status can cause serious consequences for athletes and active individuals. Hence, physically active individuals should consume a diet containing a variety of foods rich in vitamins, such as whole grains, fruits, vegetables, and lean meats. Currently, there are no specific recommendations of each vitamin for physically active individuals. Intakes of some vitamins may be increased as requirements for energy production and prevention from oxidative stress or exercised-induced problems are increased. However, vitamin intakes including supplements should not exceed ULs for the vitamins. Further research, particularly long-term studies in humans, is needed to estimate vitamin recommendations for physically active individuals and athletes.

REFERENCES

1. Otten, J.J., Hellwig, J.P., and Meyers, L.D., Eds., *Dietary Reference Intakes: The Essential Guide to Nutrient Requirements*, National Academy Press, Washington, DC, 2006, pp. 8.
2. A Food Labeling Guide: Reference Values for Nutrition Labeling. The U.S. Food and Drug Administration Website, http://www.cfsan.fda.gov/~dms/flg–7a.html. Accessed 09/28/2007. Accessed 11/10/2007.
3. Sauberlich, H.E., *Laboratory Tests for the Assessment of Nutritional Status*, 2nd ed., CRC Press, Boca Raton, FL, 1998.
4. Institute of Medicine, *Dietary Reference Intakes for Vitamin C, Vitamin E, Selenium, and Carotenoids*, National Academy Press, Washington, DC, 2000, chap. 8.

5. Institute of Medicine, *Dietary Reference Intakes for Vitamin A, Vitamin K, Arsenic, Boron, Chromium, Copper, Iodine, Iron, Manganese, Molybdenum, Nickel, Silicon, Vanadium and Zinc*, National Academy Press, Washington, DC, 2001, chap. 4.
6. DeMaever, E.M., The WHO programme of prevention and control of vitamin A deficiency, xerophthalmia and nutritional blindness, *Nutr. Health* 4, 105–12, 1986.
7. Cropper, S.S., Smith, J.L., and Groff, J.L., *Advanced Nutrition and Human Metabolism*, 4th ed., Thomson Wadsworth, Belmont, CA, 2005, pp. 326–43.
8. Underwood, B.A., Vitamin A deficiency disorders: International efforts to control a preventable "pox," *J. Nutr.* 134, 231S–6S, 2004.
9. Rodrigues, M.I., and Dohlman, C.H., Blindness in an American boy caused by unrecognized vitamin A deficiency, *Arch. Ophthalmol.* 122, 1228–9, 2004.
10. West, C.E., Eilander, A., and van Lieshout, M., Consequences of revised estimates of carotenoid bioefficacy for the dietary control of vitamin A deficiency in developing countries, *J. Nutr.* 132, 2920S–6S, 2002.
11. Stacewicz-Sapuntzakis, M., and Diwadkar-Navsariwala, V., Carotenoids, in *Nutritional Ergogenic Aids*, Wolinsky, I., and Driskell, J.A., Eds. CRC Press, Boca Raton, FL, 2004, chap. 18.
12. Institute of Medicine, *Dietary Reference Intakes for Calcium, Phosphorus, Magnesium, Vitamin D, and Fluoride*, National Academy Press, Washington, DC, 1997, chap. 7.
13. Kalman, D.S., Vitamins D and K, in *Sports Nutrition: Vitamins and Trace Elements*, Driskell, J.A., and Wolinsky, I., Eds. CRC Press, Boca Raton, FL, 2006, chap. 12.
14. Lovell, G., Vitamin D status of females in an elite gymnastics program, *Clin. J. Sport Med.* 18, 159–61, 2008.
15. Chesney, R.W., Vitamin D: Can an upper limit be defined? *J. Nutr*. 119, 1825–8, 1989.
16. Institute of Medicine, *Dietary Reference Intakes for Vitamin C, Vitamin E, Selenium, and Carotenoids*, National Academy Press, Washington, DC, 2000, chap. 6.
17. Mastaloudis, A., and Traber, M.G., Vitamin E, in *Sports Nutrition: Vitamins and Trace Elements*, Driskell, J.A., and Wolinsky, I., Eds. CRC Press, Boca Raton, FL, 2006, chap. 13.
18. National Research Council, *Recommended Dietary Allowances*, 10th ed., National Academy Press, Washington, DC, 1989, pp. 99–107.
19. Traber, M.G., Vitamin E, in *Modern Nutrition in Health and Diseases*, 9th ed., Shils, M.E., Olson, J., Shike, M., and Ross A.C., Eds., Williams and Wilkens, Baltimore, 1999, pp. 347–62.
20. U.S. Department of Agriculture, Agricultural Research Service, USDA National Nutrient Database for Standard Reference, Release 20, http://www.ars.usda.gov/ba/bhnrc/ndl. Assessed 11/16/2007.
21. Burton, G.W., Traber, M.G., Acuff, R.V., Walters, D.N., Kayden, H., Hughes, L. and Ingold, K.U., Human plasma and tissue α-tocopherol concentrations in response to supplementation with deuterated natural and synthetic vitamin E, *Am. J. Clin. Nutr.* 67, 669–84, 1998.
22. U.S. Pharmacopeia, Vitamin E, in *The United States Pharmacopeia*, 20th ed., United States Pharmacopeia Convention, Inc., Rockville, MD, 1980, pp. 846–8.
23. Evans, W.J., Vitamin E, vitamin C, and exercise, *Am. J. Clin. Nutr*. 72, 647S–52S, 2000.
24. Davies, K.J., Quintanilha, A.T., Brooks, G.A., and Packer, L., Free radicals and tissue damage produced by exercise, *Biochem. Biophys. Res. Commun.* 107, 1198–205, 1982.
25. Itoh, H., Ohkuwa, T., Yamazaki, Y., Shimoda, T., Wakayama, A., Tamura, S., et al., Vitamin E supplementation attenuates leakage of enzymes following 6 successive days of running training, *Int. J. Sports Med.* 21, 369–74, 2000.

26. Sumida, S., Tanaka, K., Kitao, H., and Nakadomo, F., Exercise-induced lipid peroxidation and leakage of enzymes before and after vitamin E supplementation, *Int. J. Biochem.* 21, 835–8, 1989.
27. Rokizki, L., Logemann, E., Huber, G., Keck, E., and Keul, J., Alpha-tocopherol supplementation in racing cyclists during extreme endurance training, *Int. J. Sport Nutr.* 4, 253–63, 1994.
28. Avery, N.G., Kaiser, J.L., Sharman, M.J., Scheett, T.P., Barnes, D.M., Gomez, A.L., et al., Effects of vitamin E supplementation on recovery from repeated bouts of resistance exercise, *J. Strength Cond. Res.* 17, 801–9, 2003.
29. Finaud, J., Lac, G., and Filaire, E., Oxidative stress: relationship with exercise and training, *Sports Med.* 36, 327–58, 2006.
30. Institute of Medicine, *Dietary Reference Intakes for Vitamin A, Vitamin K, Arsenic, Boron, Chromium, Copper, Iodine, Iron, Manganese, Molybdenum, Nickel, Silicon, Vanadium and Zinc*, National Academy Press, Washington, DC, 2001, chap. 5.
31. Craciun, A.M., Wolf, J., Knapen, M.H., Brouns, F., and Vermeer, C., Improved bone metabolism in female elite athletes after vitamin K supplementation, *Int. J. Sports Med.* 19, 479–94, 1998.
32. Al-Tamimi, E.K., and Haub, M.D., Thiamin, in *Sports Nutrition: Vitamins and Trace Elements*, Driskell, J.A., and Wolinsky, I., Eds. CRC Press, Boca Raton, FL, 2006, chap. 3.
33. Institute of Medicine, *Dietary Reference Intakes for Thiamin, Riboflavin, Niacin, Vitamin B_6, Folate, Vitamin B_{12}, Pantothenic Acid, Biotin, and Choline,* National Academy Press, Washington, DC, 2000, chap. 4.
34. Scholte, H.R., Busch, H.F.M., and Luty-Houwen, I.E.M., Vitamin-responsive pyruvate dehydrogenase deficiency in a young girl with external ophthalmoplegia, myopathy and lactic acidosis, *J. Inherited Metab. Dis.* 15, 331–4, 1992.
35. Manore, M.M., and Woolf, K., B-vitamins and exercise: Does exercise alter requirements? *Int. J. Sport Nutr. Exerc. Metab.* 16, 453–84, 2006.
36. Suzuki, M., and Itokawa, Y., Effects of thiamin supplementation on exercise-induced fatigue, *Metab. Brain Dis.* 11, 95–106, 1996.
37. Donke, D., and Nickel, B., Improvement of fine motoric movement control by elevated dosages of vitamin B_1, B_6 and B_{12} in target shooting, *Int. J. Vitam. Nutr. Res. Suppl.* 30, 198–204, 1989.
38. Webster, M.J., Scheett, T.P., Doyle, M.R., and Branz, M., The effect of a thiamin derivative on exercise performance, *Eur. J. Appl. Physiol. Occup. Physiol.* 75, 520–4, 1997.
39. Webster, M.J., Physiological and performance responses to supplementation with thiamin and pantothenic acid derivatives, *Eur. J. Appl. Physiol. Occup. Physiol.* 77, 486–91, 1998.
40. Elmadfa, I., Majchrzak, D., Rust, P., and Genser, D., The thiamin status of adult humans depends on carbohydrate intake, *Int. J. Vitam. Nutr. Res.* 71, 217–21, 2001.
41. Manore, M.M., Effect of physical activity on thiamine, riboflavin, and vitamin B-6 requirements, *Am. J. Clin. Nutr.* 72, 598S–606S, 2000.
42. Institute of Medicine, *Dietary Reference Intakes for Thiamin, Riboflavin, Niacin, Vitamin B_6, Folate, Vitamin B_{12}, Pantothenic Acid, Biotin, and Choline,* National Academy Press, Washington, DC, 2000, chap. 5.
43. Powers, H.J., Bates, C.J., Eccles, M., Brown, H. and George, E., Bicycling performance in Gambian children: Effects of supplements of riboflavin or ascorbic acid, *Hum. Nutr. Clin. Nutr.* 41, 59–69, 1987.

44. Prasad, P.A., Bamji, M.S., Lakshmi, A.V., and Satyanarayana, K., Functional impact of riboflavin supplementation in urban school children, *Nutr. Res.* 10, 275–81, 1990.
45. Suboticanee, K., Stavljenic, A., Schalch, W., and Buzina, R., Effects of pyridoxine and riboflavin supplementation on physical fitness in young adolescents, *Int. J. Vitam. Nutr.* 60, 81–8, 1990.
46. Winters, L.R., Yoon, J.S., Kalkwarf, H.J., Davies, J.C., Berkowitz, M.G., Haas, J., and Roe, D.A., Riboflavin requirements and exercise adaptation in older women, *Am. J. Clin. Nutr.* 56, 526–32, 1992.
47. Weight, L.M., Noakes, T.D., Labadarios, D., Graves, J., Jacobs, P., and Berman, P.A., Vitamin and mineral status of trained athletes including the effects of supplementation, *Am. J. Clin. Nutr.* 47, 186–91, 1988.
48. Tremblay, A., Boilard, M., Bratton, M.F., Bessette, H., and Roberge, A.B., The effects of riboflavin supplementation on nutritional status and performance of elite swimmers, *Nutr. Res.* 4, 201–8, 1984.
49. Belko, A.Z., Obarzanek, E., Roach, R., Rotter, M., Urban, G., Weinberg, S., and Roe, D.A., Effects of aerobic exercise and weight loss on riboflavin requirements of moderately obese, marginally deficient young women, *Am. J. Clin. Nutr.* 40, 553–61, 1984.
50. Belko, A.Z., Meredith, M.P., Kalkwarf, H.J., Obarzanek, E., Weinberg, S., Roach, R., et al., Effects of exercise on riboflavin requirements: Biological validation in weight reducing women, *Am. J. Clin. Nutr.* 41, 270–7, 1985.
51. National Research Council, *Recommended Dietary Allowances*, 10th ed., National Academy Press, Washington, DC, 1989, pp. 132–7.
52. Keith, R.E., and Alt, L.A., Riboflavin status of female athletes consuming normal diets, *Nutr. Res.* 11, 727–34, 1991.
53. Cropper, S.S., Smith, J.L., and Groff, J.L., *Advanced Nutrition and Human Metabolism*, 4th ed., Thomson Wadsworth, Belmont, CA, 2005, pp. 286–91.
54. Institute of Medicine, *Dietary Reference Intakes for Thiamin, Riboflavin, Niacin, Vitamin B_6, Folate, Vitamin B_{12}, Pantothenic Acid, Biotin, and Choline,* National Academy Press, Washington, DC, 2000, chap. 6.
55. Heath, E.M., Niacin, in *Sports Nutrition: Vitamins and Trace Elements*, Driskell, J.A., and Wolinsky, I., Eds. CRC Press, Boca Raton, FL, 2006, chap. 3.
56. Bergström, J., Hultman, E., Jorfeldt, L., Pernow, B., and Wahren, J., Effect of nicotinic acid on physical working capacity and on metabolism of muscle glycogen in man, *J. Appl. Physiol.* 26, 170–6, 1969.
57. Hilsendager, D., and Karpovich, P.V., Ergogenic effect of glycine and niacin separately and in combination, *Res. Q.* 35, 389–92, 1964.
58. Pernow, B., and Saltin, B., Availability of substrates and capacity for prolonged heavy exercise, *J. Appl. Physiol.* 31, 416–22, 1971.
59. Heath, E.M., Wilcox, A.R., and Quinn, C.M., Effects of nicotinic acid on respiratory exchange ratio and substrate levels during exercise, *Med. Sci. Sports Exercise* 25, 1018–23, 1993.
60. Combs, G.F. Jr., *The Vitamins: Fundamental Aspects in Nutrition and Health*, 3rd ed., Elsevier Academic Press, Burlington, MA, 2007, pp. 313–29.
61. Cropper, S.S., Smith, J.L., and Groff, J.L., *Advanced Nutrition and Human Metabolism*, 4th ed., Thomson Wadsworth, Belmont, CA, 2005, pp. 316–21.
62. Institute of Medicine, *Dietary Reference Intakes for Thiamin, Riboflavin, Niacin, Vitamin B_6, Folate, Vitamin B_{12}, Pantothenic Acid, Biotin, and Choline,* National Academy Press, Washington, DC, 2000, chap. 7.

63. Gracía-Rovés, P.M., Terrados, N., Fernández, S., and Patterson, A.M., Comparison of dietary intake and eating behavior of professional road cyclist during training and competition, *Int. J. Sport Nutr. Exerc. Metab.* 10, 92–8, 2000.
64. Paschoal, V.C.P., and Amancio, O.M.S., Nutritional status of Brazilian elite swimmers, *Int. J. Sport Nutr. Exerc. Metab.* 14, 81–94, 2004.
65. Jonnalagadda, S.S., Ziegler, P.J., and Nelson, J.A., Food preferences, dieting behaviors and body image perceptions of elite figure skaters, *Int. J. Sport Nutr. Exerc. Metab.* 14, 594–606, 2004.
66. Manore, M.M., Vitamin B_6 and exercise, *Int. J. Sport Nutr.* 4, 89–103, 1994.
67. Steen, S.N., Mayer, K., Brownell, K.D., and Wadden, T.A., Dietary intake of female collegiate heavyweight rowers, *Int. J. Sport Nutr.* 5, 223–31, 1995.
68. Rokitzki, L., Sagredos, A.N., Reuss, F., Cufi, D., and Keul, J., Assessment of vitamin B-6 status of strength and speedpower athletes, *J. Am. Coll. Nutr.* 13, 87–94, 1994.
69. Hansen, C.M., and Manore, M.M., Vitamin B_6, in *Sports Nutrition: Vitamins and Trace Elements*, Driskell, J.A., and Wolinsky, I., Eds. CRC Press, Boca Raton, FL, 2006, chap. 6.
70. Telford, R.D., Catchpole, E.A., Deakin, V., McLeay, A.C., and Plank, A.W., The effect of 7 to 8 months of vitamin/mineral supplementation on the vitamin and mineral status of athletes, *Int. J. Sport Nutr.* 2, 123–34, 1992.
71. Raczynski, G., and Szczepanska, B., Longitudinal studies on vitamin B_1 and B_6 status in Polish elite athletes, *Bio. Sport* 10, 189–94, 1993.
72. Manore, M.M., Leklem, J.E., and Walter, M.C., Vitamin B_6 metabolism as affected by exercise in trained and untrained women fed diets differing in carbohydrate and vitamin B_6 content, *Am. J. Clin. Nutr.* 46, 995–1004, 1987.
73. Dunton, N., Virk, R., and Leklem, J., The influence of vitamin B_6 supplementation and exercise to exhaustion on vitamin B_6 metabolism, *FASEB J.* 6, A1374 (abstract), 1992.
74. Grozier, P.G., Cordain, L., and Sampson, D.A., Exercise-induced changes in plasma vitamin B_6 concentrations do not vary with exercise intensity, *Am. J. Clin. Nutr.* 60, 552–8, 1994.
75. van der Beek, E.J., van Dokkum, W., Wedel, M., Schrijver, J., and van den Berg, M., Thiamin, riboflavin and vitamin B_6: Impact of restricted intake on physical performance in man, *J. Am. Coll. Nutr.* 13, 629–40, 1994.
76. van der Beek, E.J., van Dokkum, W., Schrijver, J., Wedel, M., Gaillard, A.W., Wesstra, A., et al., Thiamin, riboflavin, and vitamin B-6 and C: Impact of combined restricted intake on functional performance in man, *Am. J. Clin. Nutr.* 48, 1451–62, 1988.
77. Virk, R.S., Dunton, N.J., Young, J.C., and Leklem, J.E., Effect of vitamin B_6 supplementation on fuels, catacholamines and amino acids during exercise in men, *Med. Sci. Sports Exerc.* 31, 400–8, 1999.
78. van der Beek, E.J., Vitamin supplementation and physical exercise performance, *J. Sports Sci.* 9, 77–89, 1991.
79. Hansen, C.M., Leklem, J.E., and Shultz, T.D., Vitamin B-6 status of women with a constant intake of vitamin B-6 changes with three levels of dietary protein, *J. Nutr.* 126, 1891–901, 1996.
80. Institute of Medicine, *Dietary Reference Intakes for Thiamin, Riboflavin, Niacin, Vitamin B_6, Folate, Vitamin B_{12}, Pantothenic Acid, Biotin, and Choline,* National Academy Press, Washington, DC, 2000, chap. 8.
81. Cropper, S.S., Smith, J.L., and Groff, J.L., *Advanced Nutrition and Human Metabolism*, 4th ed., Thomson Wadsworth, Belmont, CA, 2005, pp. 301–10.
82. Oakely, G.P. Jr., Adams, M.J., and Dickinson, C.M., More folic acid for everyone, now, *J. Nutr.* 126, 751S–5S, 1996.

83. Woolf, K., and Manore, M.M., B-vitamins and exercise: Does exercise alter requirement? *Int. J. Sport Nutr. Exerc. Metab.* 16, 453–84, 2006.
84. Worme, J.D., Doubt, T.J., Singh, A., Ryan, C.J., Moses, F.M., and Deuster, P.A., Dietary patterns, gastrointestinal complaints, and nutrition knowledge of recreational triatheletes, *Am. J. Clin. Nutr.* 51, 690–7, 1990.
85. Baer, J.T., and Taper, L.J., Amenorrheic and eumenorrheic adolescent runners: Dietary intake and exercise training status, *J. Am. Diet. Assoc.* 92, 89–91, 1992.
86. Keith, R.E., O'Keeffe, K.A., Alt, L.A., and Young, K.L., Dietary status of trained female cyclists, *J. Am. Diet. Assoc.* 89, 1620–3, 1989.
87. Beshgetoor, D., and Nichols, J.F., Dietary intake and supplement use in female master cyclists and runners, *Int. J. Sport Nutr. Exerc. Metab.* 13, 166–72, 2003.
88. Beals, K.A., Eating behaviors, nutritional status and menstrual function in elite female adolescent volleyball players, *J. Am. Diet. Assoc.* 102, 1293–6, 2002.
89. Sousa, E.F., Da Costa, T.H.M., Nogueira, J.A.D., and Vivaldi, L.J., Assessment of nutrient and water intake among adolescents from sports federations in the Federal District, Brazil, *Br. J. Nutr.* published online 12/06/2007, doi:10.1017/S0007114507864841.
90. Matter, M., Stittfall, T., Graves, J., Myburgh, K., Adams, B., Jacobs, P., and Noakes, T.D., The effect of iron and folate therapy on maximal exercise performance in female marathon runners with iron and folate deficiency, *Clin. Sci.* 72, 415–22, 1987.
91. Ziegler, P., Sharp, T., Hughes, V., Evans, W., and Khoo, C.S., Nutritional status of teenage female competitive figure skaters, *J. Am. Diet. Assoc.* 101, 374–9, 2001.
92. Institute of Medicine, *Dietary Reference Intakes for Thiamin, Riboflavin, Niacin, Vitamin B_6, Folate, Vitamin B_{12}, Pantothenic Acid, Biotin, and Choline,* National Academy Press, Washington, DC, 2000, chap. 9.
93. McMartin, K.E., Vitamin B_{12}, in *Sports Nutrition: Vitamins and Trace Elements*, Driskell, J.A., and Wolinsky, I., Eds. CRC Press, Boca Raton, FL, 2006, chap. 8.
94. Tin-May-Tan, Ma-Win-May, Khin-Sann-Aung, and Mya-Tu, M., The effect of vitamin B_{12} on physical performance capacity, *Br. J. Nutr.* 40, 269–73, 1978.
95. Read, M.H., and McGuffin, L., The effect of B–complex supplementation on endurance performance, *J. Sports Med. Phys. Fitness* 23, 178–84, 1983.
96. Rodger, R.S., Fletcher, K., Fail, B.J., Rahman, H., Sviland, L., and Hamilton, P.J., Factors influencing haematological measurements in healthy adults, *J. Chronic Dis.* 40, 943–7, 1987.
97. Institute of Medicine, *Dietary Reference Intakes for Thiamin, Riboflavin, Niacin, Vitamin B_6, Folate, Vitamin B_{12}, Pantothenic Acid, Biotin, and Choline,* National Academy Press, Washington, DC, 2000, chap. 10.
98. Camporeale, G., Rodríguez-Meléndez, R., and Zempleni, J., Pantothenic acid and biotin, in *Sports Nutrition: Vitamins and Trace Elements*, Driskell, J.A., and Wolinsky, I., Eds. CRC Press, Boca Raton, FL, 2006, chap. 9.
99. Cropper, S.S., Smith, J.L., and Groff, J.L., *Advanced Nutrition and Human Metabolism*, 4th ed., Thomson Wadsworth, Belmont, CA, 2005, pp. 291–5.
100. Litoff, D., Scherzer, H., and Harrison, J., Effects of pantothenic acid supplementation on human exercise, *Med. Sci. Sports Exerc.* 17, 287, 1985.
101. Shock, N.W., and Sebrell, W.H., The effect of changes in concentration of pantothenate on the work output of perfused frog muscles, *Am. J. Physiol.* 142, 274–8, 1944.
102. Rokitzki, L., Sagredos, A., Reuss, F., Petersen, G., and Keul, J., Pantothenic acid levels in blood of athletes at rest and after aerobic exercise, *Z. Ernahrungswiss* 32, 282–8, 1993.
103. Institute of Medicine, *Dietary Reference Intakes for Thiamin, Riboflavin, Niacin, Vitamin B_6, Folate, Vitamin B_{12}, Pantothenic Acid, Biotin, and Choline,* National Academy Press, Washington, DC, 2000, chap. 11.

104. Cropper, S.S., Smith, J.L., and Groff, J.L., *Advanced Nutrition and Human Metabolism*, 4th ed., Thomson Wadsworth, Belmont, CA, 2005, pp. 295–301.
105. Institute of Medicine, *Dietary Reference Intakes for Thiamin, Riboflavin, Niacin, Vitamin B_6, Folate, Vitamin B_{12}, Pantothenic Acid, Biotin, and Choline,* National Academy Press, Washington, DC, 2000, chap. 12.
106. Zeisel, S.H., da Costa, K.A., Franklin, P.D., Alezander, E.A., Lamont, J.T., Sheard, N.F., and Beiser, A., Choline, an essential nutrient for humans, *FASEB J.* 5, 2093–8, 1991.
107. da Costa, K.A., Niculescu, M.D., Craciunescu, C.N., Fischer, L.M., and Zeisel, S.H., Choline deficiency increases lymphocyte apoptosis and DNA damage in humans, *Am. J. Clin. Nutr.* 84, 88–94, 2006.
108. Conlay, L.A., Wurtman, R.J., Blusztajn, K., Coviella, I.L., Maher, T.J., and Evoniuk, G.E., Decreased plasma choline concentrations in marathon runners, *N. Engl. J. Med.* 315, 892, 1986.
109. von Allwörden, H.N., Horn, S., Kahl, J., and Feldheim, W., The influence of lecithin on plasma choline concentrations in triathletes and adolescent runners during exercise, *Eur. J. Appl. Physiol. Occup. Physiol.* 67, 87–91, 1993.
110. Buchman, A.L., Awal, M., Jenden, D., Roch, M., and Kang, S.H., The effect of lecithin supplementation on plasma choline concentrations during a marathon, *J. Am. Coll. Nutr.* 19, 768–70, 2000.
111. Deuster, P.A. and Cooper, J.A., Choline, in *Sports Nutrition: Vitamins and Trace Elements*, Driskell, J.A., and Wolinsky, I., Eds. CRC Press, Boca Raton, FL, 2006, chap. 10.
112. Institute of Medicine, *Dietary Reference Intakes for Vitamin C, Vitamin E, Selenium, and Carotenoids*, National Academy Press, Washington, DC, 2000, chap. 5.
113. Keith, R.E., Ascorbic acid, in *Sports Nutrition: Vitamins and Trace Elements*, Driskell, J.A., and Wolinsky, I., Eds. CRC Press, Boca Raton, FL, 2006, chap. 2.
114. Cropper, S.S., Smith, J.L., and Groff, J.L., *Advanced Nutrition and Human Metabolism*, 4th ed., Thomson Wadsworth, Belmont, CA, 2005, pp. 260–75.
115. Steen, S.N. and McKinney, S., Nutritional assessment of college wrestlers, *Phys. Sportsmed.* 14, 100–14, 1986.
116. Hickson, J.F., Schrader, J., and Trischler, L.C., Dietary intakes of female basketball and gymnastics athletes, *J. Am. Diet. Assoc.* 86, 251–3, 1986.
117. Duthie, G.G., Robertson, J.D., Maughan, R.J., and Morrice, P.C., Blood antioxidant status and erythrocyte lipid peroxidation following distance running, *Arch. Biochem. Biophys.* 282, 78–83, 1990.
118. Gleeson, M., Robertson, J.D., and Maughn, R.J., Influence of exercise on ascorbic acid status in mans, *Clin. Sci.* 73, 501–5, 1987.
119. Buzina, R., and Suboticanec, K., Vitamin C physical working capacity, *Int. J. Vitam. Nutr. Res. Suppl.* 27, 157–66, 1985.
120. Johnston, C.S., Swan, P.D., and Corte, C., Substrate utilization and work efficiency during submaximal exercise in vitamin C depleted–repleted adults, *Int. J. Vitam. Nutr. Res.* 69, 41–4, 1999.
121. Babadzanjan, M.G., Kalnyn, V.R., Kossenko, S.A., and Kostina, E.I., Effect of vitamin supplements on some physiological functions of workers in electric locomotive teams, *Vopr. Pitan.* 19, 18–24, 1960.
122. Kotze, H.F., van der Walt, W.H., Rogers, G.G., and Strydom, N.B., Effects of plasma ascorbic acid levels on heat acclimatization in man, *J. Appl. Physiol.* 42, 711–6, 1977.
123. Peters, E.M., Goetzche, J.M., Grobbelaar, B., and Noakes, T.D., Vitamin C supplementation reduces the incidence of postrace symptoms of upper-respiratory infection in ultramarathon runner, *Am. J. Clin. Nutr.* 57, 170–4, 1993.

124. Thompson, D., Williams, C., MacGregor, S.J., Nicholas, C.W., McArdle, F., Jackson, M.J., and Powell, J.R., Prolonged vitamin C supplementation and recovery form demanding exercise, *Int. J. Sport Nutr. Exerc. Metab.* 11, 466–81, 2001.
125. Nieman, D.C., Peters, E.M., Henson, D.A., Nevines, E.I., and Thompson, M.M., Influence of vitamin C supplementation on cytokine changes following an ultramarathon, *J. Interferon Cytokine Res.* 20, 1029–35, 2000.
126. Petroczi, A. and Naughton, D.P., The age–gender–status profile of high performing athletes in the UK taking nutritional supplements: lessons for the future, *J. Int. Soc. Sports Nutr.* published online 01/10/2008, doi:10.1186/1550–2783–5–2.

5 Minerals—Calcium, Magnesium, Chromium, and Boron

Stella L. Volpe

CONTENTS

I. INTRODUCTION

Minerals are necessary for a number of metabolic processes in the body, and are also important in supporting growth and development. Minerals are also required in numerous reactions involved with exercise and physical activity, including energy, carbohydrate, fat and protein metabolism, oxygen transfer and delivery, and tissue repair.[1]

The mineral needs of athletes have been a topic of discussion and controversy for many years because researchers disagree whether athletes need more minerals in their diets than non-athletes or sedentary individuals. Micronutrient requirements are based on many aspects, including the intensity, duration, and frequency of the exercise, and the overall energy and nutrient intakes of the person. The purpose of this chapter is to evaluate the mineral needs of athletes.[1–3] The minerals that will be presented in this chapter are: calcium, magnesium, chromium, and boron. These minerals were chosen because there has been extensive research on them with respect to exercise or health that would impact exercise performance.

II. DIETARY REFERENCE INTAKES

The Dietary Reference Intakes (DRI) for all known vitamins and essential minerals for healthy people living in the United States were updated between 1997 and 2005.[4–8] Note that Adequate Intake (AI), Recommended Dietary Allowance (RDA), Estimated Average Requirement (EAR), and Tolerable Upper Intake Level (UL) are all under the DRI heading. The RDA is the dietary intake level that is sufficient for approximately 98% of healthy people living in the United States. The AI is a projected value that is used when the RDA cannot be established. The EAR is a value used to estimate the nutrient requirements of half of the healthy people in a group.[8] The UL is the maximum quantity of a nutrient most persons can consume without resulting in adverse side effects.[8] The DRIs for all nutrients can be found at the following website: http://www.iom.edu/Object.File/Master/21/372/0.pdf.

In most cases, if energy intakes are sufficient, the micronutrient requirements of athletes are similar to healthy, fairly active individuals; and therefore, using the DRI for evaluating nutrient needs would be suitable. Some athletes, however, may have greater requirements as a result of disproportionate losses of nutrients in sweat and urine. For these athletes, supplementation may need to be considered on an individual basis. Many athletes supplement with vitamins, minerals, and ergogenic aids on their own. The UL provides guidelines to those who supplement, which should prevent negative effects from occurring due to over-supplementation.

III. IMPORTANCE OF OBTAINING ACCURATE DIETARY INTAKE INFORMATION

Though this chapter will focus on the minerals calcium, magnesium, chromium, and boron, a total evaluation of an athlete's energy intake is necessary, because, though an athlete may consume the correct amount of micronutrients (especially if he or she is supplementing with a vitamin-mineral supplement), if energy requirements are not being met, exercise performance will still be sub-optimal. Clark et al.[9] assessed the pre- and post-season intakes of macronutrients and micronutrients in Division I female soccer players. They reported that, despite attaining total energy requirements (though carbohydrate needs were not met), vitamin E, folate, copper, and magnesium intakes were all sub-optimal (defined as < 75% of the DRI for each nutrient).

Furthermore, the actual examination of an athlete's diet must be conducted properly to ensure precision.[10] It is common for any individual, athlete or non-athlete, to under-report his or her dietary intake. As a result, it is essential that athletes are taught how to precisely report portion sizes and fluid intake, the amount and frequency of snacking, any weight management practices they may perform, and any alterations in their food patterns during and off-seasons.[10]

This chapter will provide the background of each mineral as well as studies in which the researchers have evaluated intake or used supplementation to assess their effects, if any, on exercise performance or related variables that may affect performance (e.g., body weight, metabolism, etc.).

IV. CALCIUM

A. Role of Calcium in the Human Body

Calcium is the fifth most common element and the most abundant cation in the human body; more than 99% of total body calcium is stored in the teeth and bones, with the remaining 1% distributed in the blood and muscle and intercellularly.[11] Calcium is required for numerous metabolic processes within the body including bone metabolism, muscle contraction, nerve conduction, and hormone and enzyme secretion.[4]

B. Calcium Homeostasis

Normal levels of serum calcium range from 9 to 11 mg/dL (2.2 to 2.5 mmol/L), and the body maintains tight regulation of serum calcium concentrations with three calciotropic hormones: parathyroid hormone (PTH), vitamin D, and calcitonin.[12] When serum calcium concentrations fall below 9 mg/dL, PTH sends a signal for increased production of calcitriol (produced in the kidneys), the most active form of vitamin D. Increased levels of calcitriol will result in: (1) increased renal reabsorption of calcium, (2) increased intestinal absorption of calcium (by increasing calbindin, a vitamin D-dependent protein that binds to calcium within the intestines for increase calcium absorption), and (3) increased osteoclastic (bone resorption) activity at the bone, to release more calcium in the blood, until calcium homeostasis is achieved. When serum calcium concentrations increase above 11 mg/dL, a hormone, calcitonin, will cause: (1) decreased renal reabsorption of calcium, (2) decreased intestinal calcium absorption, and (3) increased osteoblastic activity (greater bone deposition) (Figure 5.1).

Of all of calcium's roles in the body, the best known is its function in bone metabolism. Calcium is deposited (bone deposition) and removed from bone (bone resporption), which is a process known as "bone remodeling."[4] During periods of growth, bone deposition is greater than bone resorption; however, in older adults and

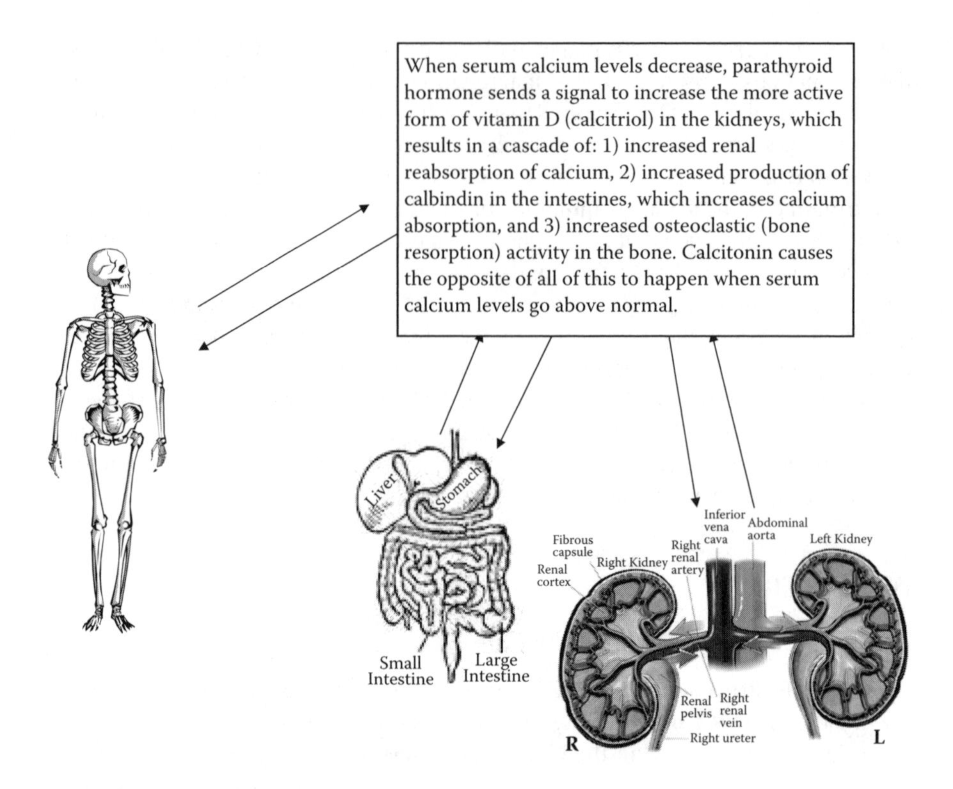

FIGURE 5.1 Calcium homeostasis.
Note: Skeleton from Microsoft PowerPoint clip art
Intestines from:
http://www.manteno.k12.il.us/webquest/elementary/LongTerm/InvasionBodySnatchers/intestin.htm
Kidneys from:
http://images.google.com/imgres?imgurl=http://www.choa.org/images/photography/kidneyguide_kidneys.jpg&imgrefurl=http://www.choa.org/default.aspx%3Fid%3D3036&h=238&w=360&sz=24&hl=en&start=16&tbnid=YBnseRkv6K184M:&tbnh=80&tbnw=121&prev=/images%3Fq%3Dkidneys%26gbv%3D2%26hl%3Den

in women who have already experienced menopause, bone resorption tends to be greater than bone deposition, which can result in osteoporosis and lead to osteoporotic ("porous bones") fractures.[4] Osteoporosis or osteopenia (generalized reduction in bone mass), however, is not a disease of the elderly or post-menopausal women only, but it can appear in young women who are experiencing amenorrhea (absence of menses), in women who have disordered eating, or a combination of both (female athlete triad). "The female athlete triad refers to the interrelationships among energy availability, menstrual function, and bone mineral density, which may have clinical manifestations including eating disorders, functional hypothalamic amenorrhea, and osteoporosis" (p. 1867).[13] For a more comprehensive view on the female athlete triad, refer to Nattiv et al.[13]

TABLE 5.1
Food Sources of Calcium

Food	Calcium (mg)
Yogurt, plain, low fat, 8 ounces (240 mL)	415
Yogurt, fruit, low fat, 8 ounces (240 mL)	245 to 384
Sardines, canned in oil, with bones, 3 ounces (90 g)	324
Cheddar cheese, shredded, 1 ½ ounces (45 mL)	306
Milk, non-fat, 8 fluid ounces (240 mL)	302
Milk, reduced fat (2% milk fat), 8 fluid ounces (240 mL)	297
Milk, whole (3.25% milk fat), 8 fluid ounces (240 mL)	291
Mozzarella, part skim 1 ½ ounces (45 g)	275
Tofu, firm, made with calcium sulfate, ½ cup (120 g)	204
Orange juice, calcium fortified, 6 fluid ounces (180 mL)	200 to 260
Salmon, pink, canned, solids with bone, 3 oz. (90 g)	181
Pudding, chocolate, instant, made w/ 2% milk, ½ cup (120 g)	153
Cottage cheese, 1% milk fat, 1 cup unpacked (240 g)	138
Spinach, cooked, ½ cup (60 g)	120
Turnip greens, boiled, ½ cup (65 g)	99
Kale, cooked, 1 cup (120 g)	94
Ice cream, vanilla, ½ cup (120 g)	85
Soy beverage, calcium fortified, 8 fluid ounces (240 mL)	80 to 500
Chinese cabbage, raw, 1 cup (120 g)	74
Tortilla, flour, ready to bake/fry, one 6" diameter (25 g)	37
Sour cream, reduced fat, cultured, 2 tablespoons (30 g)	32
Broccoli, raw, ½ cup (40 g)	21
Bread, whole wheat, 1 slice (60 g)	20
Cheese, cream, regular, 1 tablespoon (15 g)	12

From References 12 through 14.

For more information on the mineral content of other foods, refer to: http://www.nal.usda.gov/fnic/cgi-bin/nut_search.pl.

C. Calcium Requirements

The DRI for calcium was established in 1994 as an AI as 1300 mg/day for males and females 14 to 18 years of age, 1000 mg/day for men and women 19 to 50 years of age, and 1200 mg/day for men and women 51 years of age and older.[4] The UL for calcium is 2500 mg/day.[4] Various food sources of calcium are listed in Table 5.1.[14–16]

Though food is the best way to obtain any nutrient, individuals who do not consume enough calcium due to insufficient dietary intake or absorption may require calcium supplementation. There are a number of different calcium supplements; however, calcium citrate and calcium carbonate are absorbed the best. If a person does supplement, it is recommended that he or she supplements with 500 mg/day of calcium in the morning and 500 mg/day of calcium in the evening, in conjunction with 200 international units (IU) of vitamin D with each calcium dose. Two doses of calcium per day, combined with vitamin D, will maximize absorption. Calcium carbonate is best taken with meals, whereas calcium citrate can be taken with or without meals.

D. Calcium Status of Athletes

Calcium status has been assessed in a number of different types of athletes. Zalcman et al.[17] assessed the nutritional status of adventure racers, who are individuals who compete over several days, usually in teams, in a variety of events, including mountain biking, complete trekking, vertical techniques (e.g., climbing, rappelling), horseback riding, orienteering, sailing, etc. They reported low intakes of calcium in the women adventure racers.

More recently, Lovell[18] evaluated the calcium intake and serum vitamin D status of elite female gymnasts, 10 to 17 years of age. They reported that, of the 18 gymnasts evaluated, 13 had dietary calcium intakes below their recommended needs. In addition, 15 of the gymnasts had serum vitamin D levels (25-hydroxyvitamin D) that were < 75 nmol/L (> 75 nmol/L is considered optimal for bone health), and six had serum vitamin D concentrations < 50 nmol/L.[18] Though these researchers had a small sample size, the low calcium intake coupled with the below normal serum vitamin D concentrations, demonstrate an increased risk of osteoporosis and certainly impaired performance in these young athletes.

In a study of 23 nationally ranked female adolescent volleyball players, Beals[19] evaluated the nutrient intake by 3-day weighed food records, which increases the accuracy of the assessment. Beals[19] found that these athletes consumed lower energy than they expended (energy intake = 2248 + 414 kilocalories [kcal]/day, energy expenditure = 2815 kcal/day), and consumed less than the recommended intake of many micronutrients, including calcium. Beals[19] also found that a high percentage of athletes had past or present menstrual disorders (amenorrhea, oligomenorrhea, or irregular menstrual cycles). The combination of low energy and micronutrient intake and menstrual irregularities demonstrates the need for long-term studies evaluating dietary intake and nutritional status among athletes of all levels and ages, and certainly predisposes these athletes to the female athlete triad.[13]

E. Calcium Supplementation and Exercise Performance

Calcium supplementation is probably most recognized for its use to improve or maintain bone mineral density. Nonetheless, calcium supplementation has been used to evaluate its ergogenic (performance-enhancing) effects in exercisers of all ages.

Bunout et al.[20] supplemented (in a double-blind fashion) 10 men and 86 women, 70 years of age and older, who had serum vitamin D concentrations of 16 ng/mL or less, with either 800 mg/day of calcium and 400 IU of vitamin D or with 800 mg/day of calcium alone. Participants were also randomized into either a resistance training or control group and followed this regimen for 9 months. The researchers reported that the combination of calcium and vitamin D, with or without training, improved functional status and femoral bone density. In addition, the training increased muscle strength in all participants.

If older participants can benefit from calcium supplementation, what about younger individuals? Koh-Banerjee et al.[21] assessed the effects of calcium pyruvate supplementation on body composition and metabolic responses to exercise. They recruited 23 untrained woman and randomly assigned them, in a double-blind fashion, to either 5 g of calcium pyruvate or a placebo (which actually contained 2.5 g of calcium carbonate), while the participants were placed on a supervised exercise program of resistance training and walking. They found that calcium pyruvate supplementation during training did not significantly affect body composition or exercise performance, and may actually negatively impact some blood lipid concentrations. In this case, the calcium supplement used is not commonly available, and its bioavailability has not been thoroughly evaluated. In addition, the amount of calcium provided (both in the supplemented group and the placebo, were above the UL for calcium, though the researchers did not provide the amount of elemental calcium contained in either the calcium pyruvate or placebo).

Calcium supplementation combined with vitamin D may be most beneficial in older individuals who exercise, providing them with the appropriate balance of nutrients and weight-bearing activity to improve bone mineral density and functional capacity. In younger individuals, calcium supplementation may not have an ergogenic effect; however, more research is needed, using more bioavailable sources of calcium at doses below the UL to ascertain if an ergogenic effect exists.

F. Calcium Supplementation and Intake on Weight Loss

Within the last 10 years, calcium supplementation and intake has been evaluated for its impact on weight loss. A 2006 meta-analysis by Trowman and colleagues[22] reported no effects of calcium on weight loss. Their objective was to examine if there were any relationships between calcium and weight loss by reviewing and conducting a meta-analysis of randomized controlled trials of calcium supplementation in humans who were 18 years of age or older, and where body weight was the final outcome measure. Based on their criteria, 13 randomized controlled trials were incorporated in the meta-analysis. Trowman et al.[22] reported no relationship between increased intake of calcium, either via supplements or dairy products, and weight loss. In their review of the literature on calcium and weight loss, Barba and Russo[23] state that available data do not definitively support a relationship between high calcium or dairy intake and decreased body weight; however, they do support more research on the impact dairy foods have on health outside of obesity.

Nonetheless, a number of researchers have reported benefits of calcium on weight loss or fat metabolism.[24–32] Most recently, Wyatt et al.[33] reported greater weight loss and decreased waist circumference in individuals who exercised and consumed more low-fat dairy products.

V. MAGNESIUM

A. Role of Magnesium in the Human Body

Magnesium, the second most abundant intracellular divalent cation, has been recognized as a cofactor for more than 300 metabolic reactions in the body.[34–38] These processes consist of protein synthesis, adenylate cyclase synthesis, cellular energy production and storage, preservation of cellular electrolyte composition, cell growth and reproduction, deoxyribonucleic acid (DNA) and ribonucleic acid (RNA) synthesis, and stabilization of mitochondrial membranes.[36–40] Magnesium also has a vital responsibility in managing bone metabolism, nerve transmission, cardiac excitability, neuromuscular conduction, muscular contraction, vasomotor tone, and blood pressure.[36–40] Additionally, magnesium plays a major role in glucose and insulin metabolism.[41–44]

B. Measures of Magnesium Status

Because magnesium is an intracellular cation, its serum concentrations may not precisely mirror magnesium status.[45] Nonetheless, decreases in serum levels of magnesium indicate a frank deficiency, indicating that serum magnesium concentrations are specific, but not sensitive, to magnesium deficiency.[45] A more state-of-the-art measurement of magnesium status may involve measuring renal magnesium levels, where levels are measured preceding and following the administration of an intravenous magnesium load. If magnesium excretion is reduced over a period of two 24-hour measurements, a deficit exists. In addition, magnesium balance is related to calcium and potassium status, and consequently should be evaluated in combination with these two cations.[46] Despite this knowledge, most researchers still report serum magnesium concentrations to ascertain magnesium deficiency (hypomagnesemia). A comprehensive review of different methods to evaluate magnesium status will not be discussed in this chapter, but will simply be listed. The methods to assess magnesium status are serum magnesium concentrations, plasma ionized magnesium levels, intracellular magnesium concentrations, magnesium balance studies, and the magnesium tolerance test. For further information about these methods, the reader is directed to the Dietary Reference Intakes for Calcium, Phosphorus, Magnesium, Vitamin D, and Fluoride.[4]

C. Magnesium Requirements

The DRI for magnesium for adults is 310 to 420 mg/day. Intake is often below these recommendations, especially as people age.[4] Table 5.2 provides a list of some food sources of magnesium. Decreased magnesium intake has been related to an increased risk of metabolic syndrome and type 2 diabetes mellitus.[43,44] In addition, stressors such as exercise may deplete magnesium, which, together with a sub-optimal dietary magnesium intake, may negatively impact normal metabolism, exacerbate the disease state and impair exercise performance.[36]

D. Magnesium Status of Athletes

Zalcman et al.[17] also evaluated the magnesium intake of adventure athletes (18 men and 6 women). They reported inadequate intakes of magnesium, as well as calcium.

Rankinen et al.[47] evaluated the dietary intake and nutritional status of athletes (Finnish elite male ski jumpers) ($n = 21$), and compared them with age-matched controls ($n = 20$), using four-day dietary records. There were no dissimilarities between groups in age and height; though not unexpectedly, the ski jumpers had a lower mean

TABLE 5.2
Food Sources of Magnesium

Food	Magnesium (mg)
Cooked halibut, 3 ounces (100 g)	90
Dry, roasted almonds, 1 ounce (35 g)	80
Cooked spinach (originally frozen), ½ cup (60 g)	75
Instant, fortified oatmeal, prepared with water, 1 cup (240 g)	55
1 medium baked potato, with skin (300 g)	50
Smooth peanut butter, 2 tablespoons (35 g)	50
Plain, skim milk yogurt, 8 fluid ounces (240 mL)	45
Vegetarian baked beans, ½ cup (135 g)	40
Crude wheat germ, 2 tablespoons (30 g)	35
Chocolate milk, 1 cup (240 mL)	33
1 medium banana, 2.1 ounces (60 g)	30
Milk chocolate, 1.5 ounces (50 g)	28
Packed, seedless raisins, ¼ cup (45 g)	25

Adapted from: http://dietary-supplements.info.nih.gov/factsheets/magnesium.asp.

For more information on the magnesium content of other foods, refer to: http://www.nal.usda.gov/fnic/cgi-bin/nut_search.pl.

body weight and percent body fat (assessed via dual-energy x-ray absorptiometry [DEXA]). Nevertheless, energy intake was significantly lower ($p = 0.001$) in the ski jumpers compared with the control participants. Despite this disparity in energy intake, many vitamins and minerals were similar between the groups; however, vitamins D and E, zinc, and magnesium were significantly lower in the ski jumpers. Though the ski jumpers had appreciably lower intakes of these micronutrients, their biochemical markers of nutritional status were within normal limits. However, the cross-sectional nature of this and many other studies to establish nutritional status among athletes may not precisely capture deficiencies that could be occurring over time. Moreover, plasma or serum concentrations of micronutrients are not always the best measure of status.

Hassapidou and Manstrantoni[49] compared the dietary intake of elite Greek female athletes in four different sports (volleyball, middle distance running, ballet dancing, and swimming) with a non-athletic control group. They assessed dietary intake using 7-day weighed dietary records over the training season and the competitive season. Again, the use of weighed food records, especially over a week, increases the accuracy of the dietary assessment. Though micronutrient intakes did not differ between athletes and non-athletes, biochemical indices to assess status were not conducted. An additional study on dietary intake conducted in female Greek volleyball players found that these adolescent athletes did not consume recommended intakes for calcium, iron, folate, magnesium, zinc, vitamin A, and the B vitamins.[50] Neither of these groups of researchers examined nutritional status, but the lower than RIs could lead to less than optimal performance and growth in the adolescent athletes.

E. Magnesium Supplementation and Exercise Performance

Because magnesium plays an important role in so many metabolic reactions in the body, it is obvious why supplementation studies have been conducted with magnesium to evaluate its ergogenic effects. Cinar et al.[51] conducted a 4-week supplementation study to examine the impact of magnesium supplementation in exercising and sedentary individuals, compared with a control group. Thirty healthy participants, 18 to 22 years of age, were separated into the following three groups: untrained participants given 10 mg/kg/day of magnesium; participants who trained in Tae-Kwon-Do for 90 to 12 minutes per day for 5 days per week, given 10 mg/kg/day of magnesium; and a non-supplemented group who exercised the same length of time, but were not given a magnesium supplement. They reported significant increases in erythrocyte and hemoglobin concentrations in the supplemented groups, concluding that magnesium would then enhance exercise performance; however, this conclusion is too strong based on the findings, and more research would need to be performed over a longer period of time, evaluating both biochemical markers and exercise performance, to fully establish the impact of magnesium. For example, Finstad et al.[52] reported that 4 weeks of 212 mg/day of magnesium oxide improved ionized magnesium concentrations; however, exercise performance and recovery were not improved in physically active women (magnesium versus. placebo). Moreover, in a meta-analysis, Newhouse and Finstad[39] reported no effect of magnesium supplementation on exercise performance.

Perhaps magnesium supplementation may be more effective in individuals with heart disease who exercise. Pokan et al.[53] studied individuals with coronary heart disease. They based their hypothesis on previous research demonstrating that magnesium supplementation plays a role in and may improve endothelial function, exercise tolerance, and exercise-induced chest pain[41] in patients with coronary artery disease. In a double blind placebo-controlled trial, Pokan et al.[53] randomly assigned 53 males with stable coronary artery disease to either an oral magnesium (15 mmol twice per day [72 mg/day]) ($n = 28$, 61 + 9 years of age) or a placebo ($n = 25$, 58 + 10 years of age) group for 6 months. Compared with the placebo, 6 months of magnesium supplementation significantly increased intracellular magnesium levels, maximal oxygen consumption, and left ventricular heart function (as measured by ejection fraction). Based on these data, the authors concluded that magnesium supplementation is effective in improving exercise performance and heart function in men with stable coronary artery disease. A longer supplementation trial should be performed to confirm these results.

A number of researchers have confirmed the benefits of increased dietary magnesium intake or magnesium supplementation on the metabolic syndrome, insulin resistance and type 2 diabetes mellitus.[54–60] Though prevention of type 2 diabetes mellitus is extremely important, treating it is equally as important. Rodríguez-Morán and Guerrero-Romero[60] evaluated whether oral magnesium supplementation (50 mL of a magnesium chloride solution containing 50 g of magnesium chloride/1000 mL of solution) improved insulin sensitivity as well as metabolic control in individuals with both type 2 diabetes mellitus and decreased serum magnesium concentrations (< 0.74 mmol/L [<1.8 mg/dL]). Sixty-three participants qualified for this 16-week randomized, double-blind, placebo-controlled trial. To assess insulin sensitivity, homeostasis model analysis for insulin resistance (HOMA-IR) was used, while glucose concentrations and glycosylated hemoglobin (HbA1c) were used to evaluate metabolic control. At 16 weeks, the individuals who received magnesium supplementation had a significantly greater serum magnesium concentration than control subjects (0.74 + 0.10 [1.8 + 0.24 mg/dL] versus 0.65 + 0.07 mmol/L [1.58 + 0.17], p = 0.02). Those who were supplemented also significantly improved insulin sensitivity and metabolic control, based on a lower HOMA-IR index, lower fasting blood glucose levels, and lower HbA1c compared with control participants.

Though short term, this study clearly indicates the impact of magnesium supplementation on managing type 2 diabetes mellitus. Nonetheless, though this and other cited studies offer positive results of magnesium supplementation on the metabolic syndrome, insulin resistance, or type 2 diabetes mellitus, it appears that an individual must have hypomagnesemia for supplementation to be effective. This could be the reason for a lack of ergogenic effects of magnesium in many athletes; if they begin with normal serum magnesium levels, providing more through supplementation will not augment status, and hence will not affect performance.

VI. CHROMIUM

A. Role of Chromium in the Human Body and Chromium Requirements

Chromium is a required trace mineral best known for its role in potentiating the effects of insulin.[61] The DRI for chromium, which has been established as an AI, is 25 to 35 micrograms (mcg)/day for adult women and men, respectively.[7] Food sources of chromium are listed in Table 5.3.

B. Brief History of Chromium Supplementation

The popularity of chromium as a dietary supplement began in the early 1990s. It has been reported that, after calcium, chromium is the second best-selling mineral supplement on the market; in 1998, it was estimated that 10 million Americans spent a total of $150 million on chromium supplementation.[62] Chromium has been alleged to improve body composition, glucose tolerance, blood lipid levels, decrease body fat and body weight, and increase lean body mass.[61] Because picolinate, a derivative of the amino acid tryptophan, is thought to enhance the absorption of chromium into the body, chromium supplements are often sold as chromium picolinate, but other forms, such as chromium nicotinate, have also gained popularity.[61]

C. Chromium Supplementation and Exercise Performance

For athletes who are in weight-monitored sports, such as wrestling, gymnastics, and rowing, or sports where aesthetics is important (e.g., gymnastics and ice skating), chromium's use as a possible weight-loss supplement is what gained it the most recognition. However, research in overweight individuals has also been conducted. For

TABLE 5.3
Food Sources of Chromium

Food	Chromium (mcg per 100 grams of Food)
Egg yolk	183
Brewer's yeast	112
Beef	57
Cheese	56
Liver	55
Wine	45
Whole wheat bread	42
Apple peel	27
Oysters	26
Margarine	18
Spaghetti	15
Spinach	10
Peeled apple	1

Adapted from: http://www.healthyeatingclub.com/info/books-phds/books/foodfacts/html/data/data5m.html
http://dietary-supplements.info.nih.gov/factsheets/magnesium.asp
http://lpi.oregonstate.edu/infocenter/minerals/zinc/
http://dietary-supplements.info.nih.gov/factsheets/selenium.asp#h2

For more information on the mineral content of other foods, refer to: http://www.nal.usda.gov/fnic/cgi-bin/nut_search.pl.

example, Volpe et al.[63] evaluated the impact of chromium picolinate supplementation in sedentary overweight women to ascertain if chromium truly had a weight-loss effect. They performed a double-blind study in moderately obese women on body weight, body composition, and resting metabolic rate (RMR), and found that the supplementation 400 mcg/day of chromium picolinate did not result in changes in weight loss, body composition (as assessed by underwater weighing), or resting metabolic rate (assessed by indirect calorimetry) compared with women receiving an identical-looking placebo. This study was conducted in 44 women who had body mass indexes (BMIs) ranging from 27 to 41 kg/m^2, and ranged in age from 27 to 51 years. Other researchers also reported no effect of chromium supplementation on body weight or body composition in athletes (wrestlers) and non-athletes.[64,65]

Though chromium supplementation may not result in weight loss in athletes or sedentary individuals, could it act as an ergogenic aid with respect to its function in enhancing insulin signaling and insulin-mediated glucose uptake? Volek et al.[66] examined the effects of 600 mcg/day of chromium picolinate in 16 overweight men (with an average BMI = 31.1 + 3.0 kg/m^2) who were randomly assigned to either the chromium group or a placebo. The participants were supplemented or given the placebo for 4 weeks, after which they performed a supra-maximal bout of cycling ergometry to exhaust their stores of muscle glycogen. After this supra-maximal exercise bout, the researchers fed the participants with high-glycemic-index carbohydrates for the following 24 hours. Muscle biopsies were taken at rest, immediately post-exercise, and 2 and 24 hours post-exercise. Volek et al.[66] reported no differences in glucose or insulin concentrations between the groups. They concluded that 4 weeks of chromium supplementation did not augment glycogen synthesis during recovery after high-intensity exercise followed by a high-glycemic-index feeding.

Crawford et al.[67] evaluated the effects 600 mcg of niacin-bound chromium on the body composition of 20 overweight African American women. This was a cross-over design study; participants in one group received a placebo for 2 months followed by chromium supplementation for an additional 2 months, while the other group received the chromium supplementation first, followed by the placebo. The supplement resulted in significantly more fat loss, while concurrently preserving lean body mass. Though the former group did lose more body fat and preserve more lean body mass while taking the chromium supplement than the placebo, the group that took the chromium supplement first, followed by the placebo, lost more body fat and preserved more lean body mass while on the placebo versus the chromium. All study participants were placed on a diet and exercise program during the study, signifying that the resulting improvements could have stemmed from their dietary and exercise programs rather than the chromium supplementation.

In a larger study of 158 moderately obese subjects, the addition of a multi-mineral supplement, including chromium picolinate, significantly increased the rate of fat loss while maintaining lean body mass compared with a placebo.[68] This study also failed to demonstrate any specific effects of chromium picolinate because the supplement contained several other minerals that could have resulted in the significant difference. Thus, though the sample size was fairly large, it is difficult to draw solid conclusions from this study regarding the contribution that chromium picolinate made to the results.

Based on the data presented from previous studies, it does not appear that chromium (picolinate or nicotinate) has ergogenic effects on exercise performance, especially with regard to weight loss or increases in lean body mass. Research on chromium's possible impact on type 2 diabetes mellitus may be more promising, however.

VII. BORON

A. Boron Requirements and Boron Supplementation and Exercise Performance

Boron may be a vital nutrient for animals and humans but the body of scientific support has not ascertained a definitive biological function in humans, though it is essential for plants.[7,12,69] Because of this, there is no established DRI for boron.[7] Dietary boron may influence the activity of many metabolic enzymes, as well as the metabolism of steroid hormones and several micronutrients, including calcium, magnesium, and vitamin D.[7,69] (See Table 5.4 for dietary sources of boron.) Boron may also play a role in improving arthritis, plasma lipid profiles, and brain function.[69]

TABLE 5.4
Food Sources of Boron

Food	Chromium (mg per 100 grams of Food)
Raisins	4.5
Almonds, Hazelnuts	2.3
Apricots (dried)	2.1
Avocado	2.1
Walnuts	1.6
Beans (red, kidney)	1.4
Peanut Butter	1.9
Prunes	1.2
Dates	1.1
Chick Peas, Lentils	0.7
Grapes	0.5
Broccoli, Carrots	0.3
Onion	0.2

Adapted from: http://www.algaecal.com/Boron-Rich-Foods.html.

For more information on the mineral content of other foods, refer to: http://www.nal.usda.gov/fnic/cgi-bin/nut_search.pl.

Boron has been most studied for its potential effects on improving bone mineral density, and indeed, research has shown that boron supplementation can improve bone strength in some animals (e.g., chicks and rats) and bone mineral density in post-menopausal women; however, the data in rats and humans have been equivocal.[70–74] The focus of much of the research on bone mineral density and osteoporosis has focused on calcium and vitamin D; however, the ultratrace mineral boron may play a role in bone metabolism, but its role is most likely associated with its interactions with calcium, magnesium, and vitamin D.[70–74]

In one of the earlier studies, Volpe et al.[75] evaluated the effects of 3 mg/day of boron supplementation for 10 months on the bone mineral density and hormonal status of 28 college females, both athletes and non-athletes. It was a single-blind study, where participants were randomly assigned to receive boron or an identical-looking placebo; however, the participants were placed into one of four groups: boron-athletes, placebo-athletes, boron-non-athletes, placebo-non-athletes. Though some changes did occur over time, Volpe et al.[75] did not report an effect of the boron supplementation on bone mineral density, serum vitamin D concentrations, or hormonal status of any of the participants.

In the same group of 28 female participants (17 athletes, 11 non-athletes), Meacham et al.[76] evaluated the effects of boron supplementation on blood and urinary minerals. They found that the athletes consumed more boron in their diets than the sedentary participants, and that the athletes showed a slight increased bone mineral density compared with the controls (not surprisingly, since weight-bearing exercise has been shown to increase bone mineral density). However, serum phosphorus concentrations were lower in boron-supplemented participants (athletes and non-athletes) than in participants receiving the placebo, and were lower at the end of the study period than during baseline analysis. Serum magnesium concentrations were greatest in the non-athletes whose diets were supplemented with boron, and increased with time in all participants. Thus, supplementation with boron may impact the status of other minerals within the body.

In another follow-up to these same 28 participants, Meacham and colleagues[77] reported calcium excretion increased over time in all groups combined, and boron excretion increased over time in all boron-supplemented subjects. They also reported that exercise training diminished changes in serum phosphorus concentrations caused by boron supplementation. Meacham et al.[77] conclude that boron supplementation moderately affected mineral status, and exercise modified the effects of boron supplementation on serum minerals in the young women studied.

Green and Ferrando[78] were among the few researchers who evaluated 2.5 mg/day of boron supplementation for its possible effects of increasing testosterone, and hence, lean body mass, in 10 male body builders, 21 to 27 years of age, compared with a placebo (9 male body builders). After the 7-week study, they reported increases in total testosterone concentrations, lean body mass, and strength in the lesser-trained body builders; however, boron supplementation did not impact any of the variables measured, and thus did not have an ergogenic effect.

VIII. LIMITATIONS OF PREVIOUS RESEARCH

Though a great deal of research has been conducted on minerals and athletes, more is necessary. Moreover, the research that has been published has limitations, which include, but are not limited to: (1) small sample sizes, (2) variations in type of sport studied, (3) variations in levels of training and fitness of athletes researched, (4) lack of solid longitudinal data, (5) variations in methodology or study design (many have been cross-sectional), (6) variations in the types and amounts of supplementation used, and (7) some researchers used a combination of vitamin and mineral supplements, making it difficult to determine the effects of one particular vitamin or mineral.[79]

IX. FUTURE RESEARCH NEEDS

More research is required on dietary intake of the aforementioned minerals and on all minerals in a variety of athletes of all ages. A prospective study that would systematically assess the dietary intake of all types of athletes over a 2-year period would provide information on the typical dietary intake of athletes. During this prospective study, evaluation of mineral status would ascertain if the intake and status are compatible, and if not, measures can be taken to determine why. Though it is difficult to evaluate if one mineral has a significant impact over another, randomized double-blind, placebo-controlled trials on a large population of athletes can more definitively determine if supplementation (or increased intake) positively impacts exercise performance. Aside from type of athlete, sport, and gender, the impact of age on mineral intake and status in athletes would also be important to examine.

X. CONCLUSIONS

Based on the studies discussed in this chapter, athletes do appear to consume inadequate amounts of many micronutrients (and energy); however, not all athletes have impaired nutritional status, which could be a result of study design or methods of assessment, and not their true status. In addition, supplementation did not always lead to improved athletic performance. Maughan[80] stated it well in his review, "When talented, motivated and highly trained athletes meet for competition the margin between victory and defeat is usually small. When everything else is equal, nutrition can make the difference between winning and losing" (p. 87).

Economos et al.[81] published a review article evaluating 22 research studies on the nutritional intake of athletes. Based on their review, they propose an energy intake of > 50 kcal/kg/day for male athletes who train for more than 90 minutes/day, and 45 to 50 kcal/kg/day for female athletes who train for > 90 minutes/day. They also suggest that athletes who consume low-energy diets focus on sufficient intakes of iron, calcium, magnesium, zinc and vitamin B_{12}. "There is no special food that will help elite athletes perform better; the most important aspect of the diet of elite athletes is that it follows the basic guidelines for healthy eating" (p. 381).[81] In addition, athletes should work with a registered dietitian to construct nutritional and performance goals, those that will lead to consistent eating and training, and to improved performance.[79,80] With respect to the minerals reviewed for this chapter, it appears that, if energy intake is adequate, balanced, and varied, and nutritional status is within normal limits, supplementation is not warranted.[80,82] It may be warranted for athletes who restrict energy intake, participate in sports with weight restrictions, or limit certain foods and food groups.[82] Mineral supplementation, in particular calcium, magnesium, chromium and boron, does not appear to have ergogenic effects.

REFERENCES

1. Wardlaw, G.M., *Perspectives in Nutrition* 4th ed., WCB McGraw-Hill, Boston, Massachusetts, 1999.
2. Burke L., and Heeley P., Dietary supplements and nutritional ergogenic aids in sport, in *Clinical Sports Nutrition*, Burke L. and Deakin V., Eds., McGraw-Hill,. Sydney, Australia, 1994, 227–284.
3. Kimura N., Fukuwatari T., Sasaki R., Hayakawa F., and Shibata K., Vitamin intake in Japanese women college students, *J. Nutr. Sci. Vitaminol.* 49(3), 149–155, 2003.
4. Food and Nutrition Board of the Institute of Medicine. Dietary Reference Intakes for Calcium, Phosphorus, Magnesium, Vitamin D, and Fluoride. National Academy Press, Washington, DC, 1997.
5. Food and Nutrition Board of the Institute of Medicine. Dietary Reference Intakes for Thiamin, Riboflavin, Niacin, Vitamin B_6, Folate, Vitamin B_{12}, Pantothenic Acid, Biotin, and Choline. National Academy Press, Washington, DC, 1998.
6. Food and Nutrition Board of the Institute of Medicine. Dietary Reference Intakes for Vitamin C, Vitamin E, Selenium, and Carotenoids. National Academy Press, Washington, DC, 2000.
7. Food and Nutrition Board of the Institute of Medicine. Dietary Reference Intakes for Vitamin A, Vitamin K, Arsenic, Boron, Chromium, Copper, Iodine, Iron, Manganese,

Molybdenum, Nickel, Silicon, Vanadium, and Zinc. National Academy Press, Washington, DC, 2000.

8. Food and Nutrition Board of the Institute of Medicine. Dietary Reference Intakes for Water, Potassium, Sodium, Chloride, and Sulfate. National Academy Press, Washington, DC, 2005.
9. Clark M., Reed D.B., Crouse S.F., and Armstrong R.B., Pre– and post–season dietary intake, body composition, and performance indices of NCAA division I female soccer players, *Int. J. Sport. Nutr. Exerc. Metab.* 13(3), 303–319, 2003.
10. Magkos F., and Yannakoulia M., Methodology of dietary assessment in athletes: Concepts and pitfalls, *Curr. Opin. Clin. Nutr. Metab. Care.* 6(5), 539–549, 2003.
11. Weaver, C., and Heaney, R.P., Calcium, in *Modern Nutrition in Health and Disease*, 10th ed., Shils, M.E., Shike, M., Ross, A.C., Caballero, B., and Cousins R.J., Eds., Lippincott Williams & Wilkins, Philadelphia, PA, 194–210, 2006.
12. Volpe, S.L., Vitamins, minerals, and exercise, in *Sports Nutrition: A Practical Manual for Professionals*, 4th edition, Dunford M., Ed., The American Dietetic Association, Chicago, IL, 61–93, 2006.
13. Nattiv, A., Loucks, A.B., Manore, M.M., Sanborn, C.F., Sundgot–Borgen, J., Warren, M.P., American College of Sports Medicine, American College of Sports Medicine position stand. The Female Athlete Triad, *Med. Sci. Sports. Exerc.* 39(10), 1867–1882, 2007.
14. U.S. Department of Agriculture ARS. USDA Nutrient Database for Standard Reference Release 16. Nutrient Data Laboratory Home Page. 2003. http://www.nal.usda.gov/fnic/foodcomp.
15. Pennington, J., Bowes, A., Church, H., *Bowes & Church's Food Values of Portions Commonly Used,* 17th ed, Philadelphia, Lippincott Williams & Wilkins, 1998.
16. Heaney, R.P., Dowell, M.S., Rafferty, K., and Bierman, J., Bioavailability of the calcium in fortified soy imitation milk, with some observations on method, *Am. J. Clin. Nutr.* 71, 1166–1169, 2000.
17. Zalcman, I., Guarita, H.V., Juzwiak, C.R., Crispim, C.A., Antunes, H.K., Edwards, B., et al., Nutritional status of adventure racers, *Nutrition.* 23(5), 404–411, 2007.
18. Lovell, G., Vitamin D status of females in an elite gymnastics program, *Clin. J. Sport. Med.* 18(2), 159–161, 2008.
19. Beals, K.A., Eating behaviors, nutritional status, and menstrual function in elite female adolescent volleyball players, *J. Am. Diet. Assoc.* 102(9), 1293–1296, 2002.
20. Bunout, D., Barrera, G., Leiva, L., Gattas, V., de la Maza, M.P., Avendaño, M., and Hirsch, S., Effects of vitamin D supplementation and exercise training on physical performance in Chilean vitamin D deficient elderly subjects, *Exp. Gerontol.* 41(8), 746–752, 2006.
21. Koh-Banerjee, P.K., Ferreira, M.P., Greenwood, M., Bowden, R.G., Cowan, P.N., Almada, A.L., and Kreider, R.B., Effects of calcium pyruvate supplementation during training on body composition, exercise capacity, and metabolic responses to exercise, *Nutrition.* 21(3), 312–319, 2005.
22. Trowman, R., Dumville, J.C., Hahn, S., and Torgerson, D.J., A systematic review of the effects of calcium supplementation on body weight, *Br. J. Nutr.* 95(6), 1033–1038, 2006.
23. Barba, G., Russo, P., Dairy foods, dietary calcium and obesity: A short review of the evidence, *Nutr Metab. Cardiov. Disease.* 16(6), 445–451, 2006.
24. Shi, H., Dirienzo, D., and Zemel, M.B., Effects of dietary calcium on adipocyte lipid metabolism and body weight regulation in energy-restricted aP2-agouti transgenic mice, *FASEB J.* 15, 291–293, 2001.
25. Carruth, B.R., and Skinner, J.D., The role of dietary calcium and other nutrients in moderating body fat in preschool children, *Int. J. Obes.* 25, 559–566, 2001.

26. Skinner, J.D., Bounds, W., Carruth, B.R., and Ziegler, P., Longitudinal calcium intake is negatively related to children's body fat indexes, *J. Am. Diet. Assoc.* 103(12), 1626–1631, 2003.
27. Berkey, C.S., Rockett, H.R., Willett, W.C., and Colditz, G.A., Milk, dairy fat, dietary calcium, and weight gain: a longitudinal study of adolescents, *Arch. Pediat. Adolesc. Med.* 159(6), 543–550, 2005.
28. Davies, K.M., Heaney, R.P., Recker, R.R., Lappe, J.M., Barger-Lux, M.J., Rafferty, K., and Hinders, S., Calcium intake and body weight, *J. Clin. Endocrinol. Metab.* 85(12), 4635–4638, 2000.
29. Zemel, M.B., Thompson, W., Milstead, A., Morris, K., and Campbell, P., Calcium and dairy acceleration of weight and fat loss during energy restriction in obese adults, *Obes. Res.* 12(4), 582–590, 2004.
30. Melanson, E.L., Sharp, T.A., Schneider, J., Donahoo, W.T., Grunwald, G.K., and Hill, J.O., Relation between calcium intake and fat oxidation in adult humans, *Int. J. Obes.* 27, 196–203, 2003.
31. Melanson, E.L., Donahoo, W.T., Dong, F., Ida, T., and Zemel, M.B., Effect of low- and high-calcium dairy-based diets on macronutrient oxidation in humans, *Obes. Res.* 13(12), 2102–2112, 2005.
32. Boon, N., Hul, G.B., Viguerie, N., Sicard, A., Langin, D., and Saris, W.H. Effects of 3 diets with various calcium contents on 24-h energy expenditure, fat oxidation, and adipose tissue message RNA expression of lipid metabolism-related proteins, *Am. J. Clin. Nutr.* 82(6), 1244–1252, 2005.
33. Wyatt, H.R., Jortberg, B.T., Babbel, C., Garner, S., Dong, F., Grunwald, G.K., and Hill, J.O., Weight loss in a community initiative that promotes decreased energy intake and increased physical activity and dairy consumption: Calcium weighs-in, *J. Phys. Act. Health.* 5(1), 28–44, 2008.
34. Elin, R.J., Magnesium: The fifth but forgotten electrolyte, *Am. J. Clin. Pathol.* 102(5), 616–622, 1994.
35. Takaya, J., Higashino, H., and Kobayashi Y., Intracellular magnesium and insulin resistance, *Magnes. Res.* 17(2), 126–136, 2004.
36. Volpe, S.L., Magnesium in *Present Knowledge in Nutrition*, 9th edition, Bowman, B.A., and Russell, R.M., Eds., ILSI Press, Washington, DC, 400–408, 2006.
37. Bohl, C.H., and Volpe, S.L., Magnesium and exercise, *Crit. Rev. Food. Sci. Nutr.* 42(6), 533–563, 2002.
38. Volpe, S.L., Magnesium, the metabolic syndrome, insulin resistance and type 2 diabetes mellitus, *Crit. Rev. Food. Sci. Nutr.* 48(3), 293–300, 2008.
39. Newhouse, I.J., and Finstad E.W., The effects of magnesium supplementation on exercise performance, *Clin. J. Sport. Med.* 10, 195–200, 2000.
40. Rude, R.K., and Shils, M.E., Magnesium, in *Modern Nutrition in Health and Disease*, 10th ed., Shils, M.E., Shike, M., Ross, A.C., Caballero, B., and Cousins R.J., Eds., Lippincott Williams & Wilkins, Philadelphia, 223–247, 2006.
41. Chubanov, V., Gudermann, T., and Schlingmann, K.P., Essential role for TRPM6 in epithelial magnesium transport and body magnesium homeostasis, *Pflugers. Arch.* 451(1), 228–334, 2005.
42. Paolisso, G., and Barbagallo, M., Hypertension, diabetes mellitus, and insulin resistance: The role of intracellular magnesium, *Am. J. Hypertens.* 10(3), 346–355, 1997.
43. Barbagallo, M., Dominguez, L.J., Galioto, A., Ferlisi, A., Cani, C., Malfa, L., et al., Role of magnesium in insulin action, diabetes and cardio–metabolic syndrome X, *Mol. Aspects. Med.* 24(1–3), 39–52, 2003.
44. He, K., Liu, K., Daviglus, M.L., Morris, S.J., Loria, C.M., Van Horn, L., et al., Magnesium intake and incidence of metabolic syndrome among young adults, *Circulation.* 113(13), 1675–1682, 2006.

45. Murakami, K., Okubo, H., and Sasaki, S., Effect of dietary factors on incidence of type 2 diabetes: A systematic review of cohort studies, *J. Nutr. Sci. Vitaminol.* (Tokyo) 51(4), 292–310, 2005.
46. Guerrero-Romero, F., and Rodriguez-Moran, M., Hypomagnesemia is linked to low serum HDL-cholesterol irrespective of serum glucose values, *J. Diabetes Complications.* 14, 272–276, 2000.
47. Gropper, S. S., Smith, J. L., and Groff, J. L., Magnesium, in *Advanced Nutrition and Human Metabolism* (4th ed.), Thomson and Wadsworth, Belmont, CA, 2005.
48. Rankinen, T., Lyytikainen, S., Vanninen, E., Penttila, I., Rauramaa, R., and Uusitupa, M., Nutritional status of the Finnish elite ski jumpers, *Med. Sci. Sports. Exerc.* 30(11), 1592–1597, 1998.
49. Hassapidou, M.N., and Manstrantoni, A., Dietary intakes of elite female athletes in Greece, *J. Hum. Nutr. Diet.* 14(5), 391–396, 2001.
50. Papadopoulou, S.K., Papadopoulou, S.D., and Gallos, G.K., Macro– and micro–nutrient intake of adolescent Greek female volleyball players, *Int. J. Sport. Nutr. Exerc. Metab.* 12(1), 73–80, 2002.
51. Cinar, V., Nizamlioglu, M., Mogulkoc, R., and Baltaci, A.K., Effects of magnesium supplementation on blood parameters of athletes at rest and after exercise, *Biol. Trace. Elem. Res.* 115(3), 205–212, 2007.
52. Finstad, E.W., Newhouse, I.J., Lukaski, H.C., Mcauliffe, J.E., and Stewart, C.R., The effects of magnesium supplementation on exercise performance, *Med. Sci. Sports. Exerc.* 33(3), 493–498, 2001.
53. Pokan, R., Hofmann, P., von Duvillard, S.P., Smekal, G., Wonisch, M., Lettner, K., et al., Oral magnesium therapy, exercise heart rate, exercise tolerance, and myocardial function in coronary artery disease patients, *Br. J. Sports. Med.* 40(9), 773–778, 2006.
54. Kumeda, Y., and Inaba M., Metabolic syndrome and magnesium, *Clin. Calcium.* 15(11), 97–104, 2005.
55. Soltani, N., Keshavarz, M., Minaii, B., Mirershadi, F., Asl, S.Z., and Dehpour, A.R., Effects of administration of oral magnesium on plasma glucose and pathological changes in the aorta and pancreas of diabetic rats, *Clin. Exp. Pharmacol. Physiol.* 32(8), 604–610, 2005.
56. McCarty, M.F., Magnesium may mediate the favorable impact of whole grains on insulin sensitivity by acting as a mild calcium antagonist, *Med. Hypotheses.* 64(3), 619–627, 2005.
57. Lopez-Ridaura, R., Willett, W.C., Rimm, E.B., Liu, S., Stampfer, M.J., Manson, J.E., and Hu, F.B., Magnesium intake and risk of type 2 diabetes in men and women, *Diabetes Care.* 27(1), 134–140, 2004.
58. Guerrero-Romero, F., Rodríguez-Morán, M., Low serum magnesium levels and metabolic syndrome, *Acta Diabetológica.* 39, 209–213, 2002.
59. Song, Y., Manson, J.E., Buring, J.E., and Liu, S., Dietary magnesium intake in relation to plasma insulin levels and risk of type 2 diabetes in women, *Diabetes Care,* 27(1), 59–65, 2004.
60. Rodríguez-Morán, M., and Guerrero-Romero, F., Oral Magnesium supplementation improves insulin sensitivity and metabolic control in Type 2 diabetic subjects. A randomized, double–blind controlled trial, *Diabetes Care,* 26, 1147–1152, 2003.
61. Kobla, H.V., and Volpe, S.L., Chromium, exercise, and body composition, *Crit. Rev. Food. Sci. Nutr.* 40(4), 291–308, 2000.
62. Hellerstein, M.K., Is chromium supplementation effective in managing type II diabetes? *Nutr. Rev.* 56(10), 302–306, 1998.
63. Volpe, S.L., Huang, H.-W., Larpadisorn, K., and Lesser, I.I., Effect of chromium supplementation on body composition, resting metabolic rate, and selected biochemical

parameters in moderately obese women following an exercise program, *J. Am. Coll. Nutr.* 20(4), 293–306, 2001.

64. Pasman, W.J., Westerterp-Plantenga, M.S., and Saris, W.H., The effectiveness of long-term supplementation of carbohydrate, chromium, fibre and caffeine on weight maintenance, *Int. J. Obes. Rel. Met. Dis.* 21(12), 1143–1151, 1997.
65. Walker, L.S., Bemben, M.G., Bemben, D.A., and Knehans, A.W., Chromium picolinate effects on body composition and muscular performance in wrestlers, *Med. Sci. Sports Exerc.* 30(12), 1730–1737, 1998.
66. Volek, J.S., Silvestre, R., Kirwan, J.P., Sharman, M.J., Judelson, D.A., Spiering, B.A., et al., Effects of chromium supplementation on glycogen synthesis after high-intensity exercise, *Med. Sci. Sports Exerc.* 38(12), 2102–2109, 2006.
67. Crawford, V., Scheckenbach, R., and Preuss, H.G., Effects of niacin-bound chromium supplementation on body composition in overweight African-American women, *Diabetes Obes. Met.* 1, 331–337, 1999.
68. Hoeger, W.W.K., Harris, C., Long, E.M., and Hopkins, D.R., Four-week supplementation with a natural dietary compound produces favorable changes in body composition, *Adv. Ther.* 15(5), 305–313, 1998.
69. Devirian, T.A., and Volpe, S.L., The physiological effects of dietary boron, *Crit. Rev. Food. Sci. Nutr.* 43(2), 219–231, 2003.
70. Volpe, S.L., Taper, L.J., and Meacham, S., The relationship between boron and magnesium status and bone mineral density in the human: A review, *Magnes. Res.* 6(3), 291–296, 1993.
71. Kurtoğlu, F., Kurtoğlu, V., Celik, I., Keçeci, T., and Nizamlioğlu, M., Effects of dietary boron supplementation on some biochemical parameters, peripheral blood lymphocytes, splenic plasma cells and bone characteristics of broiler chicks given diets with adequate or inadequate cholecalciferol (vitamin D_3) content, *Br. Poult. Sci.* 46(1), 87–96, 2005.
72. Gallardo-Williams, M.T., Maronpot, R.R., Turner, C.H., Johnson, C.S., Harris, M.W., Jayo, M.J., and Chapin, R.E., Effects of boric acid supplementation on bone histomorphometry, metabolism, and biomechanical properties in aged female F-344 rats, *Biol. Trace. Elem. Res.* 93(1–3), 155–170, 2003.
73. Naghii, M.R., Torkaman, G., and Mofid, M., Effects of boron and calcium supplementation on mechanical properties of bone in rats, *Biofactors.* 28(3–4), 195–201, 2006.
74. Hunt, C.D., Herbel, J.L., and Nielsen, F.H., Metabolic responses of postmenopausal women to supplemental dietary boron and aluminum during usual and low magnesium intake: boron, calcium, and magnesium absorption and retention and blood mineral concentrations, *Am. J. Clin. Nutr.* 65(3), 803–813, 1997.
75. Volpe, S.L., Taper, L.J., and Meacham, S.L., The effect of boron supplementation on bone mineral density and hormonal status in college female athletes, *Med. Exerc. Nutr. Health.* 2(6), 323–330, 1993.
76. Meacham, S.L., Taper, L.J., Volpe, S.L., Effects of boron supplementation on bone mineral density and dietary, blood, and urinary calcium, phosphorus, magnesium, and boron in female athletes, *Environ. Health. Perspect.* 102(Suppl 7), 79–82, 1994.
77. Meacham, S.L., Taper, L.J., and Volpe, S.L. Effect of boron supplementation on blood and urinary calcium, magnesium, and phosphorus, and urinary boron in athletic and sedentary women, *Am. J. Clin. Nutr.* 61(2), 341–345, 1995.
78. Green, N.R., and Ferrando, A.A., Plasma boron and the effects of boron supplementation in males, *Environ. Health. Perspect.* 102(Suppl 7), 73–77, 1994.
79. Volpe, S.L., Micronutrient requirements for athletes, *Clin. Sports Med.* 26(1), 119–130, 2007.

80. Maughan R. The athlete's diet: nutritional goals and dietary strategies, *Proc. Nutr. Soc.* 61(1), 87–96, 2002.
81. Economos CD, Bortz SS, Nelson ME. Nutritional practices of elite athletes. Practical recommendations, *Sports Med.* 16(6), 381–99, 1993.
82. American College of Sports Medicine, American Dietetic Association, Dietitians of Canada. Joint Position Statement: Nutrition and athletic performance. American College of Sports Medicine, American Dietetic Association, Dietitians of Canada, *Med. Sci. Sports Exerc.* 32(12), 2130–45, 2000.

6 Hydration

Susan M. Kleiner and Douglas S. Kalman

CONTENTS

I. INTRODUCTION

The Institute of Medicine (IOM) in 2004 put forth official recommendations as to hydration needs. This official recommendation is a new step within the paradigm of Recommended Daily Intake/Allowance, as prior to 2004, the IOM stated that it was impossible to set a water recommendation.[1] Water is the largest constituent of the human body, accounting for more than 60%. Water is essential for cellular homeostasis, playing important roles in physiological and biochemical functions. Many factors impact daily hydration needs as well as our ability to hydrate.

First, as this is a text concerning nutrition and physical activity, how the body regulates and utilizes water is of importance. For example, when we exercise, core body temperature increases. This increase is coupled with heat dissipation. Heat dissipation will result in cutaneous vasodilation and change in heat transfer and exchange. If heat transfer via radiation and convection is not adequate in reducing the heat load, sweating will occur and heat will be lost by evaporation. If the water loss exceeds fluid intake, hypohydration leading to dehydration will occur.

Water is a macronutrient that is underappreciated. The IOM has created a level of water intake deemed to describe the Adequate Intake (AI). The AI is meant "to prevent deleterious, primary acute, effects of dehydration, which include metabolic and functional abnormalities" (p. 73).[1] It must be recognized that there is extreme difficulty in establishing a specific level of water intake that ensures adequate hydration and promotes optimal health under all potential conditions. Understanding the relationship between hydration states and optimal wellness along with disease relationships allows for the belief that there is a relationship between hydration and disease. Further, it is believed that hydration may play a role in the prevention of prolonged birth labor, urolithiasis, urinary tract infections, bladder cancer, constipation, pulmonary and bronchial disorders, heart disease, hypertension, venous thrombosis, and other conditions.[2,3]

The purpose of this chapter is to provide a basic fund of information as related to the aspects that affect hydration needs and fluid balance. The provision of fluid guidelines for the physically active adult and the non-active adult are included. Total lifecycle hydration is not covered herein but can be read elsewhere.[4]

II. TOPICAL OVERVIEW OF WATER

Water is an often-overlooked macronutrient. In light of the rising incidence and prevalence of overweight and obesity in developed nations, the majority of news and translation of nutrition-related research has focused on carbohydrates, protein, and fat and not hydration. The relationship between fluid intake and health is well known. A reduction in total body water stores by as little as 2% can adversely impact aerobic performance, orthostatic tolerance, and cognitive function. The body is composed of 50 to 70% water (the average of 60% is the norm in the literature) and fluid is stored or circulating. For example, muscle contains about 73% water, blood 93%, and fat mass has 10%. It is known that approximately 5–10% of total body water is turned over daily through obligatory losses (respiration, urine, and sweat). Respiratory water losses are typically recouped by the production of metabolic water formed by substrate oxidation. Fluid losses during and post-exercise also affect overall fluid balance. Thus, fluid balance is easiest thought of as wanting to achieve a balance between fluid output and intake. It has been reported that physically active adults who reside in warmer climates have daily water needs of 6 liters, with highly active populations needing even more to remain euhydrated.[5]

Water is a fluid that acts as a solvent and a transport system within the human body. It plays a central role in thermoregulation and optimal health and its acute status can affect many metabolic processes as well as physical performance and mental acuity.

Currently, the average fluid intake in the United States averages to 48 ounces per day with 19% of the fluid intake coming from foods.[6] Therefore, Americans are typically under-hydrated based on the IOM guidelines, which recommend in general that men aged 19 to 70+ consume 3.7 L/day and women aged 19 to 70+ ingest 2.7 L/d of all water sources daily (water, other liquids, and foods).

III. PROPERTIES OF WATER

Water is a multifunctional macronutrient. One of its most important functions is heat regulation (body heat). Water acts as a buffer; if there is high specific heat (the specific heat of water equals 1 when 1 kg of water is heated 1°C between 15 and 16°C).

TABLE 6.1
Daily Euhydration Variability of Total Body Water

	Liters	% Body Mass
Temperature climate	+ 0.165	+ 0.2
Heat exercise conditions	+ 0.382	+ 0.5
Daily Plasma Volume Variability		
		% Blood Volume
All conditions	+ 0.027	+ 0.6

Source: Adapted from McArdle, W.D., Katch, F.I., Katch V.L. 1999. *Sports and Exercise Nutrition*, Lippincott Williams & Wilkins, Philadelphia.[9]

The body is about 60% fluid, therefore a 70-kg man will contain ~42 kg of water throughout the body.[7] For every 1 degree rise in temperature in a 70 kg person, ~58 calories (kg-calories termed herein as calories) will be oxidized, thus the heat buffering effect of water also results in increased metabolic rate.

Thermoregulation is connected to exercise physiology (and thus physical activity) as evidenced by the evaporation of sweat, for every gram of sweat evaporated (liquid to vapor) from the skin; the body expends 0.58 calories (or 2.43 kjoules).[7,8] Therefore, we can see that water not only has high specific heat, but also assists in the transfer of heat from areas of production to dissipation. Heat transport occurs with minimal change in actual blood temperature.

Water readily transverses all cell membranes in the body. Osmotic and hydrostatic gradients dictate the movement of water. Coupled with this is that water also is affected by the activity of adenosine triphosphatase (ATPase) sodium-potassium pump (Na-K pump). Body water as a percent of body mass is distributed in the following manner (considering total body water [TBW] as 53% of total body mass): 30% cellular, 23% extracellular, 19% interstitial, 4% plasma. There is a natural daily turnover of water in the body, which can be referred to as daily euhydration variability of TBW.[9] (See Table 6.1.) When exercise is enjoyed on a regular basis by a person who previously was not engaging in activity, fluid shifts occur and plasma volume will expand. The body tightly regulates fluid balance.

IV. DEFINITION AND SYMPTOMS OF DEHYDRATION

Dehydration can be acute, perhaps following a bout of intense exercise, or chronic, resulting from less than adequate rehydration of daily water losses over a period of time. Both types of dehydration are defined as a 1% or greater loss of body weight due to fluid losses.[10,11]

Severe dehydration begins at a level of 3% or greater losses of body weight in fluid, and, as it progresses to higher levels of fluid loss, can become life threatening. Mild dehydration is defined as 1% to 2% loss of body weight due to fluid losses, and even at this lower level when chronically experienced can lead to diminished performance and morbidity.

TABLE 6.2
Symptoms of Dehydration

Early Signs	Severe Signs
Fatigue	Difficulty swallowing
Loss of appetite	Stumbling
Flushed skin	Clumsiness
Burning in stomach	Shriveled skin
Light-headedness	Sunken eyes and dim vision
Headache	Painful urination
Dry mouth	Numb skin
Dry cough	Muscle spasm
Heat intolerance	Delirium
Dark urine with a strong odor	

Early signs of dehydration include headache, fatigue, loss of appetite, flushed skin, heat intolerance, light-headedness, dry mouth and eyes, burning sensation in the stomach, and dark urine with a strong odor. Signs of more advanced, severe dehydration include difficulty swallowing, clumsiness, shriveled skin, sunken eyes and dim vision, painful urination, numb skin, muscle spasms, and delirium.[12] (See Table 6.2.)

It has been postulated that muscle cramps may be related to hydration status since muscles cramp more frequently when the body is dehydrated.[13] Heat cramps, the least serious of the three heat-related disorders (heat cramps, heat exhaustion, heat stroke) is characterized by severe cramping of the skeletal muscles that are used most heavily during exercise. It is likely that high sweat rates and dehydration disrupt the balance between the electrolytes potassium and sodium, leading to cramps. However, a cause-and-effect relationship has not been established. Recovery from exercise-associated muscle cramps requires moving the individual to a cool location (in the case of heat cramps), fluid replacement, and restoration of electrolyte balance.[14] Schwellnus, et al. however, postulate a new hypothesis unrelated to hydration status.[15] The researchers hypothesize that exercise-associated muscle cramps are caused by sustained abnormal spinal reflex activity which appears secondary to muscle fatigue. Local muscle fatigue is therefore responsible for increased muscle spindle afferent and decreased Golgi tendon organ afferent activity.

V. REGULATION OF THIRST AND HYDRATION

Thirst is subjective. The perception of being thirsty is also a subjective motivator to quench the thirst in animals and humans.[16] Regulatory systems maintain body fluid levels essential for long-term survival. Factors influencing fluid needs and urge to drink include cultural and societal habits combined with internal psychogenic drive and the regulatory controls to maintain fluid homeostasis. Regulatory control includes maintaining fluid content of various bodily compartments, the osmotic gradient of the extracellular fluids, or work with specific hormones to assist in the regulation.

When the body loses water, it is usually depleted from both the extracellular and intracellular spaces. These losses might not be equal in volume. Water and sodium chloride (NaCl), the major solute of the extracellular fluid, results in proportionately more extracellular fluid depletion than if water alone is lost. If fluid losses come from the gastrointestinal tract (i.e., diarrhea) and are of normal osmostic load (isotonic), then the depletion will be entirely from the extracellular fluid. However, if hypertonic fluid is added to the extracellular compartment, there will be an osmotic depletion of water from the intracellular compartment into the extracellular fluid, and this latter compartment will be expanded.

A range of compensatory responses can occur in synchronicity with losses from the intra- or extracellular space. Understanding the effects of vasopressin secretion, stimulation of the renin-angiotensin-aldosterone system, sympathetic activation, and reduced renal solute and water excretion is important when addressing hydration in the athlete. Hormonal responses to fluid losses however, are not solutions to returning the athlete to a euhydrated state. The only means to do this is by hydrating the individual to the tune of 600 mL per 0.46 kg of body weight lost (~1320 mL per kg weight lost). Thirst can be thought of as one component, the "vocal" component of the body's response to fluid shifts or losses.

The regulation of thirst includes osmoregulation. The osmotic pressure of the fluid (plasma osmolality) typically lies between 280–295 mosmol/kg/H20. Losses as small as 1 to 2% of body weight stimulate thirst. At this point, the athlete is already becoming dehydrated. Thirst is one response to an increase in the osmotic gradient. Changes in NaCl or glucose induce this response by not crossing across cell membranes so easily. The osmotic differences between the intracellular and extracellular spaces are what dictate the flow of fluids (higher to lower concentration occurring typically by osmosis. Osmosis is partially regulated by osmoreceptors (relative to vasopressin) in the brain and in the liver.

It is obvious that thirst regulation is multifactorial. Within the central nervous system (CNS) osmotic, ionic, hormonal, and nervous signals are integrated and impact the perception of thirst. Overcoming hypo- or dehydration following the ingestion of water or fluid involves additional pathways and factors that are beyond the scope of this chapter. If the level of hypohydration is greater that 3% of body weight loss, complete rehydration requires more than just fluid replacement from simple beverages. Food or other osmolar intake is often necessary for complete rehydration, which may require 18–24 hours.[17]

Environment can alter the thirst mechanism. Water immersion induces shifts in vascular volume and in the concentration and activity of vasopressin, renin-angiotensin II, and atrial natriuretic polypeptide, the hormones and enzymes associated with thirst and drinking.[17] Thus, in addition to the blunted thirst response associated with exercise,[18] it is likely that swimmers may have virtually no thirst response during immersion.

Taste influences hydration and beverage choice in adults and children.[19,20] Surveys show that individuals are guided by taste when they choose what and how much they drink. In children, the magnitude of rehydration is significantly affected by the flavor of the available beverage.[20]

Factors that influence urinary excretion rates and volume influence hydration status. Caffeine, based on dose response, is a diuretic. The first 1 to 3 cups (237 mL to 711 mL) of regularly caffeinated beverages (coffee, tea, cola) are typically not high enough in caffeine to act as a diuretic. However, amounts great than 114 mg to 253 mg per day (Grandjean), as often found in energy drinks, may act as a diuretic, depending on individual caffeine tolerance.[78] Alcohol is another natural diuretic. It depresses production of the antidiuretic hormone (ADH, aka vasopressin) by the pituitary gland in the brain. The kidney responds to ADH by reabsorbing water, preventing water loss. When ADH secretion is depressed, water losses increase. There is no threshold dose response for alcohol; just one drink causes a diuretic response.

The fact that disease or metabolic disorder states can impact hydration status cannot be overlooked even in the apparently healthy athlete.

VI. HYDRATION AND HEALTH AND DISEASE

Body fluid losses occur from the intra and extracellular compartments. The loss of NaCl causes greater losses from the extracellular space. In sweat, NaCl is lost at a rate of 7:1 compared with potassium.[16] Thus, fluid losses of 1–2% of body weight or greater induce the need for fluid and electrolyte replacement. However, the importance of hydration state and health or disease prevention is often overlooked. In addition, aging (advanced age) may also be a risk factor for dehydration.

Because many diseases have multifactorial origins, lifestyle, genetics, environment, and other factors including the state of hydration are worthy of examination. Mild dehydration is a factor in the development of various conditions and diseases. Conditions associated with the negative impacts of hypohydration or dehydration include alterations in amniotic fluids, prolonged labor, cystic fibrosis, renal toxicity secondary to dehydration altering how contrast agents are metabolized. The effects of chronic hypohydration or dehydration (systemic effects) include associations with (ranging from weak to mild) urinary tract infections, gallstones, constipation, hypertension, bladder and colon cancer, venous thromboembolism, cerebral infarcts, dental diseases, kidney stones, mitral valve prolapse, glaucoma, and diabetic ketoacidosis.[21] Rehydration and proper hydration assist with condition management, disease prevention, and the betterment of health. Factors that can effect hydration include: high ambient temperature, the relative humidity, high sweat losses (sweat rates), increased body temperature, exercise duration, training status of the individual, exercise intensity, high body fat percentage, underwater exercise, use of diuretic medications, and uncontrolled diabetes. The assessment of an athlete for hydration should include a review of all of the aforementioned factors.

Today, approximately 12–15% of the general population will form a kidney stone at some time.[22,23] Many factors can modify the urinary risk factors for developing stones, including age, sex, heredity, occupation, social class and affluence, geographic location and climate, and diet. Of these, diet—especially fluid intake—is the only one that can be easily changed and that has a marked effect on all urinary risk factors.[24] Stone prevalence is higher in populations with low urinary volume.[22–30] A decreased fluid intake leads to a low urine volume and increased concentrations of all stone-forming salts. The risk of stone formation is increased with urine volumes of less than 1 L/d. When fluid intake is increased to allow for urinary volumes of more than 2–2.5 L/d, without any changes in diet or other pharmacologic intervention, recurrences of all types of stones can be prevented in a large number of patients.[24–26,28]

According to Hughes and Norman, individuals at risk for urinary stone formation should consume at least 250 mL of fluid to be taken with each meal, between meals, before bedtime, and when the patient gets up at night to void. This pattern will ensure that the fluid intake is spread out over the day and that the urine is not concentrated. Patients with stones should also increase their fluid intake in hotter weather and after vigorous exercise.[24]

Several studies have discovered a direct correlation between the quantity of fluid consumed and the incidence of certain cancers.[31–34] Internationally, studies have found that urinary tract cancer subjects drink significantly less fluid than their cancer-free counterparts. The incidence of cancers of the bladder, prostate, kidney, testicle, renal pelvis, and ureter are inversely associated with water and fluid intake.

Similar findings have be made regarding colon and breast cancer.[32,33] In a population-based case-control study of the association between food groupings and colon cancer in Seattle, Washington, researchers identified a strong inverse dose–response relationship between water intake, measured as glasses of water consumed per day, and risk of colon cancer among women. Women who drank more than five glasses (no exact amount specified by authors) of water a day had a 45% decreased risk of colon cancer vs. those who consumed two or fewer glasses per day (OR for > 5 glasses/day vs. ≤ 2 glasses/day, 0.55; 95% CI, 0.31–0.99; P for trend 0.004). Among men there was a 32% decrease in risk with increasing water consumption (> 4 glasses/day vs. ≤1 glass/day), although it was not statistically significant.[32]

Acute, nonspecific diarrhea, even though transient, can cause mild to moderate dehydration that can become chronic if adequate rehydration does not occur. This can be particularly problematic during times of travel for athletes. Patients with signs or symptoms of dehydration, including dry mouth, excessive thirst, wrinkled skin, little or no urination, dizziness, or lightheadedness, should see a physician. Children with severe diarrhea or vomiting that continues for more than 24 hours should be evaluated for potential dehydration. Fluid intakes should equal 2 to 3 liters per day to avoid the hypohydration associated with acute diarrhea.[35]

Active seniors who represent the population of the "healthy elderly" still are at greater risk of dehydration. Numerous studies have demonstrated significant hypodipsia and diminished thirst sensations in the elderly.[36–38] In spite of the fact that these changes may be a normal adaptation of the aging process,[37] the consequences of dehydration in the elderly are serious and range from constipation and fecal impaction to cognitive impairment, functional decline, and death.[39] Patients with Alzheimer's disease may have additional impairment to their thirst mechanism.[40] Specific recommendations to avoid dehydration in the elderly have been published.[39–41]

The goal with each individual, whether athletic or not, is euhydration. Hydration needs have been detailed by the IOM for both genders. However, the practicality of application is hard for the everyday consumer. Easy "rule of thumb" hydration guidelines for general health are needed. Many dietitians tell their clients to shoot for a goal of drinking the equivalent in ounces of half their body weight. If you weigh

150 pounds, your beverage consumption goal per day with normal activities is 75 ounces of non-alcoholic fluid.

VII. HYDRATION AND PHYSICAL AND ATHLETIC PERFORMANCE

The consistent conclusion across multiple studies, academic societies, and training associations is that dehydration can significantly impact performance, especially in warm or hot conditions. Thus, fluid replacement guidelines have been established to minimize exertional dehydration. Dehydration is defined as a 2% loss of euhydrated body weight.[42] This negatively impacts athletic performance. Dehydration is associated with a reduction or an adverse effect on muscle strength, endurance, coordination, mental acuity, and the thermoregulatory processes.

Water losses during exercise are affected by the aforementioned parameters and, because the inter-individual variation in sweat rates are so wide, no universal recommendations are used. The closest universal rule is that for every pound of body weight lost between the initiation of exercise and the cessation, one replaces with 600 mL per 0.46 kg of body weight lost (20 ounces per pound [1.25 pints per pound; 1300 mL/kg] of body weight lost) (L. Armstrong, personal communication).

During prolonged exercise fluid and sodium losses occur. Human sweat contains 40–50 mmol sodium per liter.[42] For the most part, in the normal healthy person, large fluid losses are followed by large sodium losses. The typical sodium to potassium ratio of losses is 7:1. An athlete engaged in prolonged exercise can lose 5 liters of fluid per day with a range of 4600 to 5750 mg sodium and much smaller amounts of potassium. Heat-acclimated athletes benefit from enhanced sodium reabsorption that results in better protection of plasma volume by reducing the sodium losses. Training state of the athlete is very important when contemplating fluid needs. Salt losses do not directly impact physical performance; however, using salts in fluid replacement is proven to enhance the thirst response and aid in rehydration.

Hypohydration (1% body weight loss) also decreases the ability of athletes to perform. Athletes as a rule do not replace sweat or sodium losses enough during an event. The average marathon runner will lose up to 3% body weight and, if the run is not in a temperate climate and temperatures are more extreme, the losses could be 5%. According to Maughan, elite marathoners tend to sweat at a rate of 2 L/hour. This sweat rate exceeds intestinal absorption capability of the gut.[43,44]

A plethora of studies clearly demonstrate a negative impact of hypohydration and dehydration on athletic performance (range from 1–8% fluid losses). Studies using sports or situations designed to mimic a sport have noted a decrement in performance for soccer, basketball, running/racing, cycling, and others. In addition, better hydration is associated with lower esophageal temperature, heart rate, and ratings of perceived exertion—all factors that may impact performance.[45]

Exercise increases the metabolic rate and, as energy is converted into heat, water losses will occur. In cold climates (winter sports or outdoor sports in mild or cold climates) heat is lost via radiation and convection; as the temperature increases, the losses are noticeable as sweat. The physiological response to exercise is to expand the blood volume and to increase the sensitivity for sweating to occur. Athletes and their coaches, trainers, and nutritionists must be cognizant of changes in osmolarity.

Body temperature and the volume of the liquid being ingested, as well as the osmolarity can affect performance.

Another impact of hypohydration or dehydration that should be a concern to athletes or their training staff is the impact on cognition. The mental aspect of sports coupled with neuromuscular integration cannot be understated. The neuropsychological impacts of hydration as well as the biological mechanisms and behavioral relationships are relatively new in research. Brain behavior and cognitive assessment are also relatively new to the exercise physiology field because many new cognitive assessment tools have become available. This is despite research from the 1940s on fluid and salt intake.[46,47] A review by Lieberman found that hypohydration and dehydration were associated with increased fatigue, impaired discrimination, impaired tracking, impaired short-term memory, impaired recall and attention, while decreased arithmetic ability and a faster response time to peripheral visual stimuli were also noted.[46,47] At a deficit of only 2% loss of body weight as fluid, Gopinathan and coworkers found that subjects demonstrated significant and progressive reductions in the performance of arithmetic ability, short-term memory, and visuomotor tracking compared with the euhydrated state.[48] The applications have been tested not only in academic exercise or psychology research, but military as well. Interestingly enough, dehydration induced by heat as compared with dehydration caused by exercise elicit the same changes in cognitive performance, which indicates that dehydration is the cause, not exercise. Cognitive performance when dehydrated most often results in increased fatigue, tracking errors (vision–brain connection), and a decrease in short-term memory. Ironically, when a person is hyperhydrated, short-term memory is increased, while most of the other parameters mentioned remain neutral with no negative impacts.[49]

In practical terms, if a 150-pound (68-kg) athlete loses only 2% of his or her body weight (3 lbs; 1.4 kg), physical and mental performance can diminish.[50,51] Hence, even chronic mild dehydration (1% to 2% loss of body weight) may negatively affect athletic performance. It is in the best interest of the athlete to maintain a well-hydrated state on a regular basis, and rehydrate during and after exercise as quickly as possible to return to euhydration before the next training bout.[52]

Numerous dietary studies have demonstrated that, on average, athletes do not consume adequate fluids before, during, or after exercise.[53–60] Many athletes habitually self-induce dehydration to qualify for a designated weight class for competition.[56,57,61–64] This practice can dramatically influence exercise performance, including losses in strength, anaerobic power, anaerobic capacity, lactate threshold, and aerobic power.[61,64] Extreme cases of self-induced dehydration have resulted in death.[65]

Children are particularly at risk of dehydration in the heat, even more so than adults.[66–68] Children will rehydrate voluntarily when adequate fluids are made available.[66,67] In lieu of the current understanding that fluid needs are highly individual, the American College of Sports Medicine (ACSM) has issued generalized rather than specific hydration and rehydration guidelines in their current Position Stand on Exercise and Fluid Replacement.[69] Recommendations for prehydrating, if necessary, should include initiating beverages several hours before exercise. Beverages and snacks or small meals with sodium and salt can help stimulate thirst and retain fluids.

Fluid needs are highly individualized during exercise, based on how sweat rates and electrolyte concentrations respond to the exercise tasks, weather conditions, acclimatization, training status, and genetic predisposition, among others. The risk of dehydration and electrolyte loss is greater in prolonged exercise lasting 3 hours or more. The most practical index for customizing a fluid plan is for the individual to monitor body weight changes during training and competition-training sessions to estimate fluid losses associated with a particular task under specific weather conditions.[69]

A starting point for hydration during exercise is offered by the ACSM guidelines: marathon runners who are euhydrated at the start of the race should drink *ad libitum* from 0.4–0.8 liters/hour. The higher rates are "for faster, heavier individuals competing in warm environments, and the lower rates are for the slower, lighter persons competing in cooler environments. There is a risk that if the higher rates are employed by smaller runners, over-consumption may result. When larger runners consume the smaller amount, dehydration risk is higher. While this range is appropriate for marathon runners, it may not be appropriate for other athletes participating in other sports or events under differing conditions. Predicted sweat rates for running have been published.[69]

While the risk for dehydration during marathon events is clear, there is also a risk for hyperhydration, or hyponatremia. Care must be given to avoid emphasis on blanket recommendations that may lead to over-consumption of fluids. Current research supports the recommendation that if actual body weight and sweat loss measures are not available, thirst is the best physiological guideline for individual fluid needs during exercise.[70]

VIII. PRACTICAL MEASUREMENTS OF HYDRATION

Simply put, there is no universal standard for measuring hydration. At least 13 techniques are used for assessing hydration. Water is the body's currency, as it is the medium for circulatory function, biochemical reactions, temperature regulation, and other physiological processes. In addition, fluid turnover occurs as water is lost from fluid–electrolyte shifts, losses from the lungs, skin, and kidneys. Water is gained via food as well as fluid intake.

The types of hydration assessment methods (in the field and lab) include:

- Stable isotope dilution
- Neutron activation analysis
- Bioelectrical impedance (BIA)
- Body mass change
- Plasma osmolality
- Plasma volume change
- Urine osmolality
- Urine specific gravity
- Urine conductivity
- Urine color
- 24-hour urine volume
- Salivary flow rate (osmolality, flow rate, protein content)
- Rating of thirst

An additional practical tool used clinically is the Hydration Assessment Checklist (HA), a lengthy, in-depth assessment designed to screen for hydration problems.[71] The HA is most often used in clinical conditions and in an older population. Older adults, both in the community as well as in long-term care facilities, are often grossly underhydrated, ingesting on average less than 0.26 gallons (1 liter) daily, which is substantially lower than recommended. Of the approximately one-quarter gallon of fluid, few take in water, an essential element supporting cellular and organ health, electrolyte balance, medication absorption and distribution as well as kidney, bladder, and integumentary functioning.

The following factors have been detailed in the literature as to why one gold standard for measuring hydration is not possible:[72]

1. The physiological regulation of total body water volume (i.e., water turnover) and fluid concentrations is complex and dynamic. Renal, thirst, and sweat gland responses are involved to varying degrees, depending on the prevailing activities. Also, renal regulation of water balance (i.e., arginine vasopressin) is distinct from the regulation of tonicity.
2. The 24-hour fluid deficit varies greatly among sedentary individuals and athletes primarily due to the exercise and morphology. The deficit must be matched by food and fluid intake (the fluid portion of food is often overlooked).
3. Sodium and osmolyte consumption affect the daily water requirement. Regional customs impact the "normals" used within biochemical assessment of hydration. For example, the mean 24-hour urine osmolality in Germany is 860 mOsm/kg while in Poland it is 392 mOsm/kg and in the United States it is in the range of 280 to 295 mOsm/kg.
4. The volume and timing of fluid intake alter measurement of hydration. Pure water or hypotonic solutions ingested rapidly can cause dilute urine prior to cellular equilibrium to occur.
5. Urine samples (spot) not representing the true 24-hour void.
6. Experimental designs that differ in assessment techniques (blood vs. urine).
7. Use of stable isotopes to assess hydration. However it is not known if the isotopes are distributed throughout the body uniformly, thus the assumption used in these techniques is faulty.
8. Exercise and physical labor (as well as pregnancy labor) increases blood volume while decreasing renal blood flow and altering the glomerular filtration rate affecting hydration.
9. Changes in osmolarity and osmolality can affect the readings for hydration on certain devices (i.e., BIA).

In addition to the above, many questions exist regarding the use of plasma osmolality as a biomarker for hydration. These include questions regarding the fact that plasma osmolality varies widely depending upon the condition being tested, environment of the test, the pre-exercise hydration state, and the intervention being evaluated.

One question: is there a way to meld laboratory techniques with those in the field so that trainers, coaches and related personnel can better help athletes?

The first item to discuss is the intervention and educational sessions that athletes should receive from appropriate professionals (i.e., exercise physiologist, Registered Dietitian, Sports Nutritionist-CISSN, athletic trainer, etc.). Education is the key to preventing dehydration. Combining education with fluid stations on the field or in the general area of training, available to the athletes at specific intervals with or without *ad libitum* intake available to the athlete may make euhydration an easier goal to maintain.

The field technique using the combination of weighing the athlete before and after the training or competition and using the weight change as the guide for rehydration may just be the best standard when controlling for applicability, financial impact, and ease of education. The rehydration is 600 cc per 0.46 kg of body weight lost (1300 mL/kg). Other techniques that may be able to be used in combination with monitoring weight changes include using blood and urine testing if available. Testing for osmolality (both), sodium (both), and hematocrit levels (blood) are typical and inexpensive.

IX. THE DIFFERENCE BETWEEN WATER AND OTHER MEANS OF REHYDRATION

Normal hydration is achieved with a wide range of fluid intakes by varied humans across the lifespan. Fluid homeostasis can be challenging to maintain during physical work and heat stress. Body water composes 50–70% of body weight. Approximately 5–10% of total body water is turned over daily via obligatory losses. The greater the fluid losses (from non-emergency situations, not medical or surgical), the longer the time it will take for rehydration (4% weight loss may take up to 24 hours to rehydrate), thus prevention and use of foods or fluids that may aid in more expedient rehydration is of importance.[73]

Body water is maintained by matching daily water loss with intake. To a small degree, metabolic water production also contributes hydration (metabolic hydration yields ~250mL/day). The Food and Nutrition Board has established an adequate intake level of 3.7 L/d and 2.7 L/d for men and women respectively.[1] The Continuing Survey of Food Intakes by Individuals (CSFII) concluded that adults receive about 25% of their daily fluid intake from foods.[74]

Maintaining fluid and electrolyte balance means that active individuals need to replace the water and electrolytes lost in sweat. This requires that active individuals, regardless of age, strive to hydrate well before exercise, drink fluids throughout exercise, and rehydrate once exercise is over. As outlined by the American College of Medicine (ACSM) and the National Athletic Trainer's Association (NATA) generous amounts of fluids should be consumed 24 hours before exercise and 400–600 mL of fluid should be consumed 2 hours before exercise (this is about 6 to 10 oz).[75] During exercise, active individuals should attempt to drink ~150–350 mL (6–12 oz) of fluid every 15–20 mins. If exercise is of long duration (usually > 1 hour or 75 mins) or occurs in a hot environment, sport drinks containing carbohydrate and sodium could be used. When exercise is over, most active individuals have some level of dehydration. Drinking enough fluids to cover ~150% of the weight lost during exercise may be needed to replace fluids lost in sweat and urine. This fluid can be part of the post-exercise meal, which should also contain sodium, either in the food or beverages, since diuresis occurs (fluid losses) when only plain water is ingested. Sodium helps the rehydration process by maintaining plasma osmolality and the desire to drink.

Fluid content of foods should not be underestimated or underappreciated by health professionals. High water-content foods listed as food and percent water include: iceberg lettuce (96%), cooked squash (94%), pickle (92%), cantaloupe (90%), orange (87%), apple (86%) and pears (84%) as compared with steak (50%), Cheddar cheese (37%), white bread (36%), cookies (4%) and nuts (~2%). Therefore, including the national recommendation of five to nine fruits and vegetables in the daily diet also assists with hydration.

Pre-exercise, some athletes use beverages that contain > 100 mmol/l NaCl, which can temporarily induce hyperhydration, thus aiding in rehydration. Adding glycerol to the typical sports beverage or oral rehydration solution at a dose of 1.0 to 1.5 gm/kg/body weight also assists in inducing hyperhydration.[75]

Non-water sources of hydration include caffeinated beverages. Caffeine is stated to be a mild diuretic, however, the vast evidence indicates that caffeinated beverages and water hydrate to the same degree over a 24-hour period. Fiala et al. have noted that, although caffeine is oft rumored to be a mild diuretic, that caffeine itself can enhance exercise performance (typical dose at 5 mg/kg).[76] This study utilized 10 athletes who completed two-a-day practices (2 hr/p = 4 hr/d) for 3 consecutive days at 23°C (73°F). Utilizing a randomized double-blind design offering of caffeine rehydration agent vs. no caffeine (classic Coca-Cola® vs. its caffeine-free version), the findings revealed no evidence that caffeine intake impairs rehydration. No differential effects on urine or plasma osmolality, plasma volume, hematocrit, hemoglobin, or body weight were observed. The caffeine intake was about 244 mg caffeine/d served in ~7 cans/d of soda (~35 mg caffeine/12 oz.).[76]

On the other hand, caffeine was demonstrated to have diuretic effects in a study of 12 healthy German men and women (mean age 27 years) who were usual coffee drinkers, but abstained from drinking or eating anything containing caffeine for 5 days before the study. Six cups of coffee (642 mg caffeine/d) led to an increase in 24-hour urine excretion of 753 + 532 mL ($P < .001$), a negative fluid balance, and a decrease in body weight of 0.77 + 0.4 kg ($P < .001$). Total body water decreased by 1.1 + 1.2 kg or 2.7% ($P < .01$). However, as the subjects abstained from caffeine prior to the research, their response to caffeine as a diuretic may have been sensitized more than had they remained caffeine replete. Some research has supported the theory that caffeine tolerance in regular caffeine consumers may desensitize the individual from some of the central and peripheral effects of caffeine, although the influence is likely incomplete.[77]

Grandjean conducted a study of 18 males using a randomized crossover design with a free-living 24-hour capture design. The study tested four beverages (carbonated, caffeine caloric cola, non-caloric caffeinated cola, and coffee, and their respective effects on 24-hour hydration status. The researchers collected urine for 24 hours and analyzed for electrolytes, body weight, osmolality, hemoglobin, hematocrit, blood urea nitrogen, creatinine, and other biomarkers. The results clearly denoted no differences among the groups in any variable. Thus, we can now consider caffeine-containing beverages generally non-dehydrating and likely add to hydration.[78]

Newer research data has started to support the inclusion of small amounts of protein (PRO) with carbohydrates for hydration recovery. In 2001, 10 endurance-trained males were studied to investigate the ergogenic effects of isocaloric carbohydrate (CHO, 152.7 g) and carbohydrate-protein (112 g CHO with 40.7 g PRO) drinks ingested after a glycogen-lowering diet and exercise bout. Treatments were administered in a double-blind and counterbalanced fashion. After a glycogen-lowering diet and run, two dosages of a drink were administered with a 60-min interval between dosages. The CHO-PRO trial resulted in higher serum insulin levels (60.84 vs 30.1 mU/mL) 90 min into recovery than the CHO-only trial ($P < 0.05$). Furthermore, the time to run to exhaustion was longer during the CHO-PRO trial (540.7 ± 91.56 sec) than the CHO-only trial (446.1 ± 97.09 sec, $P < 0.05$). In conclusion, a CHO-PRO drink following glycogen-depleting exercise may facilitate a greater rate of muscle glycogen resynthesis than a CHO-only beverage, hasten the recovery process, and improve exercise endurance during a second bout of exercise performed on the same day.[78] Subsequent studies have found that adding PRO in the ratio of 1 part PRO to every 4 parts CHO has been found to induce exercise hydration on the magnitude of 15% better than the typical CHO beverage and 40% more than water alone.[80,81]

The Seifert study[81] actually concluded that, contrary to popular misconception, adding PRO to a CHO-based sports drink ... led to improved water retention by 15 % over (a CHO-only sports drink) and 40 % over plain water. In the study, cyclists exercised until they lost 2% of their body weight (through sweating) and then drank either a CHO-PRO sports drink (Accelerade™), a CHO-only sports drink (Gatorade®), or water. Over the next 3 hours, measurements were taken to determine how much of each beverage was retained in the body (vs. the amount lost through urination). The CHO-PRO sports drink was found to rehydrate the athletes 15% better than the CHO-only sports drink and 40% better than water. All three drinks emptied from the stomach and were absorbed through the intestine at the same rate. In addition, there was no difference between the CHO-PRO drink and the CHO-only drink in terms of effects on blood plasma volume. This suggests that the CHO-PRO drink resulted in increased water retention within and between cells. Therefore a CHO-PRO sports drink may be a preferable choice over plain water and a CHO-electrolyte sports drink, when rehydration and fluid retention are a concern.

An additional sports application study by Seifert[82] found that ingestion of a CHO-PRO beverage minimized muscle damage indices during skiing compared to placebo and no fluid. Thirty-one recreational skiers were separated into three groups. All three skied 12 runs, which took about 3 hours. One group drank nothing. A second group drank 6 ounces of a placebo (flavored water) after every second run. A third group drank an equal amount of the CHO-PRO sports drink (Accelerade). After the 12th run, blood samples were taken from each skier and analyzed for two biomarkers of muscle stress (myoglobin and creatine kinase). Subjects that received the CHO-PRO sports drink showed no signs of muscle damage, while indicators of muscle damage increased by 49% in subjects receiving only water.[82] Thus, it is fair to conclude that in this type of sport, using a CHO-PRO drink is more beneficial than water for maintaining skeletal integrity and hydration.

Milk, a beverage containing CHO, PRO and electrolytes, has been shown to be an effective post-exercise rehydration drink. Shirreffs and colleagues[83] compared low-fat milk alone, with an additional 20 mmol/L NaCl, a sports drink, and water on restoring fluid balance after exercise-induced hypohydration at a level of 1.8% loss of body mass in a warm environment. Urine excretion over the recovery period did not change during the milk trials, whereas there was a marked increase in output between 1 and 2 h after drinking water and the sports drink. Subjects remained in net positive fluid balance or euhydrated throughout the recovery period after drinking the milk drinks but returned to net negative fluid balance 1 h after drinking the other drinks. These results suggest that milk can be an effective post-exercise rehydration drink.

Typically, hydration and rehydration for athletes is done with a 6–8% glucose-electrolyte solution. Newer research is finding that adding just a small amount of PRO to this type of sports beverage not only enhances hydration and rehydration (or hydration maintenance) it also promotes muscle PRO synthesis (which does not happen with CHO alone), and glycogen reaccumulation while reducing markers of muscle damage. Therefore, the use of these beverages is gaining popularity for the many benefits that appear to make them superior to the typical sports beverage for during-exercise or post-exercise nutrition.

X. FLUID REPLACEMENT

This chapter discusses the importance of fluid replacement and how research shows that the volume of fluid intake generally increases when water or the beverage is flavored.[84] In general, the following fluid recommendations are used by sports nutritionists:[85,86]

- 480–600 cc Fluid: 1–2 h pre-exercise
- 300–480 cc Fluid: 15 min. pre-exercise
- 120–180 cc Fluid: every 10–15 min. during exercise
- In general, start fluid intake 24 h prior to exercise event

Fluid intake coming from food must also be considered, however, in the post-exercise recovery period, hydration is best achieved by the ingestion of either the typical glucose-electrolyte solution or a CHO-PRO mixture. However, if the exercise has a duration of less than 60–75 min, then water (can be flavored) is recommended. There are no proven ergogenic effects or benefits from vitamin or mineral enriched waters except that they provide absorbable nutrients at lower caloric costs than some foods.

The athlete may consider taking note of the volume of his or her beverage intake in order to become more familiar with how the body responds to rehydration. The athlete can personalize his or her fluid intake based upon what types of beverages result in improved recovery as measured by hydration, return to normal body weight, subsequent exercise performance, and effects on mental abilities and cognition. (See Table 6.3).

TABLE 6.3
General Fluid Guidelines around Exercise

- Drink a minimum of 1 quart (4 cups, 0.95 L) of fluid for every 1,000 kilocalories you eat every day.
- Drink at least 5 cups (1.2 L) of water every day.
- Fluids should be cool.
- For moderate exercise that lasts an hour or less, water is sufficient for replacing lost fluids. If you like flavored drinks better, then use flavored beverages.
- For intense exercise that lasts less than 1 hour and exercise lasting more than an hour, carbohydrate-electrolyte sport drinks are best. Added protein may also be beneficial.
- Drink 2 cups (474 mL) of fluid 2 hours before exercise.
- Drink 4–6 ounces (118–177 mL) every 15 to 20 min. during exercise.
- After exercise, drink 20 ounces (2½ cups .59 L) of fluid for every pound of body weight lost during exercise (1300 mL/kg)

XI. CONCLUSIONS

Exercise increases the metabolic rate. Energy production leads to heat loss, and fluid status is affected. The climate has an underappreciated effect on hydration status. In cold climates, the thermoregulatory response includes enhanced heat production by a variety of means; all result in increased fluid losses. Exercising in temperate climates is actually a little easier, as the body's accommodation response is to increase blood volume and the sweating mechanism sensitivity. Athletes and their trainers and coaches must be cognizant of physiological impacts of exercise, such as changes in body temperature and blood volume in their surrounding climate. Elevated temperature is related to blood volume reduction and performance. Maintaining fluid balance reduces the effects of climate or blood volume on hydration status.

For exercise lasting less than an hour, water or noncaloric fluid is recommended. It is not well known whether "non-intensive" exercise requires that the rehydration solution include CHO and electrolytes; most data notes no need for the calories and salts with short-term exercise bouts. However, a general fluid plan should still be followed (See Table 6.4).

If the exercise is longer in duration, maintaining hydration and rehydration is that much more important. Beverages beneficial for enhancing rehydration include CHO-electrolyte solutions and CHO-PRO beverages. Caffeinated beverages with and without calories also add to hydration and rehydration. Although, in the immediate post-exercise period, data is mounting for CHO-PRO to be the superior post-exercise rehydration and recovery beverage. Future research will focus on the multiple applications of this admixture beverage along with other potentially beneficial effects. Taste acceptance is very important for any of these beverages to actually be used by athletes; therefore, overcoming taste issues for beverages that contain PRO when used during exercise is an issue for researchers and food scientists to overcome.

In conclusion, maintaining euhydration and understanding how to rehydrate after exercise is an important aspect of sports nutrition that is underdiscussed and

TABLE 6.4
Fluid Plan

• ***Requirement:***	1 mL/kcal/day
• 2200 kcal diet	2200 mL (9 cups/day)
• 2900 kcal diet	2900 mL (12 cups/day)
• ***Additional Fluid Needs:***	
• Exercise	
• High temperature	
• Low humidity	
• High altitude	
• High fiber diet	
• Increased fluid losses (caffeine, alcohol)	

Source: Kleiner SM. 1999. Water: An essential but overlooked nutrient. *J Am Diet Assoc* 99(2):200–6. Used with permission of Elsevier, Inc.

underappreciated. All health and sports practitioners should reacquaint themselves and their patients or clients with the role of water as an important beverage for health, weight maintenance, and physical performance. Current research on the impact of drinking water on cancer and disease prevention is intriguing, but needs much more investigation before the true facts can be elucidated. Early research even raises the question of whether all water is the same for hydration,[87] encouraging major new areas of research. Further research into the use of milk as a recovery beverage for the active individual, as well as athletes, is also needed, as the average individual is unlikely to invest in an engineered recovery drink. Practitioners should further work to assist patients and clients with designing practical fluid intake strategies to ensure adequate hydration and health.

REFERENCES

1. Institute of Medicine and Food and Nutrition Board. *Dietary Reference Intakes for Water, Potassium, Sodium, Chloride and Sulfate*. Washington DC: National Academies Press, 2004.
2. Health effects of mild dehydration. 2nd International Conference on Hydration throughout Life. Dortmund, Germany. October 8–9, 2001. *Eur J Clin Nutr* 57: Supplement 2 (2003).
3. Manz F. Hydration and disease. 2007. *J Amer Coll Nutr* 26(5):535s–541s.
4. Hydration and Health Promotion. ILSI North America Conference on Hydration and Health Promotion November 29–30, 2006. *J Amer Coll Nutr* 26(5s) (2007).
5. Welch BE, Bursick ER, Iampietro PF. 1958. Relation of climate and temperature to food and water intake in man. *Metabolism* 7:141–158.
6. Bullers AC. Bottled water: Better than tap? Rockville, MD: FDA 2002. Available from: www.fda.gov/fdac/features/2002/402_h2o.html.
7. Senay LC. Water and electrolytes during physical activity. In: Wolinsky, I, eds. *Nutrition in Exercise and Sport*; 3rd edition. CRC, Boca Raton, FL. 1998. 258–273.

8. Guyton AC. *Textbook of Medical Physiology*, 8th edition. WB Saunders, Philadelphia, 1991, p. 799.
9. McArdle WD, Katch FI, Katch VL. *Sports and Exercise Nutrition*, Lippincott Williams & Wilkins, Philadelphia, 1999.
10. Kristal-Boneh E, Blusman JG, Chaemovitz C, Cassuto Y. 1988. Improved thermoregulation caused by forced water intake in human desert dwellers. *Eur J Appl Physiol* 57:220–224.
11. Brooks GA, Fahey TD. *Exercise Physiology: Human Bioenergetics and Its Applications*. New York: John Wiley & Sons, 1984.
12. Johnson WR, Buskirk ER. *Structural and Physiological Aspects of Exercise and Sport*. Princeton, NJ: Princeton Book Co, 1980.
13. Stamford B. Muscle cramps: Untying the knots. 1993. *Phys Sportsmed* 21:115–116.
14. Wilmore JH, Costill DL. *Physiology of Sport and Exercise*. Champaign, IL: Human Kinetics, 1994.
15. Schwellnus MP, Derman EW, Noakes TD. 1997. Aetiology of skeletal muscle "cramps" during exercise: A novel hypothesis. *J Sports Sci* 15:277–85.
16. McKinley, MJ, Johnson, AK. 2004. The physiological regulation of thirst and fluid intake. *News Physiol Sci* 19(1):1–6.
17. Sagawa S, Miki K, Tajima F, et al. 1992. Effect of dehydration on thirst and drinking during immersion in men. *J Appl Physiol* 72:128–134.
18. Convertino VA, Armstrong LE, Coyle EF, Mack GW, Sawka MN, Senay LC Jr, Sherman WM. 1996. American College of Sports Medicine position stand. Exercise and fluid replacement. *Med Sci Sports Exerc* 28:i–vii.
19. Weissman AM. 1997. Bottled water use in an immigrant community: A public health issue? *Am J Public Health* 87:1379–1380.
20. Meyer F, Bar-Or O, Passe D, Salsberg A. 1994 Hypohydration in children during exercise in the heat: Effect on thirst, drink preferences and rehydration. *Int J Sport Nutr* 4:22–35.
21. Manz F. 2007. Hydration and disease. *J Amer Coll Nutr* 26(5):535s–541s.
22. Curhan GC, Curhan SG. 1994. Dietary factors and kidney stone formation. *Comp Ther* 20:485–9.
23. Goldfarb S. 1990. The role of diet in the pathogenesis and therapy of nephrolithiasis. *Endocrinol Metab Clinics NA* 19:805–20.
24. Hughes J, Norman RW. 1992. Diet and calcium stones. *Can Med Assoc J* 146:137–43.
25. Borghi L, Meschi T, Amato F, Briganti A, Novarini A, Giannini A. 1996. Urinary volume, water and recurrences in idiopathic calcium nephrolithiasis: A 5-year randomized prospective study. *J Urol* 155:839–43.
26. Iguchi M, Umekawa T, Ishikawa Y, Katayama Y, Kodama M, Takada M, et al. 1990. Clinical effects of prophylactic dietary treatment on renal stones. *J Urol* 144:229–32.
27. Pin NT, Ling NY, Siang LH. 1992. Dehydration from outdoor work and urinary stones in a tropical environment. *Occup Med* 42:30–2.
28. Embon OM, Rose GA, Rosenbaum T. 1990. Chronic dehydration stone disease. *Br J Urol* 66:357–62.
29. Hiatt RA, Ettinger B, Caan B, Quesenberry CP, Jr., Duncan D, Citron JT. 1996 Randomized controlled trial of a low animal PRO, high fiber diet in the prevention of recurrent calcium oxalate kidney stones. *Am J Epidemiol* 144:25–33.
30. Ackermann D. 1990. Prophylaxis in idiopathic calcium urolithiasis. *Urolog Res* 18 Suppl 1:S37–40.
31. Bitterman WA, Farhadian H, Abu Samra C, Lerner D, Amoun H, Krapf D, Makov UE. 1991. Environmental and nutritional factors significantly associated with cancer of the urinary tract among different ethnic groups. *Urol Clin NA* 18:501–8.

32. Shannon J, White E, Shattuck AL, Potter JD. 1996. Relationship of food groups and water intake to colon cancer risk. *Cancer Epidemiol, Biomark Prev* 5:495–502.
33. Stookey JD, Belderson PE, Russell JM, Barker ME. 1997. Correspondence re: J. Shannon et al., Relationship of food groups and water intake to colon cancer risk. *Cancer Epidemiol, Biomark Prev* 5: 495–502; 6:657–8.
34. Wilkens LR, Kadir MM, Kolonel LN, Nomura AM, Hankin JH. 1996. Risk factors for lower urinary tract cancer: the role of total fluid consumption, nitrites and nitrosamines, and selected foods. *Cancer Epidemiol, Biomark Prev* 5:161–6.
35. Brownlee HJ, Jr. 1990. Family practitioner's guide to patient self-treatment of acute diarrhea. *Am J Med* 88:27S–29S.
36. Dauterman KW, Bennett RG, Greenough WB 3rd, Redett RJ, Gillespie JA, Applebaum G, Schoenfeld CN. 1995. Plasma specific gravity for identifying hypovolaemia. *J Diarrhoeal Dis Res* 13:33–38.
37. Mack GW, Weseman CA, Langhans GW, Scherzer H, Gillen CM, Nadel ER. 1994. Body fluid balance in dehydrated healthy older men: Thirst and renal osmoregulation. *J Appl Physiol* 76:1615–1623.
38. Ayus JC, Arieff AI. 1996. Abnormalities of water metabolism in the elderly. *Semin Nephrol* 16:277–88.
39. Sansevero AC. 1997. Dehydration in the elderly: Strategies for prevention and management. *Nurse Pract* 22:41–42,51–57,63–72.
40. Albert SG, Nakra BR, Grossberg GT, Caminal ER. 1994. Drinking behavior and vasopressin responses to hyperosmolality in Alzheimer's disease. *Int Psychogeriat* 6:79–86.
41. Weinberg AD, Minaker KL. 1995. Dehydraton. Evaluation and management in older adults. *JAMA* 274:1552–1556.
42. Sharp RL. 2006. Role of sodium in fluid homeostasis with exercise. *J Amer Coll Nutr* 25:231s–239s.
43. Whiting PH, Maughan RL. 1984. Dehydration and serum biochemical changes in marathon runners. *Eur J Appl Physiol* 52:183.
44. Maughan RJ. 1991. Fluid and electrolyte loss and replacement in exercise. *J Sports Sci* 9:117.
45. Murray B. 2006. Hydration and physical performance. *J Amer Coll Nutr* 26(5): 542s–548s.
46. Grandjean AC. 2006. Dehydration and cognitive performance. *J Amer Coll Nutr* 26(5): 549s–554s.
47. Lieberman HR. 2006. Hydration and Cognition: A critical review and recommendations for future research. *J Amer Coll Nutr* 26(5): 555s–561s.
48. Gopinathan PM, Pichan G, Sharma VM. 1988. Role of dehydration in heat stress-induced variations in mental performance. *Arch Environ Hlth* 43:15–7.
49. Cian C, Koulmann N, Barraud P, Raphel C, Jimeniz C, Meli B. 2000 . Influence of variations on body hydration on cognitive function: Effect of hyperhydration, heat stress, and exercise-induced dehydration. *J Psychophysiol* 14:29–36.
50. Torranin C, Smith DP, Byrd RJ. 1979. The effect of acute thermal dehydration and rapid rehydration on isometric and isotonic endurance. *J Sports Med Phys Fit* 19:1–9.
51. Greenleaf JE. The body's need for fluids. In: Haskell W, Scala J, Whittam J, eds. Nutrition and athletic performance. *Proceedings of the Conference on Nutritional Determinants in Athletic Performance*. Palo Alto, CA: Bull Publishing Company, 1982.
52. Kleiner, SM. 1999. Water: an essential but overlooked nutrient. *J Am Diet Assoc* 99(2):200–6.
53. Burke LM. 1997 Fluid balance during team sports. *J Sports Sci* 15:287–95.
54. Wiita BG, Stombaugh IA. 1996 Nutrition knowledge, eating practices, and health of adolescent female runners: A 3-year longitudinal study. *Int J Sport Nutr* 6:414–25.

55. Steen SN, Mayer K, Brownell KD, Wadden TA. Dietary intake of female collegiate heavyweight rowers. *Int J Sport Nutr* 1995 5:225–31.
56. Kleiner SM, Bazzarre TL, Ainsworth BE. 1994. Nutritional status of nationally ranked elite bodybuilders. *Int J Sport Nutr* 4:54–69.
57. Kleiner SM, Bazzarre TL, Litchford MD. 1990. Metabolic profiles, diet, and health practices of championship male and female bodybuilders. *J Am Diet Assoc* 90:962–967.
58. Gabel KA, Aldous A, Edgington C. 1995. Dietary intake of two elite male cyclists during 10–day, 2,050-mile ride. *Int J Sport Nutr* 5:56–61.
59. Eden BD, Abernethy PJ. 1994. Nutritional intake during an ultraendurance running race. *Int J Sport Nutr* 4:166–74.
60. Iuliano S, Naughton G, Collier G, Carlson J. 1998. Examination of the self–selected fluid intake practices by junior athletes during a simulated duathlon event. *Int J Sport Nutr* 8:10–23.
61. Fogelholm M. 1994. Effects of bodyweight reduction on sports performance. *Sports Med* 18:249–267.
62. Fogelholm GM, Koskinen R, Laakso J, Rankinen T, Ruokonen I. 1993. Gradual and rapid weight loss: Effects on nutrition and performance in male athletes. *Med Sci Sports Exerc* 25:371–7.
63. Tarnopolsky MA, Cipriano N, Woodcroft C, Pulkkinen WJ, Robinson DC, Henderson JM, MacDougall JD. 1996. Effects of rapid weight loss and wrestling on muscle glycogen concentration. *Clin J Sport Med* 6:78–84.
64. Webster S, Rutt R, Weltman A. 1990. Physiological effects of a weight loss regimen practiced by college wrestlers. *Med Sci Sports Exerc* 22:229–234.
65. CDC. Prevention. *Morbidity and Mortality Weekly Report* 1998:105–108.
66. Meyer F, Bar-Or O, Passe D, Salsberg A. 1994. Hypohydration in children during exercise in the heat: Effect on thirst, drink preferences and rehydration. *Int J Sport Nutr* 4:22–35.
67. Meyer F, Bar-Or O, MacDougall D, Heigenhauser GJF. 1995. Drink composition and the electrolyte balance of children exercising in the heat. *Med Sci Sports Exerc* 27:882–887.
68. American Academy of Pediatrics 1982. Committee on Sports Medicine Position Paper: Climatic heat stress and the exercising child. *Pediatrics* 69:808–809.
69. Sawka MN, Burke LM, Eichner ER, Maughan RJ, Montain SJ, Stachenfeld NS. 2007. Position Stand: Exercise and fluid replacement. *Med Sci Sports Exerc* 39:2:377–390.
70. Beltrami F, Hew-Butler T, Noakes T. 2008. Drinking policies and exercise-associated hyponatraemia: Is anyone still promoting overdrinking? *Br J Sports Med* Apr 23. (Epub ahead of print).
71. Zembrzuski CD. 1997. Hydration assessment checklist. *Geriat Nursing* 18(1):20–26.
72. Armstrong LE. 2006. Assessing hydration status: The elusive gold standard. *J Amer Coll Nutr* 26(5):575s–584s.
73. Kenefick RW, Sawka M. 2006. Hydration at the work site. *J Amer Coll Nutr* 26(5):597s–603s.
74. Heller KE, Sohn W, Burt BA, Eklund SA. 1999. Water consumption in the United States in 1995–1996 and implications for water fluoridation policy. *J Publ Health Dent* 59:3–11.
75. Shirreffs SM, Armstrong LE, Cheuvront SN. 2004. Fluid and electrolyte needs for preparation and recovery from training and competition. *J Sports Sci*. 22:57–63.
76. Fiala, K.A., D.J. Casa, and M.W. Roti. 2004. Rehydration with a caffeinated beverage during the nonexercise periods of 3 consecutive days of 2-a-day practices. *Int. J. Sport Nutr. Exerc. Metab.* 14:419–429.
77. Watson J, Deary I, Kerr D. 2002. Central and peripheral effects of sustained caffeine use: tolerance is incomplete. *Br J Clin Pharmacol* Oct 54(4):400–6.

78. Grandjean AC, Reimers KJ, Bannick KE, Haven MC. 2000. The effect of caffeinated, non-caffeinated, caloric and non-caloric beverages on hydration. *J Amer Coll Nutr* 19(5):591–600.
79. Niles ES, Lachowetz T, Garfi J, Sullivan W, Smith JC, Leyh BP, Headley SA. 2001. CHO-PRO drink improves time to exhaustion after recovery from endurance exercise. *J Exercise Physiol-online* 4(1).
80. Ivy JL, Goforth HW Jr, Damon BM, McCauley TR, Parsons EC, Price TB. 2002. Early postexercise muscle glycogen recovery is enhanced with a CHO-PRO supplement. *J Appl Physiol*. Oct 93(4):1337–44.
81. Seifert JG, Harmon J, DeClercq P. 2006. PRO added to a sports drink improves fluid retention. *Int J Sports Nutr Exerc Metab* 16: 420–429,.
82. Seifert JG, Kipp RW, Amann M, Gazal O. 2005. Muscle damage, fluid ingestion, and energy supplementation during recreational alpine skiing. *Int J Sports Nut Exer Metab* 15: 528–536.
83. Shirreffs SM, Watson P, Maughan RJ. 2007. Milk as an effective post-exercise rehydration drink. *Br J Nutr* Jul 98(1):173–80. Epub Apr 26.
84. Minehan MR, Riley MD, Burke LM. 2002. Effect of flavor and awareness of kilojoule content of drinks on preference and fluid balance in team sports. *Int J Sports Nutr Exerc Metab* 12:81–92.
85. Pivarnik, JM. Water and electrolytes during exercise. In: *Nutrition in Exercise and Sport*, Hickson J and Wolinsky I, eds. CRC Press, Boca Raton, FL 1989.
86. McArdle WD, Katch FI, Katch VL. *Sports & Exercise Nutrition*. Lippincott Williams & Wilkins. 1999 Pages 275–276
87. Kleiner SM, Krieger DR, Schwartz HI, Kalman D, Feldman S, Lou L. 2007. A double blind comparator trial of the effects of H2ULTRA water vs. tap, distilled and mineral water on rehydration after exercise in healthy male volunteers. *J Am Diet Assoc* 107(8):A30.

7 Weight Management

Richard B. Kreider and Colin D. Wilborn

CONTENTS

I. INTRODUCTION

It is commonly believed that a calorie is a calorie. Consequently, many believe that weight management is simply a problem of balancing caloric intake with energy expenditure. However, this is not always the case. Weight management involves a proper mix of dietary influences and exercise regimens. Many individuals who work out are trying to gain muscle weight to improve their physique, increase strength, enhance performance, or slow the aging process. While gaining weight is too easy for many of us, some athletes have difficulty gaining weight or maintaining it throughout a competitive season. Additionally, it is much harder to gain the right type of weight (i.e., muscle). Also, many athletes and recreationalists would like to lose fat weight safely and healthily. This leads many athletes to consume too many or too few calories based on their needs. Thus, weight management includes an understanding of key concepts, macronutrient composition, and nutritional supplements.

II. WEIGHT MANAGEMENT CONCEPTS

A. Energy Balance

1. Energy Intake and Expenditure

"Energy balance" is a catchphrase that is commonly used by exercise physiologists, nutritionists, and dieticians. It refers to the number of calories (energy) that we take in and whether it is above or below the amount we need to live. Depending on which side of the scale this falls, it will determine whether we are gaining or losing weight.

Energy is consumed in the diet through protein, carbohydrate, and fat intake. In the presence of excess calories, the body will subsequently convert and store them as triglycerides in adipose tissue. Over time, if this process continues, obesity results. Obesity as defined by some as a body mass index (BMI) greater than 30. However, because BMI is not an accurate reflection of adipose mass,[1] it may not be the best objective measure of obesity. Obesity results as a consequence of increasing both the size and number of adipocytes.[2,3]

As stated, the overconsumption of macronutrients contributes to obesity. However, not all macronutrients contribute to obesity in an equal manner. For instance, a high-fat meal that results in a positive energy balance will stimulate fat storage without a subsequent match in fat oxidation.[4,5] Furthermore, the deposition of excess dietary triglycerides into adipose tissue is associated with a very low metabolic cost (0–2%).[6] In contrast, Flatt et al. reported that the conversion of carbohydrate into fat is an energy-requiring process in which 25% of the energy content is lost as heat.[7] Of the three macronutrients, protein requires the most metabolic cost to be converted to and subsequently stored as fat. In studies involving twins, energy intake and obesity has been explored. Authors studying both monozygotic and dizygotic twins reported that there may be macronutrient-specific familial influences, but not conclusively.[8] Also, greater-than-average caloric intake was associated with increased levels of body fat, despite likely genetic influences on both phenotypes.[8] However, the authors concluded by stating that more research is needed to determine the genetic influence on energy intake. Finally, Tholin et al. studied genetic and environmental influences on eating behavior in a large cohort of monozygotic and dizygotic twins. The study concluded that genetic factors are of great importance of in the eating behavior in young adult male twins.[9]

In conclusion, it has been reported that the increase in the prevalence of obesity has concomitantly occurred with an increase in portion sizes of foods that we consume.[10] Furthermore, it has been shown that eating low-energy-dense foods such as fruits and vegetables helps sustain satiety while concurrently reducing energy intake, which appears to be a more effective weight loss strategy than fat reduction and decreased portion sizes.[10] Energy expenditure, also known as physical activity, is one of the two components of the energy balance equation.[11] Both energy intake and energy expenditure are profoundly important when discussing the etiology of obesity. Energy expenditure is composed of three categories: basal metabolic rate, thermic effect of food, and physical activity. Physical activity can also be broken down into two distinct sub-classes. The first is activity thermogenesis, which is volitional exercise. The second category is coined non-activity exercise thermogenesis, which is all of the activity that one performs that is not related to "sporting-like" exercise.[12] Examples of this include fidgeting, housework, etc.

It should be noted that non-activity exercise thermogenesis is often difficult to quantify. Activity thermogenesis accounts for approximately 15–50% of total daily expenditure in the sedentary to very active population respectively.[13] It further has been estimated that spontaneous minor activity performed during the day can account for 20% of the differences of energy expenditure in a 24-hour time frame.[14] Equally important, Castaneda et al. reports that minimal amounts of spontaneous physical activity are a major predictor of accumulating fat mass during overfeeding in humans.[15] An inverse association between physical activity and weight as a result of epidemiological studies has also been shown.[16] Similarly, Meredith et al.[17] reported a negative association between aerobic exercise at 65–80% maximal oxygen (VO_{2max}) uptake and body composition. Additionally, a meta-analysis demonstrated that weight training as well as aerobic exercise is effective in facilitating weight loss, but also can increase or maintain lean mass.[18] Thus, adding physical activity to promote weight loss encourages favorable changes in body composition. Sedentary lifestyle is commonly mentioned as a significant cause of the mounting prevalence of obesity.

In a study by Slentz et al.[19] researchers reaffirmed what many have already suspected. If individuals partake in a modest exercise program similar to those suggested by the Centers for Disease Control and the American College of Sports Medicine, significant increases in visceral fat can be avoided and exercise that is a modest increase beyond their recommendations can facilitate significant decreases in visceral, subcutaneous, and total abdominal fat without changes in daily dietary intake. In a study published in 2005, researchers looked at the comparison of monozygotic twins in relation to lipoprotein and weight variation between vigorously active and sedentary siblings. The authors reported vigorous exercise could possibly reduce genetic influences on body mass index.[20] Therefore, it is of critical importance to investigate energy expenditure in relation to obesity, especially when it has been reported that approximately 22–29% of adults report that they engage in no leisure-time physical activity.[13]

2. Diet-Induced Thermogenesis

While there is no doubt that a major contributing factor to the obesity epidemic is a lack of exercise, recent research has also shown that frequency of eating, as well as carbohydrate, fats, and protein have varying physiological and thermogenic effects.[21,22] In other words, a calorie may not be a calorie and the types of carbohydrate, proteins, and fats one consumes in the diet may influence the propensity to gain or lose weight. For example, different types of carbohydrate affect insulin levels to a greater degree than others. High-glycemic index (GI) carbohydrates increase glucose and insulin levels to a greater degree than low- to moderate-GI carbohydrates. Over time, consuming a diet rich in high-GI foods may serve to reduce insulin sensitivity.[23] Reductions in insulin sensitivity (i.e., increased insulin resistance) have been implicated as a possible causative factor for diabetes and obesity.[23,24] Consequently, consuming fewer high-GI foods or reducing carbohydrate availability in the diet have been shown to improve insulin sensitivity and promote greater weight loss.[25]

The type of carbohydrate consumed may also directly influence thermogenic properties. For example, Schwartz and colleagues[26,27] evaluated the effects of consuming a meal containing fructose (low-GI carbohydrate) versus glucose (high-GI carbohydrate) on glucose, insulin, and energy expenditure. As expected, the researchers found that ingesting the meal containing glucose as the source of carbohydrate promoted a higher glucose and insulin level than when fructose was used as the carbohydrate source. Interestingly, the researchers found that carbohydrate oxidation and thermogenesis was higher after consuming the fructose-containing meal in comparison with glucose. In other words, the type of carbohydrate consumed during a meal may influence the thermogenic effect of the meal.[28] This may be one reason that people tend to lose more weight when placed on diets in which the carbohydrate source is primarily low- to moderate-GI foods compared with high-GI carbohydrates.[24]

The amount of fat in the diet also appears to influence thermogenesis.[29] Research has indicated that high-carbohydrate/low-fat diets appear to promote a greater thermogenesis than high-fat/low-carbohydrate diets. For example, Maffeis and colleagues[30] compared the effects of ingesting a high-carbohydrate meal (68% carbohydrate, 20% fat, 12% protein) versus a high-fat meal (40% carbohydrate, 48% fat, 12% protein) on substrate oxidation, thermogenesis, and fat storage in obese children. Results revealed that consuming a high-fat meal promoted less of a thermogenic effect and a greater fat storage than the high-carbohydrate meal. Similarly, Westerterp et al.[31,32] evaluated the effects in consuming high-carbohydrate, high-protein diet (60% carbohydrate, 10% fat, 30% protein) compared with a high-fat diet (30% carbohydrate, 60% fat, 10% protein) on diet-induced thermogenesis. Results revealed that carbohydrate oxidation and energy expenditure was greater when consuming the high-carbohydrate, high-protein diet (14.6% versus 10.5% of energy intake). These findings and others suggest that a high-carbohydrate diet promotes greater thermogenesis than a high-fat diet.

While there is evidence that carbohydrate is more thermogenic than fat, there is also evidence that protein is the king of thermogenesis. Protein, in fact, may play a significant role in weight management.[33] For example, Jequier[34] reported that intravenously administered nutrient-induced thermogenesis was approximately 6–8% of energy infused with carbohydrate and 2–3% of energy infused with fat. However, thermogenesis was 30–40% of energy infused following amino acid administration. Robinson and colleagues[35] compared the thermogenic effects of consuming isocaloric amounts of high-carbohydrate and high-protein meals. The researchers found that the thermic response of consuming high-protein meals was significantly greater than when consuming a high-carbohydrate meal (9.6% versus 5.7%). Further, the greater energy expenditure could be attributed to a greater nitrogen turnover (protein metabolism).

If protein consumption has a greater thermic effect than carbohydrate and fat, then people would theoretically gain less weight if fed a hypercaloric diet consisting of a higher amount of protein compared with carbohydrate or fat. In support of this theory, Webb and Annis[36] overfed subjects for 30 days by 1000 calories as provided from a normal mixed American diet, 60% of calories as carbohydrate, or 70% of calories provided by protein. The researchers found that subjects who added 1000 calories of mixed calories and high carbohydrate gained approximately 6 pounds of body weight whereas the subjects who consumed the high-protein diet gained only 3.9 pounds. The researchers attributed the lesser amount of weight gain to extra calories expended from protein thermogenesis.

Johnston and coworkers,[37] evaluated the effects of ingesting a high-protein meal on thermogenesis. Subjects were fed a control diet for 2 days followed by ingesting either a high-protein or high-carbohydrate diet for 1 day. Resting energy expenditure was determined following a 10-hour fast and 2.5 hours after ingesting breakfast, lunch, and dinner. After 28 or 56 days, subjects repeated the experiment following the alternate diet. Results revealed that energy expenditure was 100% greater 2.5 hours after ingesting the high-protein meals in comparison with the high-carbohydrate meals. In addition, nitrogen balance was significantly greater when ingesting the high-protein diet. These findings and others indicate that protein is a more thermogenic macronutrient than fat and carbohydrate.

Leidy et al. evaluated the effects of acute and chronic consumption of higher dietary protein on energy expenditure, macronutrient use, and appetite.[38] Thirty-eight women chronically consuming a 750 kcal/d energy-deficient diet with a protein content of 30% or 18% for 9 weeks were tested. With chronic diet groups combined, high protein led to lower respiratory exchange ratio, lower carbohydrate oxidation, and higher fat oxidation compared with the lower protein group. High protein also led to reduced self-reported postprandial hunger and desire to eat. The authors concluded that during weight loss, thermogenesis and protein use appear to be influenced by chronic protein intake.

B. Weight Loss

To promote weight loss, dietitians generally recommend that people reduce caloric intake by about 500 calories per day while increasing energy expenditure through exercise. One of the primary ways dietitians recommend reducing caloric intake is by cutting fat from the diet or replacing fat with carbohydrate.[39–41] This approach has been reported to be effective; however, it has recently been criticized for a several reasons. First, the amount of fat in the diet of Americans has declined from about 40–45% to 30–35% over the last 10–20 years.[24] Nevertheless, the incidence of obesity has reached epidemic proportions.[24] The increased incidence of obesity is believed to be due to a combination of overeating, a lack of exercise, and an increased consumption of high-GI carbohydrates, which has been shown to decrease insulin sensitivity.[24,41–43] Second, research has shown that people who follow a high-carbohydrate, low-fat, and low-protein diet typically lose a significant amount of muscle mass.[42] Muscle mass has been positively correlated with resting energy expenditure.[44,45] Weight loss associated with decreases in muscle mass have been shown to decrease resting energy expenditure and thereby make it difficult to maintain weight loss. As a result, people who lose weight often regain the weight lost within 1–2 years.[42,46] Increasing dietary availability of protein and incorporating a resistance training program while dieting has been reported to help maintain muscle mass, resting energy expenditure,[47] and lipid oxidation.[48] Theoretically, this should allow an individual to maintain weight loss to a better degree over time. There is also an emerging body of evidence indicating that ingesting a moderate- to high-protein, low-fat diet promotes greater weight loss than a high-carbohydrate, low-fat diet. The reason for this greater weight loss efficacy may be related in part to the thermogenic properties of protein.

C. Weight Gain

In addition to proper training, nutrition plays a key role in promoting muscle hypertrophy. This involves: (1) making sure you are eating enough calories of the proper types of energy nutrients; (2) proper timing of nutrient intake; and (3) choosing effective sports supplements that will help to increase muscle mass. The most common method of promoting weight gain is to maintain a slightly hypercaloric diet (e.g, 500–1,000 kcals/day higher than energy balance). To determine how much food (calories) needs to be eaten on a daily basis, two pieces of information need to be determined: the resting energy expenditure and the activity factor. Resting energy expenditure (REE) is the amount of energy needed to sustain resting metabolic rate. In simple terms, it represents the fewest amount of calories that you need to eat on a daily basis to maintain resting metabolic functions. REE does not include energy expenditure from daily living activities such as work or a structured exercise program. Generally, the heavier and taller you are, the greater the daily REE, while age decreases REE. For example, if you had a 30-year-old female who was 66 inches tall (168 cm) and weighed 150 lbs (68 kg), her REE would be approximately 1482 kcal/day. Likewise, if you had a 25-year-old male who was 72 inches tall (183 cm) and weighed 195 lbs (89 kg), his estimated REE would be 2036 kcal/day. This would represent the minimum number of calories needed to maintain resting energy expenditure levels. Additional calories must be added for energy expenditure from work, exercise, and nonexercise activity thermogenesis (NEAT) in order to estimate the number of calories needed to energy balance (i.e., body weight).

D. Weight Maintenance

Numerous diets can help people lose weight. However, the challenge is to maintain weight once it is lost. In our Curves research, we have found that women can maintain weight loss for up to a year if they continue to exercise, eat a well-balanced diet, and apply one basic principle to weight management. This is to monitor body weight and to follow a high-protein 1200 kcal/day diet for only 2–3 days if they gain 3 pounds of body weight. This basic principle allows people to eat a normal healthy diet most of the time while needing to cut back on calories only every once in a while if they gain weight. The same principle can be implemented for men following a 1600 kcal/day diet. Some of the dietary supplements discussed above can also help stimulate energy expenditure or curb appetite. The main goal, though, is to not allow oneself to regain weight once lost, which has proven to be difficult.[49]

III. DIETARY MACRONUTRIENT COMPOSITION

A. High Carbohydrate Diets

1. Glycemic Index of Carbohydrates

The GI measures the rate of absorption and digestion of carbohydrates and their effect on blood sugar levels. When you consume a high-GI food, blood glucose and insulin levels increase, promoting storage of the glucose into the liver and muscle.[50] The rise in insulin levels serves to increase carbohydrate oxidation while suppressing fat utilization. For example, ingesting high-GI foods will result in a rapid increase in blood sugar. Raising the blood sugar levels rapidly can result in rebound hypoglycemia because the body releases a hormone (insulin) to bring the blood sugar levels back down to normal. Sometimes the body "over-compensates" with insulin and releases too much too rapidly. This can result in hypoglycemia or low blood sugar. Hypoglycemia can cause light-headedness, weakness, and tachycardia (elevated heart rate) until the low blood sugar level is corrected. Ingestion of high-GI foods and drinks prior to and during exercise should be avoided. Table 7.1 provides the GI of a list of foods.

The sugars found in most sports drinks are glucose, fructose, and sucrose. Sucrose is a disaccharide composed of glucose and fructose. Fructose is absorbed more slowly when compared with glucose and therefore does not create the rapid swings in blood sugar levels that may occur when ingesting high-GI foods. Ingesting a low-GI carbohydrate about 45 min prior to exercise may result in a more stable blood sugar level during the early stages of prolonged exercise.[51] However, when either fructose or glucose is ingested immediately before or during exercise, there appears to be no difference in blood sugar and carbohydrate metabolism. Furthermore, neither fructose nor glucose is better at sparing muscle glycogen.[52] One drawback to the

TABLE 7.1
Glycemic Index of Common Foods

High Glycemic > 85	Medium Glycemic 60–85	Low Gylcemic < 60
Glucose*	Banana	Fructose
Sucrose	Grapes	Dates
Syrup	Oatmeal	Figs
Honey	Orange juice	Applesauce
Bagel	Pasta	Ice cream
Candy	Rice	Milk
Molasses	Corn	Yogurt
Potatoes	Baked beans	Vegetable soups
Raisins	Potato chips	Fruits

*Glucose is the baseline = 100

slow absorption of fructose is its tendency to draw water into the intestines. This can result in cramping and diarrhea. Therefore, athletes should be cautious when consuming fructose for the first time.

A number of studies have evaluated the effects of ingesting various forms of carbohydrate on performance. In one study,[53] cyclists who ingested a low-GI meal 30 min prior to exercise had lower blood glucose and insulin levels than subjects ingesting a high-GI meal. In addition, cycling time to exhaustion was increased by 59% after ingesting the low-GI meal. These findings suggest that ingesting a low-GI meal prior to exercise would be advantageous from a metabolic and performance standpoint. However, other studies have reported that blood glucose levels were maintained better during high-intensity exercise in subjects who ingested high-GI foods rather than low-GI foods with no significant effects on endurance performance.[54,55] In support of this latter contention, research conducted in our lab evaluated the effects of ingesting different types of carbohydrate gels on endurance cycling performance.[56]

In a double-blind, randomized, and crossover study design, subjects ingested either a placebo, a high-GI carbohydrate gel (sucrose) or a low- to moderate-GI gel (honey) prior to and during a cycling time trial lasting about 3 hours. Results revealed that ingestion of both carbohydrate gels improved performance with no adverse effects from ingesting the higher-GI gel. These findings indicate that it really doesn't matter which type of carbohydrate is ingested prior to or during exercise. Although ingesting low-GI foods or drinks may result in a more controlled release of blood sugar into the blood prior to exercise, there just is not enough evidence to recommend that athletes will improve their performance during prolonged exercise when they ingest low-GI foods or drinks.[57–59]

For people trying to lose weight or promote health, it makes sense to consume low-GI carbohydrates in the diet instead of high-GI carbohydrates. In this regard, the metabolic effects of carbohydrates differ based on the GI. Consumption of high-GI foods causes a greater increase in insulin, carbohydrate storage, and carbohydrate utilization in comparison with consuming low-GI carbohydrates. High-GI diets have been associated with obesity, diabetes, and heart disease. Short-term intervention trials suggest that simply replacing high-GI foods with low-GI foods promotes weight loss and improves insulin sensitivity.[24,58] For this reason, a growing number of obesity researchers recommend that people consume a moderate- to high-carbohydrate diet consisting primarily of low-GI foods. Athletes should also consume the majority of carbohydrates in their diet in the form of low- to moderate-GI foods, except that carbohydrate intake during and following exercise should consist of high-GI foods.

For the athlete, however, some additional points need to be made. First, research has shown that exercise training improves insulin sensitivity and helps individuals manage body weight.[50] Therefore, people who engage in habitual exercise training may not benefit as much from a low-GI diet as sedentary individuals or diabetics. It is also possible that the potential negative effects on health of consuming high-GI foods may be of less concern in trained individuals. Second, research has indicated that ingesting high-GI foods with protein after exercise is important to enhance protein and glycogen synthesis. The increased protein and glycogen synthesis is believed to be due in part to an increase in insulin levels. Therefore, it is our view that healthy athletes should not restrict intake of high-GI carbohydrates following exercise. There is also evidence that ingesting a low- to moderate-GI carbohydrate prior to exercise may improve carbohydrate availability and reduce protein degradation during exercise. In addition, most sports drinks and sports gels are high-GI carbohydrates. Research has consistently shown that ingestion of sports drinks or sport gels during exercise may enhance prolonged exercise performance.[60–63] Based on this research, we suggest the following dietary guidelines for athletes in consideration of the GI:

- Maintain an isoenergetic diet consisting of high carbohydrate (5–8 g/kg/day), moderate protein (1.5–2.0 g/kg/day), and low fat (0.5–1.5 g/kg/day) during training.
- Consume low- to moderate-GI carbohydrates during pre-exercise meals and for snacks in between meals.
- Consume moderate- to high-GI carbohydrates during prolonged exercise, depending on tolerance.
- Consume moderate- to high-GI carbohydrates with protein during post-workout snacks and meals.
- Replacing high-GI foods with low-GI foods during low-calorie dieting phases may assist in weight loss.

B. High Protein Diets

There is also evidence that consuming a low calorie diet with a greater percentage of protein than traditionally recommended promotes greater weight loss (with or without resistance training).[64] For example, Piatti and coworkers[65] evaluated the effects on weight reduction, insulin sensitivity, and protein status in overweight females of ingesting a low-calorie diet (800 kcal/day) consisting of either high-protein content (35% carbohydrate, 45% protein, and 20% fat) or high-carbohydrate content (60% carbohydrate, 20% protein, and 20% fat) for 21 days. Results revealed that subjects lost a similar amount of weight in both groups. However, subjects consuming the high-protein diet maintained protein balance to a greater degree, lost less muscle mass, and experienced an increase in insulin sensitivity in comparison with subjects on the high-carbohydrate diet. Skov and colleagues[66] evaluated the effects on weight loss in 65 overweight men and women of consuming a high-carbohydrate (58% carbohydrate 12% protein, 30% fat) or high protein (carbohydrate 45%, protein 25%, fat 30%) diet for 6 months compared with controls. Results revealed that subjects consuming the high-protein diet lost 8.1 pounds (3.6 kg) more weight and 7.3 pound (3.3 Kg) more fat than subjects ingesting the high-carbohydrate diet. In addition, subjects ingesting the high-protein diet experienced a significant reduction in fasting triglycerides and free fatty acids. In companion papers, these researchers reported that increasing dietary intake of protein had no adverse effects on kidney function or bone.[67,68] The researchers concluded that replacing carbohydrate with protein is an effective and safe means of promoting weight loss in obese subjects.

In another study, Baba and associates[69] evaluated the effects on weight loss, energy expenditure, insulin, and blood lipids of ingesting a hypocaloric high-carbohydrate (58% carbohydrate, 12% protein, and 30% fat) or high-protein (% carbohydrate, 45% protein, and 30% fat) in 13 obese subjects who had elevated insulin levels diet for 28 days. The researchers reported that weight loss was greater (18.3 versus 13.2 pounds) and resting energy expenditure and insulin levels were maintained to a greater degree in the high-protein group. Parker and coworkers[70] evaluated the effects of ingesting a high- or low-protein weight loss diet on body composition, glucose, and insulin levels in 54 obese subjects with type II diabetes. In this study, subjects ingested a 1600 kcal/day high-carbohydrate (55% carbohydrate, 16% protein, 26% fat) or high-protein (42% carbohydrate, 28% protein, 28% fat) for 8 weeks. The researchers reported that subjects lost an average of 11.4 pounds during the dietary intervention. Females ingesting the high-protein diet lost significantly more total (11.7 [5.3 kg] versus 6.2 [3.2 kg] pounds) and abdominal fat (2.9 [1.3 kg] versus 1.5 [.68 kg] pounds) compared with those following a high-carbohydrate diet. Although similar trends were observed, no differences were observed between types of diets in fat loss among men. Collectively, these findings suggest that consumption of a high-protein, low-fat diet may promote greater weight loss or maintenance of lean tissues and metabolic rate than high-carbohydrate, low-fat diets.

Although high-protein, low-carbohydrate weight loss diets have been criticized (particularly if they increase dietary fat intake), there is accumulating evidence that they may be more effective in promoting weight loss and maintaining muscle mass and resting energy expenditure than high-carbohydrate weight-loss diets.[71] One possible reason for the greater efficacy of high-protein, low-fat diets is that protein has greater thermogenic effects than carbohydrate and fat. To lose fat weight, the recommendation is to: (1) reduce caloric intake by 500 calories per day; (2) consume primarily low- to moderate-GI carbohydrates; (3) participate in a strength training program (30–60 minutes, 3–4 times per week); and, (4) consume a relatively low-fat (20–30% of calories), moderate-carbohydrate (35–45% of calories), high-protein (20–40% of calories) diet. While this may not be advantageous for endurance athletes involved in intense exercise training, an emerging body of evidence suggests this approach may be more effective in promoting fat loss than traditional high-carbohydrate, low-fat diets.

C. Diet Foods

Most of the products in this category represent low-fat, low-carbohydrate, high-protein food alternatives. They typically consist of prepackaged bars, meal replacement powders (MRP) or ready to drink (RTD) supplements. They are designed to provide convenient foods or snacks to help people follow a particular low- or high-calorie diet plan. In the scientific literature, diets that provide between 420 and 1000 calories per day are known as very low-calorie diets (VLCDs). Pre-packaged food, MRPs, or RTDs are often provided in VLCD plans to help people cut calories. In most cases, VLCD plans recommend behavioral modification and that people start a general exercise program. In addition, these foods can be added to existing diet plans to increase caloric intake if weight gain is desired.

Research on the safety and efficacy of people maintaining VLCDs generally indicate that they can promote weight loss. For example, Hoie et al.[72] reported that maintaining a VLCD for 8 weeks promoted a 12.7 kg (12.6%) loss in total body mass, a 9.5 kg loss in body fat (23.8%), and a 3.2 kg (5.2%) loss in lean body mass in 127 overweight volunteers. Leutholtz and colleagues[73] reported that addition of a exercise training program (900 kcal/week) while maintaining a VLCD (420 kcal/d for 12 weeks) resulted in similar preservation of lean body mass at 40 and 60% of the heart rate reserve (HRR). Kern and coworkers[74] reported that a medically supervised weight loss program involving behavioral modification and VLCD promoted a 23 kg weight loss and that 61% of subjects maintained at least 50% of the weight loss at 12 and 18 months follow-up. These findings and others indicate that VLCDs (typically using MRPs or RTDs) can be effective particularly as part of an exercise and behavioral modification program. Most people appear to maintain at least half of the initial weight lost for 1–2 years. However, recidivism rates are relatively high in 2- to 5-year follow-up studies. Therefore, although these diets may help people lose weight in the short term, it is essential people who use them follow good diet and exercise practices to maintain the weight loss.

IV. WEIGHT MANAGEMENT SUPPLEMENTS

A. Fat Blockers

A number of weight-loss products claim to help suppress appetite, reduce cravings for foods, and interfere with fat absorption. The theoretical rationale of these supplements is simple. If you're not hungry or do not crave food, then you won't be tempted to overeat and it will be easier to stay on a diet. Additionally, if you block fat absorption, less fat (and fewer calories) will be stored in the body. After reviewing these types of supplements, we found five types of nutrients or supplements typically sold to suppress appetite and cravings or block fat absorption as follows.

1. Fiber

One of the oldest and most common methods of suppressing the appetite is to eat a high-fiber diet. Ingesting high-fiber foods (fruits, vegetables) or fiber supplements increases the feeling of fullness (satiety). They typically allow you to feel full while ingesting fewer calories. Theoretically, maintaining a high-fiber diet may serve to help decrease the amount of food you eat. In addition, high-fiber diets or supplements have also been purported to help lower cholesterol and blood pressure as well as help diabetics manage glucose and insulin levels. Some of the research conducted on high-fiber diets indicates that they provide some benefit, particularly in diabetic populations. For example, Raben et al.[75] reported that subjects maintaining a low-fat (26%), high-fiber (3.9 g/MJ) diet for 11 weeks lost 1.3 kg of weight and 1.6 kg of fat. Other studies report either no significant effects or modest amounts of fat loss. Collectively, these findings suggest that maintaining a high-fiber diet may have some health benefit but do not appear to promote marked weight or fat loss.

2. *Gymnema sylvestre*

Gymnema sylvestre is purported to affect glucose and fat metabolism as well as inhibit sweet cravings. In support of these contentions, some recent data have been published by Shigematsu and colleagues[76,77] indicating that short- and long-term oral supplementation of *Gymnema sylvestre* in rats fed normal and high-fat diets may have some positive effects on fat metabolism, blood lipid levels, and weight gain or fat deposition. Although these findings are interesting, we are aware of no published studies that have evaluated the effects of *Gymnema sylvestre* supplementation on lipid metabolism or body composition in humans. Consequently, more research is needed before conclusions can be drawn.

3. Chitosan

Chitosan has been marketed as a weight-loss supplement for several years. It is purported to inhibit fat absorption and lower cholesterol. Several animal studies report decreased fat absorption, increased fecal fat content, and lower cholesterol following chitosan feedings.[78,79] However, the effects in humans appear to be less impressive. For example, although there are some data suggesting that chitosan supplementation may lower blood lipids in humans,[80] other studies report no effects on fecal fat content[81] or body composition alterations[82,83] when administered to people following their normal diet. It seems that people may be prone to eat more when they know they are taking a fat-blocking supplement, much as people tend to eat more when they consume low-fat foods. Whether chitosan may promote greater amounts of fat loss when people are put on a controlled diet is unclear.

B. Thermogenics

Thermogenics are supplements designed to stimulate metabolism, thereby increasing energy expenditure and promoting weight loss. They typically contain the "ECA" stack of ephedra alkaloids (e.g., Ma Haung, 1R,2S Nor-ephedrine HCl, *Sida cordifolia*), caffeine (e.g., Gaurana, Bissey Nut, Kola) and aspirin/salicin (e.g., willow bark extract). More recently, other potentially thermogenic nutrients have been added to various thermogenic formulations. For example, thermogenic supplements may also contain synephrine (e.g., *Citrus aurantium*, bitter orange), calcium and sodium phosphate, thyroid stimulators (e.g., guggulsterones, L-tyrosine, iodine), cayenne and black pepper, ginger root.

A significant amount of research has evaluated the safety and efficacy of some of these thermogenic nutrients. For example, Boozer et al.[84] reported that 8 weeks of ephedrine (72 mg/d) and caffeine (240 mg/d) supplementation promoted a 4.0 kg loss in body mass and a 2.1% loss in body fat with minor side effects. Molnar and associates[85] reported that overweight children treated for 20 weeks with ephedrine and caffeine observed a 14.4% loss in body mass and a 6.6% decrease in body fat with no differences in side effects. Interestingly, Greenway and colleagues[86] reported that ephedra and caffeine supplementation was a more cost-effective treatment for reducing weight, cardiac risk, and LDL cholesterol than several weight-loss drugs (fenfluramine with mazindol or phentermine). Finally, Nazar and coworkers[87] reported that 4 weeks of phosphate supplementation increased resting metabolic rate by 12–19%. Less is known about the safety and efficacy of synephrine, thyroid stimulators, cayenne or black pepper, and ginger root. Since the FDA banned the provision of ephedra in dietary supplements, most thermogenic supplements contain a combination of green tea extract, gaurana (naturally occurring caffeine), or willow bark (a naturally occurring form of aspirin). It is our recommendation that you consult with your physician before considering use of any thermogenic supplement that may contain various central nervous system stimulants. Nevertheless, research has shown that use of various types of thermogenic-based supplements can promote weight loss.

C. Lypolytic Nutrients

A number of nutrients have been purported to increase fat metabolism (lipolysis). The following briefly describes the theoretical rationale and reported effects of the most common lypolytic nutrients and herbs found in weight loss supplements. Other purported lypolytic nutrients are described in Table 7.2.

1. Betaine

Betaine is a compound involved in the metabolism of choline and homocysteine. A number of studies have evaluated the effects of betaine feedings on liver metabolism, fat metabolism, and fat deposition in animals.[93,94] There has also been interest in determining whether betaine supplementation may help lower homocysteine levels, which have recently been identified as a marker of risk to heart disease.[95] For this reason, betaine supplements have been marketed as a supplement designed to promote heart health as well as weight loss. Although the potential theoretical rationale of betaine supplementation is interesting, it is currently unclear whether betaine supplementation may serve as an effective weight-loss supplement in humans.

2. Calcium Pyruvate

Calcium pyruvate is another supplement that hit the scene about 5 or 6 years ago with great promise. The theoretical rationale was based on studies from the early 1990s that reported that calcium pyruvate supplementation (16–25 g/d with or without dihydroxyacetone phosphate [DHAP]) promoted fat loss in overweight or obese patients

TABLE 7.2
Other Purported Weight Loss Supplements.

Nutrient	Theoretical Ergogenic Value
Cayenne (Capsaicin)	Capsaicin promotes thermogenesis, reduces hunger, and may trigger fat breakdown. Many weight-loss supplements contain various peppers.[88,89]
Citrus aurantium	A naturally occurring source of synephrine. Through its stimulation of specific adrenergic receptors (β-3, but not β-1, β-2 or α-1), synephrine is theorized to stimulate fat metabolism without the negative cardiovascular side effects.May have stimulant properties that can assist in increasing metabolism and/or fat oxidation.
5-HTP	5-Hydroxytryptophan (5-HTP) is an amino acid that is the intermediate step between tryptophan and serotonin. It is believed to be an appetite suppressant and cause weight loss. [90]
Sesamin	Sesamin is a naturally occurring lignan that is present in pure sesame oil. Sesamin has been suggested to serve as a fat oxidizer.
Hoodia Gordonii	*Hoodia Gordonii* is believed to be a powerful appetite suppressant with some anecdotal evidence. A number of weight loss supplements contain Hoodia, although more research is needed.
Glycomacropeptides	Glycomacropeptides are low molecular weight peptides found in specially processed whey proteins. Stimulate the release of CCK (cholecystokinin), a hormone that signals the brain when one is full. Thus, they might have appetite suppression capabilities.
Phosphatidylserine	One of the best known and most effective ways to lower excess cortisol levels is with the nutrient Phosphatidylserine. Lower cortisol levels are associated with weight loss.
Evodiamine	This herbal extract is a mild stimulant that has shown positive energy and diuretic characteristics. Evodiamine also has the unique ability to significantly elevate the production of body heat and increase resting core temperature.[91]
Tetradecylthioacetic Acid	Tetradecylthioacetic acid (TTA) is a non-beta-oxidizable fatty acid analog that potently regulates lipid homeostasis.
Phaseolus vulgaris Extract	The key ingredient to look for in a Carb Blocker type product is *Phaseolus vulgaris* extract because this is the ingredient that has been shown to block the absorption of carbohydrates in the digestive tract.
Guggul Lipids	Guggul has long been known to normalize lipid metabolism.
Octopamine	Octopamine HCl, also known as Norsynephrine HCl is an interesting compound is that it is a naturally occurring β3 adrenergic agonist.
Salvia sclarea	*Salvia sclarea* is also the primary ingredient in Norambrolide, an ingredient claimed by the herbal-supplement industry to promote fat catabolism and therefore weight loss.
Yohimbine	Increases testosterone levels, improving muscle mass and strength. Purported to raise levels of norepinephrine to stimulate metabolism and cause weight loss.[92]

following a medically supervised weight-loss program.[96–98] Although the mechanism for these findings was unclear, the researchers speculated that it might be related to appetite suppression or altered carbohydrate and fat metabolism. Because calcium pyruvate is very expensive, several studies have attempted to determine whether ingesting smaller amounts of calcium pyruvate (6–10 g/d) affect body composition in untrained and trained populations. Results of these studies are mixed. Kalman and colleagues[99] reported that calcium pyruvate supplementation (6 g/d for 6 weeks) significantly decreased body weight (–1.2 kg), body fat (–2.5 kg), and percent body fat (–2.7%). However, Stone and colleagues,[100] reported that pyruvate supplementation did not affect hydrostatically determined body composition during 5 weeks of in-season college football training. In our study,[101] we found that 30 days of calcium pyruvate supplementation (10 g/d) in moderately overweight females participating in supervised exercise program produced only a modest change in body fat (–0.3 kg). Although some supportive data indicates that calcium pyruvate supplementation may enhance fat loss when taken at high doses (6–16 g/d), there is no evidence that ingesting the doses typically found in pyruvate supplements (0.5–2 g/d) has any affect on body composition.

3. Carnitine

Carnitine serves as an important transporter of fatty acids from the cytosol into the mitochondria of the cell. Theoretically, increasing cellular levels of carnitine would thereby enhance transport of fats into the mitochondria and fat metabolism. For this reason, L-carnitine has been one of the most common nutrients found in various weight-loss supplements. Over the years, a number of studies have been conducted on the effects of L-carnitine supplementation on fat metabolism, exercise capacity and body composition. Although some data shows that L-carnitine supplementation may be beneficial for some patient populations, most well controlled studies indicate that L-carnitine supplementation does not affect muscle carnitine content, fat metabolism, or weight loss in overweight or trained subjects.[102] For example, Villani et al.[103] reported that L-carnitine supplementation (2 g/d for 8 weeks) did not affect weight loss, body composition, or markers of fat metabolism in overweight women. In our view, although there may be some therapeutic and ergogenic value to L-carnitine supplementation (e.g., to enhance tolerance to training), it appears to have little value as a fat-loss supplement. This may be due, in part, to the manner in which carnitine is ingested. New fat-melt tablets have been reported to have better bioavailability and absorption characteristics, which may enhance the impact on fat oxidation.

4. Chromium

Interest in chromium as a potential body composition modifier emanated from studies suggesting that chromium may enhance insulin sensitivity and glucose disposal in diabetics. Initial studies reported that chromium supplementation during resistance training improved fat loss and gains in lean body mass as determined by skinfold measurements.[104] However, recent studies using more accurate methods of assessing body composition have mostly reported no effects on body composition in healthy nondiabetic individuals. For example, Walker and colleagues[105] reported that chromium supplementation (200 μg/d for 14 weeks) did not affect body composition alterations in healthy wrestlers during training. Likewise, Lukaski and associates[106] reported that 8 weeks of chromium supplementation during resistance training did not affect strength or dual energy x-ray absorptiometry (DEXA) determined body composition changes. However, Crawford and coworkers[107] reported that niacin bound chromium supplementation (600 μg/d for 8-wks) promoted a significant loss in body fat and maintenance in muscle mass in 20 overweight African-American women following a modest diet and exercise program. It is our view that, although most studies indicate that short-term (4–12 weeks) chromium supplementation (200–400 μg/d) does not appear to significantly affect body composition in athletes undergoing training, there may be some benefit in diabetics or overweight populations that deserves additional study.

5. Forskolin (*Coleus forskholii*)

Forskolin is another relatively new weight loss supplement to hit the scene. Forskolin is a plant native to India that has been used for centuries in traditional Ayurvedic medicine, primarily to treat skin disorders and respiratory problems.[108] Considerable research has evaluated the physiological and potential medical applications of forskolin over the past 25 years. It has been reported to reduce blood pressure, increase the heart's ability to contract, help inhibit platelet aggregation, improve lung function, and aid in the treatment of glaucoma.[108,109] With regard to weight loss, forskolin has been reported to increase cyclic AMP and thereby stimulate fat metabolism. [110,111] Theoretically, forskolin may therefore serve as an effective weight loss supplement. In support of this theory, Sabinsa Corporation (the principle source for forskolin in the U.S.) reported that forskolin supplementation (250 mg of a 10% forskolin extract taken twice daily for 8 weeks) administered in an open label manner to six overweight females promoted a 7.25 lb loss in body weight and a 7.7% decrease in bioelectrical impedance (BIA) determined body fat.[112] Although this was not a placebo-controlled, double-blind study and BIA is not the most accurate method of assessing body composition, these preliminary findings provide some support to contentions that forskolin supplementation may promote fat loss. However, additional well-controlled research is needed before any conclusions can be made.

6. Conjugated Linoleic Acids (CLA)

CLA are essential fatty acids that have been reported to possess significant health benefits in animals. In terms of weight loss, CLA feedings to animals have been reported to markedly decrease body fat accumulation.[113,114] Consequently, CLA has been marketed as a health and weight-loss supplement since the mid 1990s. Although basic research in animals is very promising, the effect of CLA supplementation in humans is less clear.[115] Some data suggest that CLA supplementation may modestly promote fat loss or increases in lean mass.[116–119] However, the majority of studies indicate that CLA supplementation (1.7–12 g/d for 4 weeks–6 months) has limited to no effects on body composition alterations in untrained or trained populations.[119–124]

Recent longer-term CLA studies have shown more promising results. Consequently, CLA supplementation may have promise to promote general health as well as help manage body composition.

7. Dehydroepiandrosterone (DHEA) and 7-Keto DHEA

Dehydroepiandrosterone (DHEA) and its sulfated conjugate DHEAs represent the most abundant adrenal steroids in circulation.[125] Although DHEA is considered a weak androgen, it can be converted to the more potent androgens testosterone and dihydrotestosterone in tissues. In addition, DHEAs can be converted into androstenedione and testosterone. DHEA levels have been reported to decline with age in humans,[126] a decline that has been associated with increased fat accumulation and risk to heart disease.[127] Because DHEA is a naturally occurring compound, it has been suggested that dietary supplementation of DHEA may help maintain DHEA availability, maintain or increase testosterone levels, reduce body fat accumulation, or reduce risk to heart disease as one ages.[125,127] Although animal studies have generally supported this theory, the effects of DHEA supplementation on body composition in human trials have been mixed. For example, Nestler and coworkers[128] reported that DHEA supplementation (1,600 mg/d for 28 days) in untrained healthy males promoted a 31% reduction in percentage of body fat. However, Vogiatzi and associates[129] reported that DHEA supplementation (40 mg/d for 8 weeks) had no effect on body weight, percent body fat, or serum lipid levels in obese adolescents. More recently, 7-keto DHEA has been marketed as a potentially more effective form of DHEA. 7-keto DHEA is a precursor to DHEA that is believed to possess anabolic and lypolytic properties. Although a number of studies have evaluated the physiological effects of 7-keto DHEA on a variety of mechanisms, it is currently unclear whether 7-keto DHEA affects body composition alterations during training. However, additional research is needed before definitive conclusions can be made.

8. *Garcinia cambogia* (HCA)

HCA is a nutrient that has been hypothesized to increase fat oxidation by inhibiting citrate lyase and lipogenesis. Theoretically, this may lead to greater fat burning and weight loss over time. Although there is some evidence that HCA may increase fat metabolism in animal studies, there is little to no evidence showing that HCA supplementation affects body composition in humans. For example, Ishihara et al.[130] reported that HCA supplementation spared carbohydrate utilization and promoted lipid oxidation during exercise in mice. However, Kriketos and associates[131] reported that HCA supplementation (3 g/d for 3 days) did not affect resting or post-exercise energy expenditure or markers of lipolysis in healthy men. Likewise, Heymsfield and coworkers[132] reported that HCA supplementation (1.5 g/d for 12 weeks) while maintaining a low-fat, high-fiber diet did not promote greater weight or fat loss than subjects on placebo. Finally, Mattes and colleagues[133] reported that HCA supplementation (2.4 g/d for 12 weeks) did not affect appetite, energy intake, or weight loss. These findings suggest that HCA supplementation does not appear to promote fat loss in humans.

9. Phosphatidyl Choline (Lecithin)

Phosphatidyl choline (PC) is considered an essential nutrient that is needed for cell membrane integrity and to facilitate the movement of fats in and out of cells. It is also a component of the neurotransmitter acetylcholine, and is needed for normal brain functioning, particularly in infants. For this reason, PC has been purported as a potentially effective supplement to promote fat loss as well as improve neuromuscular function. Some data from animal studies supports the potential value of PC as a weight loss supplement.[134] There has also been some interest in determining the potential ergogenic value of choline supplementation during endurance exercise.[135] However, it is currently unclear whether PC supplementation affects body composition in humans.

D. Psychotropic Herbs

This is a relatively new type of weight-loss-supplement category. Such herbs often contain elements such as St. John's wort, kava, ginkgo biloba, ginseng, and L-tyrosine. More recently, *Hoodia gordonii* has been marketed as a powerful appetite suppressant. They are believed to serve as naturally occurring antidepressants, relaxants, and mental stimulants. The theoretical rationale regarding weight loss is that they may help people fight depression or maintain mental alertness while dieting. Although a number of studies support their potential role as naturally occurring psychotropics or stimulants, the potential value in promoting weight loss is unclear.

1. *Hoodia gordonii*

Hoodia (hoodia, xhooba, khoba, Ghaap, hoodia cactus, South African desert cactus) is a cactus-like plant that grows primarily in the deserts of South Africa, Botswana, Namibia, and Angola. In the last few years, hoodia has been heavily marketed for weight loss and has become immensely popular. The plant has been eaten for centuries by the Kalahari bushmen living in the area, reportedly to prevent hunger during long journeys. South African researchers applied for a patent for the use of this compound as a diet aid and licensed it to a British pharmaceutical company. According to recent CBS and BBC news reports, companies have spent millions of dollars in research on Hoodia and conducted a study of its effects on human volunteers. In one study, they report that obese volunteers who took Hoodia ended up eating about 1000 calories per day less than those who did not take the supplement. However, no clinical research has been published that assessed the effectiveness of Hoodia on appetite suppression and weight loss.

E. Diuretics

The theoretical basis for use of herbal diuretics primarily stems from several studies that have evaluated the effects of various herbal compounds on markers of diuresis in rats. For example, Grases and colleagues[136] evaluated the effects of infusion of seven different herbs (*Verbena officinalis, Lithospermum officinale, Taraxacum officinale* [dandelion], *Equisetum arvense, Arctostaphylos uva-ursi, Arctium lappa, and Silene saxifraga*) on markers of kidney stone formation and diuresis in female rats. The researchers reported that although more effective substances were available, infusion of these herbs promoted some beneficial effects on diuresis and risk factors of kidney stone formation. Beaux and colleagues[137] reported that administration of aqueous extracts of *Sambucus nigra* and *Arctostaphylos uva-ursi* and hydroalcohol extracts of *Orthosiphon stamineus* and *Hieracium pilosella* to rats increased urine output. Additionally, they reported that *O. stamineus* and *S. nigra* increased urinary sodium excretion. Similarly, Hao and colleagues[138] reported that oral ingestion of linialoling (KLP) increased diuresis and urine volume in rats. Hnatyszyn and coworkers[139] reported that oral ingestion of 400 mg/kg of *Phyllanthus sellowianus* Muell. Arg (Euphorbiaceae) increased urine output in test animals with no apparent side effects. Collectively, these studies provide some scientific basis that certain herbs may possess diuretic properties—at least in animals.

It is currently less clear whether herbal diuretics can effectively promote diuresis and weight loss in humans. To our knowledge, researchers from the University of Utah who presented a pair of research papers at the 2001 American College of Sports Medicine meeting were the first to examine this relationship. In this regard, Dolan and colleagues[140] and Crosby and colleagues[141] evaluated the effects of diuretic medicines and herbs on weight loss, dehydration, and metabolic rate. Their rationale was based on observations from pilot work indicating that diuretic-induced dehydration (3–5%) served to decrease resting metabolic rate (RMR). To further examine this relationship, these researchers evaluated the effects of administering furosemide (a common diuretic medicine) and dietary supplements containing the herb pamabron and dandelion or horsetail extract on markers of hydration and energy expenditure in 14 healthy female subjects. In the first study,[140] the subjects spent 2 days and nights in the laboratory. On the first night, subjects were administered 1 mg/kg of furosemide. Dietary intake and sleep times were controlled. Markers of dehydration, urine output, resting energy expenditure, and respiratory exchange ratio (a marker of carbohydrate and fat metabolism) were obtained on the 2 subsequent mornings following administration of the diuretic. Subjects repeated the experiment on a separate occasion without receiving the diuretic in order to provide a control trial. Results revealed that, in comparison with the control trial, furosemide administration promoted a significant amount of dehydration (–3.1%), greater urine output, a decrease in mean resting energy expenditure (control 1304 vs. diuretic 1253 kcal/day), and a higher respiratory exchange ratio (control 0.94 vs. diuretic 0.98). These findings suggested that diuretic-induced dehydration served to decrease resting energy expenditure and fat oxidation in these subjects.

Although more research is needed, it appears that short-term use of herbal diuretics may mildly promote diuresis, leading to marginal amounts of fluid and weight loss (about 0.5–1 lbs [.22–.45 Kg] in the first day). Whether prolonged use of herbal diuretics may be more beneficial in promoting weight loss is not clear. Nevertheless, claims that herbal diuretics can "shred off" undesired water weight appear to be based more on hype than on available scientific evidence.

F. Weight Gain and Muscle Mass

The last thing we consider when working with athletes trying to gain muscle mass is use of dietary supplements. Even then, we recommend them only after the athlete is incorporating the principles above and will recommend only supplements research has shown to be effective in promoting lean mass during training. If you are an athlete competing in a sport, one also has to consider whether the nutrients or supplements are permissible to be used or provided to the athlete. The U.S. National Collegiate Athletic Association (NCAA), for example, has a list of supplements that are permissible and non-permissible for a team to provide to their athletes. Athletes can take the supplements on the non-permissible list but they have to purchase them on their own. Care should also be taken to ensure there are no banned substances in a particular nutritional supplement for an athlete. While there are numerous supplements available, we typically recommend only a few.

1. Protein

Research has indicated that athletes undergoing intense training may need additional protein in their diet to meet protein needs (i.e., 1.5–2.0 grams/day). Athletes who do not ingest enough protein may slow recovery and training adaptations.[142] Although not completely necessary, we have found that commercially available carbohydrate and protein supplements offer a convenient way to ensure that an athlete is meeting carbohydrate and protein needs.[143] However, ingesting additional protein beyond that necessary to meet protein needs does not appear to promote additional gains in strength and muscle mass.

The research focus over recent years has been to determine whether different types of protein (e.g., whey, casein, soy, colostrum, etc.) may have varying effects on the physiological, hormonal, or immunological responses to training. Different types of protein offer some advantages over others. For example, whey and soy protein have a very high proportion of essential amino acids (EAA), are digested at a faster rate, and lead to greater increases in protein synthesis than other forms of protein. We typically recommend that athletes wanting to gain muscle mass ingest 10–20 grams of a fast-digesting protein (i.e., whey) several times throughout the day to sustain protein synthesis. In addition, they should consume a dairy product (yogurt, skim milk, etc.), milk protein, or a combination of whey and casein prior to going to bed to provide both fast- (whey) and slow- (casein) digesting proteins. In this way, EAA is provided for protein synthesis (whey) as well as prolonged release of amino acids (casein), which can reduce catabolism during prolonged fasting periods. Ingesting protein with additional leucine or glutamine can also provide some benefits in optimizing protein synthesis and maintaining a healthy immune system particularly during heavy training periods.

Finally, timing of protein intake is critical. Therefore, we typically will have athletes ingest a carbohydrate/protein shake or bar within 30 minutes after workouts and competition. Preferably, the protein should be whey that can quickly release EAA into the blood and promote post-exercise protein synthesis or be a good source of leucine and glutamine.[144]

2. Creatine

Creatine is one of the most effective nutritional supplements available to athletes to increase high intensity exercise capacity and muscle mass during training. Numerous studies have indicated that creatine supplementation increases body mass or muscle mass during training.[145–149] Gains are typically 2–5 (0.9 to 2.2 kg) pounds greater than controls during 4–12 weeks of training.[146,147] The gains in muscle mass appear to be a result of an improved ability to perform high-intensity exercise, enabling an athlete to train harder and thereby promote greater training adaptations.[150] In addition, many cellular level changes have been shown to occur as a result of creatine supplementation.[151] We have found that adding 5–8 grams of creatine to vitamin- and mineral-fortified carbohydrate/protein shakes during intentional weight-gain periods is the most effective way to promote gains in muscle mass. For example, most of our initial creatine studies added 5–8 grams of creatine to a typical carbohydrate/protein meal replacement shake.[152,153]

Athletes ingesting three carbohydate/protein/creatine shakes a day during 4–12 weeks of heavy resistance and conditioning training gained 5–8 pounds of muscle mass (about 2.5–3.5 kg). These gains were significantly greater than training without nutritional supplementation (controls), ingesting iso-energetic amounts of carbohydrate, or ingesting isoenergetic and hypercaloric amounts of carbohydrate and protein supplements. While we now don't believe it necessary to ingest as much creatine as we utilized in these initial studies (i.e., 20–25 grams/day following the initial loading period), this approach did promote the greatest gains in strength and muscle mass during training. Consequently, when athletes want to gain muscle mass, we usually recommend they take 2–3 carbohydrate/protein shakes per day with 1 small teaspoon of creatine (about 3–5 grams) during heavy resistance training until their goal weight is achieved. In our experience, this has proven to be a highly effective way of promoting gains in muscle mass during training both in the clinical research trials we have conducted and from practical experience working with athletes needing to gain weight.

3. β-hydroxy β-methylbutyrate (β-HMB)

In addition to protein and creatine, some of our athletes have also added calcium β-HMB to their weight-gain nutritional strategies. HMB is a metabolite of the amino acid leucine. Leucine and metabolites of leucine have been reported to inhibit protein degradation.[154,155] Research has shown that adding HMB to animal feed promoted greater gains in fat-free mass and lower body fat. In humans, supplementing the diet with 1.5–3 grams/day of calcium HMB has been reported to increase muscle mass and strength in untrained subjects initiating training[156–158] and in the elderly.[159] Gains in muscle mass are typically 0.5–1 kg greater than controls during 3–6 weeks of training. There is also recent evidence that HMB supplementation may delay the onset of anaerobic threshold[160] and strength gains during training.[161] In addition, there is evidence that HMB supplementation may lessen the catabolic effects after performing a 20-km run[162] and following eccentrically induced muscle damage.[163] Thus, HMB may help athletes recover from intense training. Finally, there is evidence that co-ingesting HMB with creatine[164] promoted greater gains in strength and muscle mass in comparison with supplementing the diet with a placebo and creatine alone. In support of this theory, Nissen and colleagues[165] conducted a meta-analysis on various nutritional strategies purported to promote increases in muscle mass and found that creatine and HMB were the only strategies that were found to significantly increase lean muscle mass during training.

However, it should be noted that not all studies support contentions that HMB supplementation increases fat-free mass during training. We conducted two studies on HMB.[166,167] In the first study,[166] HMB (3 grams/day) was added to a low-carbohydrate sports drink and compared with the same drink containing a placebo, creatine, or a combination of creatine with HMB. We found no significant effects of HMB supplementation on training adaptations when taken alone or with creatine. In a follow-up study, we added 3 or 6 grams/day of HMB to a vitamin- and mineral-fortified carbohydrate and protein MRP supplement. Subjects supplemented with the MRP three times per day during resistance training. We found a slight increase in mean fat-free mass (up to 0.9 kg) but these differences were not significantly different among groups. It should also be noted that the gains observed were not nearly as impressive as we had seen when adding creatine to MRPs. Other studies support these findings in that they report no significant effects of HMB supplementation on muscle hypertrophy during training.[161,168–170] The discrepancy in results in untrained versus trained subjects may be due to a greater variability in response of HMB supplementation among athletes.[166,167,170] Consequently, while there are some advantages from HMB supplementation described in the literature, the effects on body composition is unclear, particularly in trained subjects. For this reason, we do not recommend that our athletes take HMB. If athletes want to try it, we tell them they should do so only after first implementing the other previously described strategies.

4. Beta-Alanine

While the three sports supplements mentioned have quite a few scientific studies supporting their effectiveness in increasing lean body mass, the sports supplement beta-alanine is relatively new and promising but does not yet have multiple scientific studies supporting its muscle-building potential. One study that was recently published by Hoffman et al.[171] is very promising and provides some scientific evidence for adding beta-alanine supplementation for those wishing to increase lean body mass. In this study, collegiate football players participating in a 10-week resistance training program ingested a placebo, creatine, or creatine plus beta-alanine. The most interesting finding from this study was that the creatine plus beta-alanine resulted in significant increases in lean body mass as compared with the placebo- and creatine-only groups. Because this is the only study showing potential for beta-alanine supplementation for increasing lean body mass, one must avoid making any definite conclusions about the effectiveness of this supplement until more studies are conducted that demonstrate similar findings. Also, future studies investigating the effects of beta-alanine alone (without combining it with creatine) will be very interesting. Be on the lookout, as this supplement is becoming very popular and may become the “new” creatine in the years to come.

V. FUTURE RESEARCH NEEDS

The clinical study of weight management in athletes has many hurdles and roadblocks to overcome. The difficulty in the study of dietary intervention is simply compliance. Without a controlled environment, such as that of a hospital, researchers are left to rely on dietary recall. One of the primary issues in weight management research is that of diet records. Over the last several years, the importance of evaluation of nutritional intervention with exercise has come to be a top priority. However, one the largest sources of error is dietary recall. In a perfect world, researchers could monitor all food intake for their study participants. This is logistically impossible, unless your participants are in-house. Thus, all conventional methods of dietary adherence depend on subjects' reports. Most labs lack independent biochemical, physiological, or genetic measures of dietary intake. Therefore, we do not know if subjects actually follow the diets being tested and compared. We also know that most subjects in weight-loss studies under-report their energy intake and its components.[172] The sad reality is that we do not actually know if the results of any current diet trials are valid or reliable. Winkler[173] has identified three ways in which researchers can help control diet intervention studies: (1) biomarkers of intake for energy, macro- and micronutrients and other food components relevant to weight gain or loss; (2) field measuring instruments that are cheap, rapid, painless, non-intrusive, and self-administrable; and (3) electronic data transmission systems that preclude subjects' ability to misreport. Nonetheless, several areas of research are needed:

Studies that investigate biological mechanisms underlying weight loss and weight gain in athletes (neuroendocrine, endocrine, and gastrointestinal function, muscle and adipocyte biology, etc.)

Studies to elucidate the role of energy expenditure during weight management, including voluntary physical activity, thermic effect of feeding, nonexercise-activity thermogenesis, sympathetic/parasympathetic nervous system function

Studies of the effects of age-related changes on responses to weight maintenance interventions, including effects on body composition, metabolic regulation, and other physiologic responses

Studies of dietary strategies to enhance long-term weight maintenance (such as meal replacements, alterations in nutrient density or macronutrient composition)

Studies using approved or investigational weight managment agents to enhance weight maintenance

Clinical studies evaluating the impact of differing types, intensity, and frequency of physical activity on long-term weight maintenance

VI. CONCLUSIONS

Many athletes seek to improve performance by improving body composition. Weight management is paramount for optimal performance. Most people can increase muscle mass if they incorporate basic training and nutritional practices. We believe that this can best be accomplished if athletes determine their body composition so that results can be monitored; engage in heavy resistance training; consume a slightly hypercaloric diet with sufficient protein; properly time nutrient intake; and, consider using only dietary supplements that research has shown to be effective in promoting significantly greater gains in muscle mass during training. While there are many dietary supplements purported to promote gains in muscle mass, our experience and research has indicated that ingesting a quality carbohydrate/protein supplement containing a high proportion of EAA as well as creatine in the manner described is highly effective in optimizing muscle-mass gains during training. If one is engaged in heavy training, adding leucine, glutamine, and possibly HMB to the post-exercise nutritional regimen may also help optimize recovery and/or help the athlete tolerate heavy training demands.

It is necessary for some athletes to lose weight. To lose fat weight, our recommendation is to reduce caloric intake by 500 calories per day, consume primarily low- to moderate-GI carbohydrates, participate in a strength-training program (30–60 minutes, 3–4 times per week), and consume a relatively low-fat (20–30% of calories), moderate-carbohydrate (35–45% of calories), high-protein (20–40% of calories) diet. In addition, numerous nutritional and herbal products are marketed to promote weight loss. Most have a theoretical basis for use but little data supporting safety and efficacy in weight loss in humans. A number are heavily marketed despite data indicating that they do not affect body composition in humans at the dosages recommended. The available research suggests that the most effective weight-loss supplements appear to be those that help individuals manage a low-caloric diet (e.g., diet foods, MRPs, RTDs) and thermogenic supplements. High-fiber diets may also help manage weight loss but to a lesser degree. There is good theoretical rationale and some supportive data indicating that phosphate, green tea extract, pyruvate/DHAP (at high doses), and long-term use of CLA may offer some benefit to weight loss. Remember that the best way to increase fat metabolism and promote weight loss is through exercise and eating a well balanced but slightly hypocaloric diet.

REFERENCES

1. Clement, K., and Ferre, P. 2003. Genetics and the pathophysiology of obesity, *Pediatr. Res.* 53, 721–5.
2. Spiegelman, B.M., and Flier, J.S. 2001. Obesity and the regulation of energy balance, *Cell.* 104, 531–43.
3. Knittle, J.L., Timmers, K., Ginsberg-Fellner, F., Brown, R.E., and Katz, D.P. 1979. The growth of adipose tissue in children and adolescents: Cross-sectional and longitudinal studies of adipose cell number and size, *J. Clin. Invest.* 63, 239–46.
4. Flatt, J.P., Ravussin, E., Acheson, K.J., and Jequier, E. 1985. Effects of dietary fat on postprandial substrate oxidation and on carbohydrate and fat balances, *J. Clin. Invest.* 76, 1019–24.
5. Schutz, Y., Flatt, J.P., and Jequier, E. 1989. Failure of dietary fat intake to promote fat oxidation: a factor favoring the development of obesity, *Am. J. Clin. Nutr.* 50, 307–14.
6. Jequier, E., and Tappy, L. 1999. Regulation of body weight in humans, *Physiol. Rev.* 79, 451–80.
7. Flatt, J.P., *The Biochemistry of Energy Expenditure*, Libbey, London, 1980, pp. 211–218.
8. Faith, M., Rha, S.S., Neale, M.C., and Allison, D. 1999. Evidence for genetic influences on human energy intake: Results from a twin study using measured observations, *Behav. Genet.* 29, 145–54.
9. Tholin, S., Rasmussen, F., Tynelius, P., and Karlsson, J. 2005. Genetic and environmental influences on eating behavior: the Swedish Young Male Twins Study, *Am. J. Clin. Nutr.* 81, 564–9.

10. Ello-Martin, J.A., Ledikwe, J., and Rolls, B.J. 2005. The influence of food portion size and energy density on energy intake: Implications for weight management, *Am. J. Clin Nutr.* 82, 236S–241S.
11. Bray, G., *Contemporary Diagnosis and Management of Obesity and The Metabolic Syndrome*, Handbooks in Health Care, Newtown, PA , 2003; pp. 240–262.
12. Levine, J.A., and Kotz, C.M. 2005. NEAT—non-exercise activity thermogenesis—egocentric and geocentric environmental factors vs. biological regulation, *Acta Physiol Scand.* 184, 309–18.
13. Hill, J., Saris, W., and Levine, J.A., *The Handbook of Obesity: Etiology and Pathophysiology,* 2nd ed., Marcel Dekker Inc., New York, 2004.
14. Dauncey, M.J. 1990. Activity and energy expenditure, *Can. J. Physiol. Pharmacol.* 68, 17–27.
15. Castaneda, T.R., Jurgens, H., Wiedmer, P., Pfluger, P., Diano, S., Horvath, T.L., et al. 2005. Obesity and the neuroendocrine control of energy homeostasis: The role of spontaneous locomotor activity, *J. Nutr.* 135, 1314–9.
16. DiPietro, L. 1995. Physical activity, body weight, and adiposity: An epidemiologic perspective, *Exerc. Sport Sci. Rev.* 23, 275–303.
17. Meredith, C.N., Zackin, M.J., Frontera, W.R., and Evans, W.J. 1987. Body composition and aerobic capacity in young and middle-aged endurance-trained men, *Med. Sci. Sports Exerc.* 19, 557–63.
18. Ballor, D.L., and Keesey, R.E. 1991. A meta-analysis of the factors affecting exercise-induced changes in body mass, fat mass and fat-free mass in males and females, *Int. J. Obes.* 15, 717–26.
19. Slentz, C.A., Aiken, L.B., Houmard, J.A., Bales, C.W., Johnson, J.L., Tanner, C.J., et al. 2005. Inactivity, exercise and visceral fat. STRRIDE: A randomized, controlled study of exercise intensity and amount, *J. Appl. Physiol.* 99, 1613–8.
20. Williams, P.T., Blanche, P.J., and Krauss, R.M. 2005. Behavioral versus genetic correlates of lipoproteins and adiposity in identical twins discordant for exercise, *Circulation.* 112, 350–6.
21. Hermsdorff, H.H., Volp, A.C., and Bressan, J. 2007. Macronutrient profile affects diet-induced thermogenesis and energy intake, *Arch. Latinoam Nutr.* 57, 33–42.
22. Smeets, A.J., and Westerterp-Plantenga, M.S. 2008. Acute effects on metabolism and appetite profile of one meal difference in the lower range of meal frequency, *Br. J. Nutr.* 99, 1316–21.
23. Marques-Lopes, I., Ansorena, D., Astiasaran, I., Forga, L., and Martinez, J.A. 2001. Postprandial de novo lipogenesis and metabolic changes induced by a high-carbohydrate, low-fat meal in lean and overweight men, *Am. J. Clin.Nutr.* 73, 253–61.
24. Brand–Miller, J.C., Holt, S. Pawlak, D.B., and McMillan, J. 2002. Glycemic index and obesity, *Am. J. Clin. Nutr.* 76, 281S–5S.
25. Abete, I., Parra, D., and Martinez, J.A. 2008. Energy-restricted diets based on a distinct food selection affecting the glycemic index induce different weight loss and oxidative response, *Clin. Nutr.,* Feb. 26 (Epub ahead of print).
26. Schwarz, J.M., Schutz, Y., Fr(idevaux, F., Acheson, K.J., Jeanpretre, N., Schneider, H., et al. 1989. Thermogenesis in men and women induced by fructose vs glucose added to a meal, *Am. J. Clin. Nutr.* 49, 667–74.
27. Schwarz, J., Schutz, Y., Piolino, V., Schneider, H., Felber, J.P., and Jequier, E. 1992. Thermogenesis in obese women: Effect of fructose vs. glucose added to a meal, *Am. J. Physiol.* 262, E394–401.
28. Keogh, J.B., Lau, C.W., Noakes, M., Bowen, J., and Clifton, P.M. 2007. Effects of meals with high soluble fibre, high amylose barley variant on glucose, insulin, satiety and thermic effect of food in healthy lean women, *Eur. J. Clin. Nutr.* 61, 597–604.

29. Rasmussen, L.G., Larsen, T.M., Mortensen, P.K., Due, A., and Astrup, A. 2007. Effect on 24-h energy expenditure of a moderate-fat diet high in monounsaturated fatty acids compared with that of a low-fat, carbohydrate-rich diet: A 6-mo controlled dietary intervention trial, *Am. J. Clin. Nutr.* 85, 1014–22.
30. Maffeis, C., Schutz, Y., Grezzani, A., Provera, S., Piacentini, G., and Tato, L. 2001. Meal-induced thermogenesis and obesity: Is a fat meal a risk factor for fat gain in children? *J. Clin. Endocrinol. Metab.* 86, 214–9.
31. Westerterp, K.R., Wilson, S.A., and Rolland, V. 1999. Diet induced thermogenesis measured over 24 h in a respiration chamber: effect of diet composition, *Int. J. Obes. Relat. Metab. Disord.* 23, 287–92.
32. Westerterp-Plantenga, M.S., Rolland, V., Wilson, S.A., and Westerterp, K.R. 1999. Satiety related to 24 h diet-induced thermogenesis during high protein/carbohydrate vs. high fat diets measured in a respiration chamber, *Eur. J. Clin. Nutr.* 53, 495–502.
33. Paddon-Jones, D., Westman, E., Mattes, R.D., Wolfe, R.R., Astrup, A., and Westerterp-Plantenga, M. 2008. Protein, weight management, and satiety, *Am. J. Clin. Nutr.* 87, 1558S–61S.
34. Jequier, E. 1984. Thermogenesis induced by nutrient administration in man, *Infusionsther Klin. Ernahr.* 11, 184–8.
35. Robinson, S., Jaccard, C., Persaud, C., Jackson, A.A., Jequier, E., and Schutz, Y. 1990. Protein turnover and thermogenesis in response to high-protein and high-carbohydrate feeding in men, *Am. J. Clin. Nutr.* 52, 72–80.
36. Webb, P., and Annis, J.F. 1983. Adaptation to overeating in lean and overweight men and women, *Hum. Nutr. Clin. Nutr.* 37, 117–31.
37. Johnston, C.S., Day, C.S., and Swan, P.D. 2002. Postprandial thermogenesis is increased 100% on a high-protein, low-fat diet versus a high-carbohydrate, low-fat diet in healthy, young women, *J. Am. Coll. Nutr.* 21, 55–61.
38. Leidy, H.J., Mattes, R.D., and Campbell, W.W. 2007. Effects of acute and chronic protein intake on metabolism, appetite, and ghrelin during weight loss, *Obesity (Silver Spring).* 15, 1215–25.
39. Position of Dietitians of Canada, the American Dietetic Association, and the American College of Sports Medicine: Nutrition and Athletic Performance. 2000. *Can. J. Diet. Pract. Res.* 61, 176–92.
40. Position of the American Dietetic Association, Dietitians of Canada, and the American College of Sports Medicine: Nutrition and athletic performance 2000. *J. Am. Diet. Assoc.* 100, 1543–56.
41. Jequier, E. 2002. Pathways to obesity, *Int. J. Obes. Relat. Metab. Disord.* 26 Suppl 2, S12–7.
42. Reaven, G.M. 2000. Diet and Syndrome X, *Curr. Atheroscler. Rep.* 2, 503–7.
43. Gaesser, G.A. 2007. Carbohydrate quantity and quality in relation to body mass index, *J. Am. Diet. Assoc.* 107, 1768–80.
44. Pouw, E., Schols, A., Deutz, N.E., and Wouters, E.F. 1998. Plasma and muscle amino acid levels in relation to resting energy expenditure and inflammation in stable chronic obstructive pulmonary disease, *Am. J. Respir. Crit. Care Med.* 158, 797–801.
45. Schrauwen, P., Schaart, G., Saris, W.H., Slieker, L.J., Glatz, J.F., Vidal, H., and Blaak, E.E. 2000. The effect of weight reduction on skeletal muscle UCP2 and UCP3 mRNA expression and UCP3 protein content in Type II diabetic subjects, *Diabetologia* 43, 1408–16.
46. Poirier, P., and Despres, J.P. 2001. Exercise in weight management of obesity, *Cardiol. Clin.* 19, 459–70.
47. Geliebter, A., Maher, M.M., Gerace, L., Gutin, B., Heymsfield, S.B., and Hashim, S.A. 1997. Effects of strength or aerobic training on body composition, resting metabolic rate, and peak oxygen consumption in obese dieting subjects, *Am. J. Clin. Nutr.* 66, 557–63.

48. Berggren, J.R., Boyle, K.E., Chapman, W., and Houmard, J.A. 2008. Skeletal muscle lipid oxidation and obesity: Influence of weight loss and exercise, *Am. J. Physiol. Endocrinol. Metab.* 294, E726–32.
49. Weiss, E., Galuska, D., Kettel Khan, L., Gillespie, C., and Serdula, M. 2007. Weight regain in U.S. adults who experienced substantial weight loss, 1999–2002, *Am. J. Prev. Med.* 33, 34–40.
50. Murakami, C., Myoga, K., Kasai, R., Ohtani, K., Kurokawa, T., Ishibashi, S., et al. 1993. Screening of plant constituents for effect on glucose transport activity in Ehrlich ascites tumour cells, *Chem. Pharm. Bull. (Tokyo).* 41, 2129–31.
51. Guezennec, C.Y. 1995. Oxidation rates, complex carbohydrates and exercise, *Sports Med.* 19, 365–372.
52. Williams, M., *Nutrition for Health Fitness & Sport*, 6th ed., McGraw-Hill, Dubuque, IA, 2002, p. 251.
53. DeMarco, H.M., Sucher, K.P., Cisar, C.J., and Butterfield, G.E. 1996. 1999. Pre-exercise carbohydrate meals: Application of glycemic index, *Med. Sci. Sports Exerc.* 31, 164–70.
54. Febbraio, M.A., and Stewart, K.L. 1996. CHO feeding before prolonged exercise: Effect of glycemic index on muscle glycogenolysis and exercise performance, *J. Appl. Physiol.* 81, 1115–20.
55. Wee, S.L., Williams, C., Gray, S., and Horabin, J. 1999. Influence of high and low glycemic index meals on endurance running capacity, *Med. Sci. Sports Exerc.* 31, 393–9.
56. Earnest, C.P., Lancaster, S.L., Rasmussen, C.J., Kerksick, C.M., Lucia, A., Greenwood, M.C., et al. 2004. Low vs. high glycemic index carbohydrate gel ingestion during simulated 64-km cycling time trial performance, *J. Strength Cond Res.* 18, 466–72.
57. Burke, L.M., Collier, G.R., and Hargreaves, M. 1998. Glycemic index—a new tool in sport nutrition? *Int. J. Sport Nutr.* 8, 401–15.
58. Walberg-Rankin, J. 1997. Glycemic index and exercise metabolism, *Sports Sci. Exchange.* 10, 1–7.
59. Walton, P., and Rhodes, E.C. 1997. Glycaemic index and optimal performance, *Sports Med.* 23, 164–72.
60. Ali, A., Williams, C., Nicholas, C.W., and Foskett, A. 2007. The influence of carbohydrate–electrolyte ingestion on soccer skill performance, *Med. Sci. Sports Exerc.* 39, 1969–76.
61. Currell, K., and Jeukendrup, A.E. 2008. Superior endurance performance with ingestion of multiple transportable carbohydrates, *Med. Sci. Sports Exerc.* 40, 275–81.
62. Stevenson, E.J., Williams, C., Mash, L.E., Phillips, B., and Nute, M.L. 2006. Influence of high-carbohydrate mixed meals with different glycemic indexes on substrate utilization during subsequent exercise in women, *Am. J. Clin. Nutr.* 84, 354–60.
63. Wallis, G.A., Dawson, R., Achten, J., Webber, J., and Jeukendrup, A.E. 2006. Metabolic response to carbohydrate ingestion during exercise in males and females, *Am. J. Physiol. Endocrinol. Metab.* 290, E708–15.
64. Kushner, R.F., and Doerfler, B. 2008. Low-carbohydrate, high-protein diets revisited, *Curr. Opin. Gastroenterol.* 24, 198–203.
65. Piatti, P.M., Monti, F., Fermo, I., Baruffaldi, L., Nasser, R., Santambrogio, G., et al. 1994. Hypocaloric high-protein diet improves glucose oxidation and spares lean body mass: Comparison to hypocaloric high-carbohydrate diet, *Metabolism.* 43, 1481–7.
66. Skov, A.R., Toubro, S., Ronn, B., Holm, L., and Astrup, A. 1999. Randomized trial on protein vs. carbohydrate in ad libitum fat reduced diet for the treatment of obesity, *Int. J. Obes. Relat. Metab. Disord.* 23, 528–36.

67. Skov, A.R., Haulrik, N., Toubro, S., Molgaard, C., and Astrup, A. 2002. Effect of protein intake on bone mineralization during weight loss: A 6-month trial, *Obes. Res.* 10, 432–8.
68. Skov, A.R., Toubro, S., Bulow, J., Krabbe, K., Parving, H.H., and Astrup, A. 1999. Changes in renal function during weight loss induced by high vs. low-protein low-fat diets in overweight subjects, *Int. J. Obes. Relat. Metab. Disord.* 23, 1170–7.
69. Baba, N.H., Sawaya, S., Torbay, N., Habbal, Z., Azar, S., and Hashim, S. 1999. High protein vs. high carbohydrate hypoenergetic diet for the treatment of obese hyperinsulinemic subjects, *Int. J. Obes. Relat. Metab. Disord.* 23, 1202–6.
70. Parker, B., Noakes, M., Luscombe, N., and Clifton, P. 2002. Effect of a high-protein, high-monounsaturated fat weight loss diet on glycemic control and lipid levels in type 2 diabetes, *Diabetes Care.* 25, 425–30.
71. Krieger, J.W., Sitren, H.S., Daniels, M., and Langkamp-Henken, B. 2006. Effects of variation in protein and carbohydrate intake on body mass and composition during energy restriction: A meta-regression, *Am. J. Clin. Nutr.* 83, 260–74.
72. Hoie, L.H., Bruusgaard, D., and Thom, E. 1993. Reduction of body mass and change in body composition on a very low calorie diet, *Int. J. Obes. Relat. Metab. Disord.* 17, 17–20.
73. Leutholtz, B.C., Keyser, R.E., Heusner, W., Wendt, V.E., and Rosen, L. 1995. Exercise training and severe caloric restriction: effect on lean body mass in the obese, *Arch. Phys. Med. Rehabil.* 76, 65–70.
74. Kern, P.A., Trozzolino, L., Wolfe, G., and Purdy, L. 1994. Combined use of behavior modification and very low-calorie diet in weight loss and weight maintenance, *Am. J. Med. Sci.* 307, 325–8.
75. Raben, A., Jensen, N.D., Marckmann, P., Sandstrom, B., and Astrup, A.V. 1997. Spontaneous weight loss in young subjects of normal weight after 11 weeks of unrestricted intake of a low-fat/high-fiber diet, *Ugeskr. Laeger* 159, 1448–53.
76. Shigematsu, N., Asano, R., Shimosaka, M., and Okazaki, M. 2001. Effect of administration with the extract of *Gymnema sylvestre* R. Br. leaves on lipid metabolism in rats, *Biol. Pharm. Bull.* 24, 713–7.
77. Shigematsu, N., Asano, R., Shimosaka, M., and Okazaki, M. 2001. Effect of long term administration with *Gymnema sylvestre* R. BR. on plasma and liver lipid in rats, *Biol. Pharm. Bull.* 24, 643–9.
78. Gallaher, C.M., Munion, J., Hesslink, R., Jr., Wise, J., and Gallaher, D.D. 2000. Cholesterol reduction by glucomannan and chitosan is mediated by changes in cholesterol absorption and bile acid and fat excretion in rats, *J. Nutr.* 130, 2753–9.
79. Chiang, M.T., Yao, H.T., and Chen, H.C. 2000. Effect of dietary chitosans with different viscosity on plasma lipids and lipid peroxidation in rats fed on a diet enriched with cholesterol, *Biosci. Biotechnol. Biochem.* 64, 965–71.
80. Wuolijoki, E., Hirvela, T., and Ylitalo, P. 1999. Decrease in serum LDL cholesterol with microcrystalline chitosan, *Methods Find. Exp. Clin. Pharmacol.* 21, 357–61.
81. Guerciolini, R., Radu-Radulescu, L., Boldrin, M., Dallas, J., and Moore, R. 2001. Comparative evaluation of fecal fat excretion induced by orlistat and chitosan, *Obes. Res.* 9, 364–7.
82. Pittler, M.H., Abbot, N.C., Harkness, E.F., and Ernst, E. 1999. Randomized, double-blind trial of chitosan for body weight reduction, *Eur. J. Clin. Nutr.* 53, 379–81.
83. Ho, S.C., Tai, E.S., Eng, P.H., Tan, C.E., and Fok, A.C. 2001. In the absence of dietary surveillance, chitosan does not reduce plasma lipids or obesity in hypercholesterolaemic obese Asian subjects, *Singapore Med. J.* 42, 6–10.
84. Boozer, C.N., Nasser, J.A., Heymsfield, S.B., Wang, V., Chen, G., and Solomon, J.L. 2001. An herbal supplement containing Ma Huang-Guarana for weight loss: A randomized, double-blind trial, *Int. J. Obes. Relat. Metab. Disord.* 25, 316–24.

85. Molnar, D., Torok, K., Erhardt, E., and Jeges, S. 2000. Safety and efficacy of treatment with an ephedrine/caffeine mixture: The first double-blind placebo-controlled pilot study in adolescents, *Int. J. Obes. Relat. Metab. Disord.* 24, 1573–8.
86. Greenway, F.L., Ryan, D.H., Bray, G.A., Rood, J.C., Tucker, E.W., and Smith, S.R. 1999. Pharmaceutical cost savings of treating obesity with weight loss medications, *Obes. Res.* 7, 523–31.
87. Nazar, K., Kaciuba-Uscilko, H., Szczepanik, J., Zemba, A.W., Kruk, B., Chwalbinska-Moneta, J., et al. 1996. Phosphate supplementation prevents a decrease of triiodothyronine and increases resting metabolic rate during low energy diet, *J. Physiol. Pharmacol.* 47, 373–83.
88. Westerterp-Plantenga, M.S., Smeets, A., and Lejeune, M.P. 2005. Sensory and gastrointestinal satiety effects of capsaicin on food intake, *Int. J. Obes. (Lond).* 29, 682–8.
89. Yoshioka, M., St.-Pierre, S., Drapeau, V., Dionne, I., Doucet, E., Suzuki, M., and Tremblay, A. 1999. Effects of red pepper on appetite and energy intake, *Br. J. Nutr.* 82, 115–23.
90. Cangiano, C., Laviano, A., Del Ben, M., Preziosa, I., Angelico, F., Cascino, A., and Rossi-Fanelli, F. 1998. Effects of oral 5-hydroxy-tryptophan on energy intake and macronutrient selection in non-insulin dependent diabetic patients, *Int. J. Obes. Relat. Metab. Disord.* 22, 648–54.
91. Kobayashi, Y., Nakano, Y., Kizaki, M., Hoshikuma, K., Yokoo, Y., and Kamiya, T. 2001. Capsaicin-like anti-obese activities of evodiamine from fruits of Evodia rutaecarpa, a vanilloid receptor agonist, *Planta Med.* 67, 628–33.
92. Kucio, C., Jonderko, K., and Piskorska, D. 1991. Does yohimbine act as a slimming drug? *Isr. J. Med. Sci.* 27, 550–6.
93. Garcia Neto, M., Pesti, G.M., and Bakalli, R.I. 2000. Influence of dietary protein level on the broiler chicken's response to methionine and betaine supplements, *Poult. Sci.* 79, 1478–84.
94. Overland, M., Rorvik, K.A., and Skrede, A. 1999. Effect of trimethylamine oxide and betaine in swine diets on growth performance, carcass characteristics, nutrient digestibility, and sensory quality of pork, *J. Anim. Sci.* 77, 2143–53.
95. Brouwer, I.A., Verhoef, P., and Urgert, R. 2000. Betaine supplementation and plasma homocysteine in healthy volunteers, *Arch. Intern. Med.* 160, 2546–7.
96. Stanko, R.T., Tietze, D.L., and Arch, J.E. 1992. Body composition, energy utilization, and nitrogen metabolism with a severely restricted diet supplemented with dihydroxyacetone and pyruvate, *Am. J. Clin. Nutr.* 55, 771–6.
97. Stanko, R.T., Reynolds, H.R., Hoyson, R., Janosky, J.E., and Wolf, R. 1994. Pyruvate supplementation of a low–cholesterol, low–fat diet: effects on plasma lipid concentrations and body composition in hyperlipidemic patients, *Am. J. Clin. Nutr.* 59, 423–7.
98. Stanko, R.T., and Arch, J.E. 1996. Inhibition of regain in body weight and fat with addition of 3-carbon compounds to the diet with hyperenergetic refeeding after weight reduction, *Int. J. Obes. Relat. Metab. Disord.* 20, 925–30.
99. Kalman, D., Colker, C.M., Wilets, I., Roufs, J.B., and Antonio, J. 1999. The effects of pyruvate supplementation on body composition in overweight individuals, *Nutrition* 15, 337–40.
100. Stone, M.H., Sanborn, K., Smith, L.L., O'Bryant, H.S., Hoke, T., Utter, A.C., et al. 1999. Effects of in-season (5 weeks) creatine and pyruvate supplementation on anaerobic performance and body composition in American football players, *Int. J. Sport Nutr.* 9, 146–65.
101. Kreider, R., Koh, P., Ferreira, M., Cowan, P., and Almada, A. 1998. Effects of pyruvate supplementation during training on body composition and metabolic responses to exercise, *Med. Sci. Sports Exerc.* 30, S62 (abstract).

102. Brass, E.P. 2000. Supplemental carnitine and exercise, *Am. J. Clin. Nutr.* 72, 618S–23S.
103. Villani, R.G., Gannon, J., Self, M., and Rich, P.A. 2000. L-Carnitine supplementation combined with aerobic training does not promote weight loss in moderately obese women, *Int. J. Sport Nutr. Exerc. Metab.* 10, 199–207.
104. Kreider, R.B. 1999. Dietary supplements and the promotion of muscle growth with resistance exercise, *Sports Med.* 27, 97–110.
105. Walker, L.S., Bemben, M.G., Bemben, D.A., and Knehans, A.W. 1998. Chromium picolinate effects on body composition and muscular performance in wrestlers, *Med. Sci. Sports Exerc.* 30, 1730–7.
106. Lukaski, H.C., Bolonchuk, W.W., Siders, W.A., and Milne, D.B. 1996. Chromium supplementation and resistance training: effects on body composition, strength, and trace element status of men, *Am. J. Clin. Nutr.* 63, 954–65.
107. Crawford, V., Scheckenbach, R., and Preuss, H.G. 1999. Effects of niacin-bound chromium supplementation on body composition in overweight African-American women, *Diabetes Obes. Metab.* 1, 331–7.
108. Ammon, H.P., and Muller, A.B. 1985. Forskolin: From an ayurvedic remedy to a modern agent, *Planta Med.* 473–7.
109. de Souza, N.J., Dohadwalla, A.N., and Reden, J. 1983. Forskolin: A labdane diterpenoid with antihypertensive, positive inotropic, platelet aggregation inhibitory, and adenylate cyclase activating properties, *Med. Res. Rev.* 3, 201–19.
110. Seamon, K.B., Padgett, W., and Daly, J.W. 1981. Forskolin: Unique diterpene activator of adenylate cyclase in membranes and in intact cells, *Proc. Natl. Acad. Sci. USA.* 78, 3363–7.
111. Litosch, I., Hudson, T.H., Mills, I., Li, S.Y., and Fain, J.N. 1982. Forskolin as an activator of cyclic AMP accumulation and lipolysis in rat adipocytes, *Mol. Pharmacol.* 22, 109–15.
112. Badmaev, V., Majeed, M., Conte, A.A., and Parker, J.E. Diterpene forskolin (*Coleus forskohlii*, Benth.): A possible new compound for reduction of body weight by increasing lean body mass; Sabinsa Corporation: Piscataway, NJ, 2001. http://www.forslean.com/clinical_studies.html.
113. Pariza, M.W., Park, Y., and Cook, M.E. 1999. Conjugated linoleic acid and the control of cancer and obesity, *Toxicol. Sci.* 52, 107–10.
114. MacDonald, H.B. 2000. Conjugated linoleic acid and disease prevention: A review of current knowledge, *J. Am. Coll. Nutr.* 19, 111S–8S.
115. Larsen, T.M., Toubro, S., Gudmundsen, O., and Astrup, A. 2006. Conjugated linoleic acid supplementation for 1 y does not prevent weight or body fat regain, *Am. J. Clin. Nutr.* 83, 606–12.
116. Thom, E. A pilot study with the aim of studying the efficacy and tolerability of Tonalin CLA on the body composition in humans, Technical Report. Medstat. Research Limited, Lillestram, Norway, July, 1997.
117. Lowery, L.M., Appicelli, P.A., and Lemon, P.W.R. 1998. Conjugated linoleic acid enhances muscle size and strength gains in novice bodybuilders, *Med. Sci. Sports Exerc.* 30, S182.
118. Riserus, U., Berglund, L., and Vessby, B. 2001. Conjugated linoleic acid (CLA) reduced abdominal adipose tissue in obese middle-aged men with signs of the metabolic syndrome: A randomised controlled trial, *Int. J. Obes. Relat. Metab. Disord.* 25, 1129–35.
119. Blankson, H., Stakkestad, J.A., Fagertun, H., Thom, E., Wadstein, J., and Gudmundsen, O. 2000. Conjugated linoleic acid reduces body fat mass in overweight and obese humans, *J. Nutr.* 130, 2943–8.
120. Beuker, F., Haak, H., and Schwietz, H. In "CLA and body styling," Symposium: Vitamine und Zusatzstoffe, Jena, 1999; pp 229–237.

121. Von Loeffelholz, C., Von Loeffelholz, B.A., Von Loeffelholz, B., and Jahreis, G. 1999. Influence of conjugated linoleic acid (CLA) supplementation on body composition and strength in bodybuilders, *Jena.* 7, 238–43.
122. Zambell, K.L., Keim, N.L., Van Loan, M.D., Gale, B., Benito, P., Kelley, D.S., and Nelson, G.J. 2000. Conjugated linoleic acid supplementation in humans: Effects on body composition and energy expenditure, *Lipids.* 35, 777–82.
123. Medina, E.A., Horn, W.F., Keim, N.L., Havel, P.J., Benito, P., Kelley, D.S., et al. 2000. Conjugated linoleic acid supplementation in humans: Effects on circulating leptin concentrations and appetite, *Lipids.* 35, 783–8.
124. Kreider, R.B., Ferreira, M., Greenwood, M., Wilson, M., and Almada, A.L. 2002. Effects of conjugated linoleic acid supplementation during resistance training on body composition, bone density, strength, and selected hematological markers, *J. Strength Cond. Res.* 16, 325–34.
125. Ebeling, P., and Koivisto, V.A. 1994. Physiological importance of dehydroepiandrosterone, *Lancet.* 343, 1479–81.
126. Denti, L., Pasolini, G., Sanfelici, L., Ablondi, F., Freddi, M., Benedetti, R., and Valenti, G. 1997. Effects of aging on dehydroepiandrosterone sulfate in relation to fasting insulin levels and body composition assessed by bioimpedance analysis, *Metabolism.* 46, 826–32.
127. De Pergola, G., Zamboni, M., Sciaraffia, M., Turcato, E., Pannacciulli, N., Armellini, F., et al. 1996. Body fat accumulation is possibly responsible for lower dehydroepiandrosterone circulating levels in premenopausal obese women, *Int. J. Obes. Relat. Metab. Disord.* 20, 1105–10.
128. Nestler, J.E., Barlascini, C.O., Clore, J.N., and Blackard, W.G. 1988. Dehydroepiandrosterone reduces serum low density lipoprotein levels and body fat but does not alter insulin sensitivity in normal men, *J. Clin. Endocrinol. Metab.* 66, 57–61.
129. Vogiatzi, M.G., Boeck, M.A., Vlachopapadopoulou, E., el-Rashid, R., and New, M.I. 1996. Dehydroepiandrosterone in morbidly obese adolescents: Effects on weight, body composition, lipids, and insulin resistance, *Metabolism.* 45, 1011–5.
130. Ishihara, K., Oyaizu, S., Onuki, K., Lim, K., and Fushiki, T. 2000. Chronic (β)-hydroxycitrate administration spares carbohydrate utilization and promotes lipid oxidation during exercise in mice, *J. Nutr.* 130, 2990–5.
131. Kriketos, A.D., Thompson, H.R., Greene, H., and Hill, J.O. 1999. (β)-Hydroxycitric acid does not affect energy expenditure and substrate oxidation in adult males in a postabsorptive state, *Int. J. Obes. Relat. Metab. Disord.* 23, 867–73.
132. Heymsfield, S.B., Allison, D.B., Vasselli, J.R., Pietrobelli, A., Greenfield, D., and Nunez, C. 1998. *Garcinia cambogia* (hydroxycitric acid) as a potential antiobesity agent: A randomized controlled trial, *JAMA.* 280, 1596–600.
133. Mattes, R.D., and Bormann, L. 2000. Effects of (β)-hydroxycitric acid on appetitive variables, *Physiol. Behav.* 71, 87–94.
134. Rama Rao, S.V., Sunder, G.S., Reddy, M.R., Praharaj, N.K., Raju, M.V., and Panda, A. 2001. Effect of supplementary choline on the performance of broiler breeders fed on different energy sources, *Br. Poult. Sci.* 42, 362–7.
135. Buchman, A.L., Awal, M., Jenden, D., Roch, M., and Kang, S.H. 2000. The effect of lecithin supplementation on plasma choline concentrations during a marathon, *J. Am. Coll. Nutr.* 19, 768–70.
136. Grases, F., Melero, G., Costa-Bauza, A., Prieto, R., and March, J.G. 1994. Urolithiasis and phytotherapy, *Int. Urol. Nephrol.* 26, 507–11.
137. Beaux, D., Fleurentin, J., and Mortier, F. 1999. Effect of extracts of *Orthosiphon stamineus Benth*, *Hieracium pilosella* L., *Sambucus nigra* L., and *Arctostaphylos uva-ursi* (L.) Spreng. in rats, *Phytother. Res.* 13, 222–5.

138. Hao, M., Li, C., and Xu, Y. 1997. Diuretic effect of liniaoling (KLP), *Zhongguo Zhong Yao Za Zhi.* 22, 747–50, 765.
139. Hnatyszyn, O., Mino, J., Gorzalczany, S., Opezzo, J., Ferraro, G., Coussio, J., and Acevedo, C. 1999. Diuretic activity of an aqueous extract of *Phyllanthus sellowianus*, *Phytomedicine.* 6, 177–9.
140. Dolan, R.L., Crosby, E.C., Leutkemeir, M.J., Barton, R.G., and Askew, E.W. 2001. The effects of diuretics on resting metabolic rate and subsequent shifts in respiratory exchange ratios, *Med. Sci. Sports Exerc.* 33, S163.
141. Crosby, E.C., Dolan, R.L., Benson, J.E., Leutkemeir, M.J., Barton, R.G., and Askew, E.W. 2001. Herbal diuretic induced dehydration and resting metabolic rate, *Med. Sci. Sports Exerc.* 33, S163.
142. Kreider, R.B. 1999. Dietary supplements and the promotion of muscle growth with resistance exercise, *Sports Med.* 27, 97–110.
143. Tang, J.E., Manolakos, J.J., Kujbida, G.W., Lysecki, P.J., Moore, D.R., and Phillips, S.M. 2007. Minimal whey protein with carbohydrate stimulates muscle protein synthesis following resistance exercise in trained young men, *Appl. Physiol. Nutr. Metab.* 32, 1132–8.
144. Willoughby, D.S., Stout, J.R., and Wilborn, C.D. 2007. Effects of resistance training and protein plus amino acid supplementation on muscle anabolism, mass, and strength, *Amino Acids.* 32, 467–77.
145. Cribb, P.J., and Hayes, A. 2006. Effects of supplement timing and resistance exercise on skeletal muscle hypertrophy, *Med. Sci. Sports Exerc.* 38, 1918–25.
146. Kreider, R. Creatine supplementation in exercise and sport. In *Energy-Yielding Macronutrients and Energy Metabolism in Sports Nutrition*, Driskell, J., and Wolinsky, I., Eds., CRC Press, Boca Raton, FL, 1999, pp. 213–42.
147. Kreider, R.B. 2003. Effects of creatine supplementation on performance and training adaptations, *Mol. Cell Biochem.* 244, 89–94.
148. Kreider, R.B., Ferreira, M., Wilson, M., Grindstaff, P., Plisk, S., Reinardy, J., et al. 1998. Effects of creatine supplementation on body composition, strength, and sprint performance, *Med. Sci. Sports Exerc.* 30, 73–82.
149. Williams, M.H., and Branch, J.D. 1998. Creatine supplementation and exercise performance: An update, *J. Am. Coll Nutr.* 17, 216–34.
150. Kraemer, W.J., and Volek, J.S. 1999. Creatine supplementation. Its role in human performance, *Clin. Sports Med.* 18, 651–66.
151. Olsen, S., Aagaard, P., Kadi, F., Tufekovic, G., Verney, J., Olesen, J. L., et al. 2006. Creatine supplementation augments the increase in satellite cell and myonuclei number in human skeletal muscle induced by strength training, *J. Physiol.* 573, 525–34.
152. Kreider, R.B., Klesges, B., Harmon, K., Grindstaff, P., Ramsey, L., Bullen, D., et al. 1996. Effects of ingesting supplements designed to promote lean tissue accretion on body composition during resistance training, *Int. J. Sport Nutr.* 6, 234–46.
153. Kreider, R.B., Klesges, R.C., Lotz, D., Davis, M., Cantler, E., Harmon-Clayton, K., et al. 1999. Effects of nutritional supplementation during off-season college football training on body composition and strength, *J. Exerc. Physiol.* 2, 24–39.
154. Nair, K.S., Schwartz, R.G., and Welle, S. 1992. Leucine as a regulator of whole body and skeletal muscle protein metabolism in humans, *Am. J. Physiol.* 263, E928–34.
155. Wilson, G.J., Wilson, J.M., and Manninen, A.H. 2008. Effects of beta-hydroxy-beta-methylbutyrate (HMB) on exercise performance and body composition across varying levels of age, sex, and training experience: A review, *Nutr. Metab. (London).* 5, 1.
156. Gallagher, P.M., Carrithers, J.A., Godard, M.P., Schulze, K.E., and Trappe, S.W. 2000. Beta-hydroxy-beta-methylbutyrate ingestion, Part I: Effects on strength and fat free mass, *Med. Sci. Sports Exerc.* 32, 2109–15.

157. Nissen, S., Sharp, R., Ray, M., Rathmacher, J.A., Rice, D., Fuller, J.C., Jr., et al. 1996. Effect of leucine metabolite beta-hydroxy-beta-methylbutyrate on muscle metabolism during resistance-exercise training, *J. Appl. Physiol.* 81, 2095–104.
158. Panton, L.B., Rathmacher, J.A., Baier, S., and Nissen, S. 2000. Nutritional supplementation of the leucine metabolite beta-hydroxy-beta-methylbutyrate (hmb) during resistance training, *Nutrition.* 16, 734–9.
159. Vukovich, M.D., Stubbs, N.B., and Bohlken, R.M. 2001. Body composition in 70-year-old adults responds to dietary beta-hydroxy-beta-methylbutyrate similarly to that of young adults, *J. Nutr.* 131, 2049–52.
160. Vukovich, M.D., and Dreifort, G.D. 2001. Effect of beta-hydroxy beta-methylbutyrate on the onset of blood lactate accumulation and peak in endurance-trained cyclists, *J. Strength Cond. Res.* 15, 491–7.
161. Thomson, J.S. 2004. Beta-hydroxy-beta-methylbutyrate (HMB) supplementation of resistance trained men, *Asia Pac. J. Clin. Nutr.* 13, S59.
162. Knitter, A.E., Panton, L., Rathmacher, J.A., Petersen, A., and Sharp, R. 2000. Effects of beta-hydroxy-beta-methylbutyrate on muscle damage after a prolonged run, *J. Appl. Physiol.* 89, 1340–4.
163. van Someren, K.A., Edwards, A.J., and Howatson, G. 2005. Supplementation with beta-hydroxy-beta-methylbutyrate (HMB) and alpha-ketoisocaproic acid (KIC) reduces signs and symptoms of exercise-induced muscle damage in man, *Int. J. Sport Nutr. Exerc. Metab.* 15, 413–24.
164. Jowko, E., Ostaszewski, P., Jank, M., Sacharuk, J., Zieniewicz, A., Wilczak, J., and Nissen, S. 2001. Creatine and beta-hydroxy-beta-methylbutyrate (HMB) additively increase lean body mass and muscle strength during a weight-training program, *Nutrition.* 17, 558–66.
165. Nissen, S.L., and Sharp, R.L. 2003. Effect of dietary supplements on lean mass and strength gains with resistance exercise: A meta-analysis, *J. Appl. Physiol.* 94, 651–9.
166. Kreider, R., Ferreira, M., Greenwood, M., Wilson, M., Grindstaff, P., Plisk, S., et al. 2000. Effects of calcium B-HMB supplementation during training on markers of catabolism, body composition, strength and sprint performance, *J. Exerc. Physiol.* 3(4), 48–59.
167. Kreider, R.B., Ferreira, M., Wilson, M., and Almada, A.L. 1999. Effects of calcium beta-hydroxy-beta-methylbutyrate (HMB) supplementation during resistance-training on markers of catabolism, body composition and strength, *Int. J. Sports Med.* 20, 503–9.
168. Ransone, J., Neighbors, K., Lefavi, R., and Chromiak, J. 2003. The effect of beta-hydroxy beta-methylbutyrate on muscular strength and body composition in collegiate football players, *J. Strength Cond. Res.* 17, 34–9.
169. O'Connor, D.M., and Crowe, M.J. 2003. Effects of beta-hydroxy-beta-methylbutyrate and creatine monohydrate supplementation on the aerobic and anaerobic capacity of highly trained athletes, *J. Sports Med. Phys. Fitness* 43, 64–8.
170. Slater, G., Jenkins, D., Logan, P., Lee, H., Vukovich, M., Rathmacher, J.A., and Hahn, A.G. 2001. Beta-hydroxy-beta-methylbutyrate (HMB) supplementation does not affect changes in strength or body composition during resistance training in trained men, *Int. J. Sport Nutr. Exerc. Metab.* 11, 384–96.
171. Hoffman, J., Ratamess, N., Kang, J., Mangine, G., Faigenbaum, A., and Stout, J. 2006. Effect of creatine and beta-alanine supplementation on performance and endocrine responses in strength/power athletes, *Int. J. Sport Nutr. Exerc. Metab.* 16, 430–46.
172. Pikholz, C., Swinburn, B., and Metcalf, P. 2004. Under-reporting of energy intake in the 1997 National Nutrition Survey, *N. Z. Med. J.* 117, U1079.
173. Winkler, J., 2005. The fundamental flaw in obesity research. *Obes. Rev.* 6, 199–202.

8 Endurance Performance

Ellen J. Coleman

CONTENTS

I. INTRODUCTION

Endurance events include a wide variety of competitions, including marathon runs, Olympic distance triathlons, cross country skiing races, and long road races and mountain cycling events. Ultra-endurance events involve races that last from 4 to 24 hours and include running > 30 to 100 miles (48 to 160 km), cycling > 100 to 300 miles (160 to 480 km), and triathlons ranging from the half-Ironman distance to the full Ironman distance of a 2.4-mile (38-km) swim, 112-mile (179-km) bike ride, and 26.2-mile (42-km) marathon run. Multistage ultra-endurance events involve competing over consecutive days, such as the Tour de France bicycle race (~2,500 miles or 4,000 km over 22 days), the Race Across America (RAAM) cycling event (3,000 miles or 4,800 km), and the Australian Sidney to Melbourne foot race (628 miles or 1005 km).

Endurance athletes have unique nutrient demands due to their high energy expenditures and must cope with a variety of practical hurdles to achieve their fuel and fluid goals.

II. EXERCISE METABOLISM

The predominant energy system for endurance athletes is the aerobic energy system with brief, intermittent involvement of anaerobic energy systems. During prolonged exercise, the oxidative metabolism of carbohydrate and fat provide the vast majority of ATP for muscle contraction.[1]

Fat oxidation reaches its peak during prolonged exercise at ~65% of VO_{2max}.[2] During moderate-intensity exercise in endurance-trained people, plasma fatty acids and intramuscular triglycerides contribute equally to fat oxidation.[2] In a typical ultra-endurance event such as a half-Ironman triathlon or ultrarun, the exercise intensity averages about 65% of VO_{2max} or less and lipids are the primary fuel source.[1]

In a high-intensity endurance event such as a marathon, the exercise intensity is often 75% of VO_{2max} or more and carbohydrate, primarily muscle glycogen, is the primary fuel source. Although amino acid oxidation occurs to a limited extent during endurance exercise, carbohydrate and lipid are the most important oxidative substrates.[1]

The utilization of muscle glycogen is the most rapid during the early stages of exercise and is related to exercise intensity. As muscle glycogen declines during continued exercise, blood glucose becomes more important as a carbohydrate fuel source. Muscle glucose uptake increases in conjunction with increases in exercise intensity and duration. The glycogenolysis of liver glycogen initially supplies the majority of blood glucose. As the exercise duration increases and liver glycogen declines, the contribution of blood glucose from gluconeogenesis increases. Hypoglycemia occurs when the liver glucose output can no longer keep up with muscle glucose uptake during prolonged exercise.[1]

Fatigue during prolonged exercise is often, but not always, associated with muscle glycogen depletion and/or hypoglycemia. Thus, nutritional strategies that optimize carbohydrate availability before, during, and after exercise are recommended to improve endurance performance.[1,2]

Nutritional strategies to increase the availability and utilization of fat (e.g. fat loading and caffeine ingestion) have also been proposed to benefit endurance athletes by slowing the rate of carbohydrate utilization.

III. ENERGY EXPENDITURE AND INTAKE

The energy expenditure for an endurance athlete depends on the athlete's weight, age, and gender and the intensity, duration, and type of activity.[3] To meet energy demands, these athletes often need to eat meals and snacks continuously throughout the day.[4,5]

Endurance athletes should consume adequate energy and carbohydrate during training to maintain a desirable training intensity and so maximize training adaptations. They should practice adjusting their fueling strategies based on the workout intensity, duration, and environmental conditions. Testing specific foods and fluids before, during, and after training sessions also allows the athlete to determine effective fueling strategies for competition.[4–6]

Burke and colleagues reported that elite male ultra-endurance triathletes consumed an average of 4079 calories/day during a weekly training schedule of 8.1 miles (13 km) of swimming, 202 miles (323 km) of cycling, and 47 miles (75 km) of running.[7] The authors also reported that male marathon runners consumed an average of 3570 calories per day during training while running 91.6 miles per week.[7] Fudge and colleagues reported an average energy intake of 3152 calories and energy expenditure of 3478 calories in elite endurance Kenyan distance runners during heavy training.[8]

Garcia-Roves and associates reported that elite male cyclists consumed 5333 calories per day during training and 5452 calories per day while racing.[9] Martin and associates reported that elite female cyclists consumed 3261 calories per day during training and 3540 calories per day while racing. Most but not all of the female cyclists modulated energy intake based on energy expenditure.[10]

Nutrient needs for competition are often higher than during training, especially for multiple-day events. In ultra-endurance events lasting up to 24 hours, it isn't necessary or practical to meet total energy expenditure.[11]

Kimber and colleagues calculated a mean energy expenditure of 10,036 calories for male athletes and 8570 calories for female athletes during the New Zealand Ironman triathlon. The authors reported a mean energy intake of 3940 calories for the male triathletes and 3115 calories for the female triathletes.[12] When adjusted for fat-free mass, total energy expenditure was similar between genders. The triathletes' average energy expenditure was significantly greater than their average energy intake, creating a substantial energy deficit for both men (5973 calories) and women (5213 calories). This indicates that the triathletes obtained a large amount (59%) of their energy during the Ironman from endogenous fuel stores.[12]

Glace and colleagues found that male ultrarunners consumed 6047 calories during a 100-mile (160-km) trail run.[13] The authors calculated a mean energy expenditure of 13,560 calories, thus creating an energy deficit of 7513 calories in 24.3 hours.[13] In another study, Glace and associates found that male and female ultrarunners consumed 7022 calories during a 100-mile trail run in the heat.[14] The authors calculated a mean energy expenditure of 9538 calories, thus creating an energy deficit of 2516 calories in 26.2 hours.[14]

Saris and colleagues calculated a mean daily energy expenditure of 6069 calories and a mean daily energy intake of 5785 calories for five male cyclists competing in the Tour de France.[15] Gabel and colleagues reported a mean energy intake of 7125 calories/day for two elite male cyclists during a 10-day, 2050-mile (3280-km) ride on the original Pony Express Trail.[16] Garcia-Roves and associates reported a mean energy intake of 5595 calories per day for 10 elite male cyclists during the Tour de Spain.[17]

Eden and Abernathy reported a mean energy intake of 5952 calories/day for a male ultradistance runner who completed the Australian Sidney to Melbourne foot race 628 miles or 1005 km) in 8.5 days.[18] O'Connor reported an energy intake of about 6000 calories per day for a male ultradistance runner who completed a 9126

TABLE 8.1
Calorie Intake

Event	Gender	Calorie intake/day
Elite ultra-endurance triathletes[7]	M	4079
Marathon runners[7]	M	3570
Elite Kenyan distance runners[8]	M	3478
Elite road cyclists[9]	M	5333 training 5452 racing
Elite road cyclists[10]	F	3261 training 3540 racing
New Zealand Ironman triathlon[12]	M	3940
New Zealand Ironman triathlon[12]	F	3115
Ultrarunners[13]	M	6047 (24.3 hours)
Ultrarunners[14]	M and F	7022 (26.2 hours)
Tour de France cyclists[15]	M	5785
Pony Express Trail cyclists[16]	M	7125
Tour de Spain cyclists[17]	M	5595
Sidney to Melbourne run[19]	M	5952
Run around Australia[11]	M	~6000
RAAM Cyclist[20]	M	8429
RAAM Cyclist[21] 4th place finish	M	9612
RAAM Cyclist[22] 1st place finish	F	7950

mile (14,602 km) run around Australia in 191 days.[11] During a 2-week portion of the run, Hill and Davies estimated the runner's daily energy expenditure to be 6321 calories using the doubly labeled water technique.[19]

Lindeman reported a mean energy intake of 8429 calories/day for a male cyclist competing in the RAAM who finished in 10 days, 7 hours, and 53 minutes after riding as much 22 hours per day.[20] Knechtle and associates reported a mean energy intake of 9612 calories per day for a male cyclist who completed the RAAM in fourth place after 9 days, 16 hours, and 45 minutes.[21] Clark and colleagues reported a mean energy intake of 7950 calories/day for a female cyclist who won the RAAM in 12 days, 6 hours, and 21 minutes.[22] For a summary of these figures, see Table 8.1.

IV. MACRONUTRIENTS

A. Carbohydrate

Adequate carbohydrate stores (muscle and liver glycogen and blood glucose) are critical for optimum endurance performance. Consuming adequate carbohydrate on a daily basis is necessary to meet the fuel requirements of the athlete's training program as well as replenish muscle and liver glycogen between training sessions and competitive events.[2,5]

It is apparent that a high carbohydrate intake acutely enhances recovery and improves endurance performance over 24 to 72 hours.[5] Fallowfield and Williams reported that a high-carbohydrate diet (8.8 g/kg/day) restored endurance capacity within 22.5 hours of recovery between training sessions.[23] An isocaloric diet containing less carbohydrate (5.8 g/kg/day) was associated with decreased endurance.[23]

Although a high carbohydrate intake promotes greater recovery of muscle glycogen, only a handful of studies show chronic improvements in training outcomes over 11 to 28 days.[5] Achten and colleagues found that a high-carbohydrate diet (8.5 g/kg/day) allowed better maintenance of physical performance and mood state during 11 days of intensified running training compared with a moderate carbohydrate diet (5.4 g/kg/day).[24] Simonsen and colleagues found that a diet containing 10 g of carbohydrate/kg/day promoted greater muscle glycogen content and power output during training than a diet containing 5 g of carbohydrate/kg/day over 4 weeks of intense twice-daily rowing training.[25]

Until research shows otherwise, the evidence from studies of acute carbohydrate intake and performance remain the best estimate of the chronic carbohydrate needs of endurance athletes.[5] Overwhelming evidence indicates that carbohydrate supplementation before and during exercise improves endurance performance.[5] The use of short-term dietary and training strategies to increase muscle glycogen stores (e.g. carbohydrate loading) also improve performance.[5] Thus, a high-carbohydrate diet is still the best recommendation for endurance athletes.[5]

Endurance athletes engaged in moderate-duration, low-intensity training should consume 5 to 7 g of carbohydrate/kg/day.[5,26] During moderate to heavy endurance training, athletes should consume 7 to 12 g of carbohydrate/kg/day.[5,26] Athletes participating in extreme endurance training for 4 to 6 hours per day should consume 10 to 12 g of carbohydrate/kg/day.[5,26] These general recommendations should be fine-tuned with consideration of the athlete's total energy needs, specific training needs, and feedback from their training performance.[5]

Daily carbohydrate recommendations[5,26] are as follows:

- Low intensity training: 5 to 7 g of carbohydrate/kg/day
- Heavy endurance training: 7 to 12 g of carbohydrate/kg/day
- Extreme endurance training (4 to 6 hours per day): 10 to 12 g of carbohydrate/kg/day

Results of dietary surveys of serious male endurance athletes published between 1990 and 1999 suggest they are consuming an appropriate amount of carbohydrate—7.6 g/kg/day.[5] Results of dietary surveys of serious female endurance athletes published between 1990 and 1999 suggest they are less likely to consume adequate dietary carbohydrate due to lower energy intakes—5.7 g/kg/day.[5]

Burke and colleagues found that male ultra-endurance triathletes consumed 9 g of carbohydrate/kg/day during training.[7] These authors also reported that male marathon runners consumed 8 g of carbohydrate/kg/day during training. Fudge and colleagues reported that elite endurance Kenyan distance runners consumed 9 g of carbohydrate/kg/day during heavy training.[8]

Garcia-Roves and associates reported that elite male cyclists consumed 11 g of carbohydrate/kg/day during heavy training and 12 g/kg/day during racing.[9] Martin and associates reported that elite female cyclists consumed 9 g of carbohydrate/kg/day during heavy training and 9.9 g/kg/day during racing.[10]

A study of Tour de France male cyclists by Saris and colleagues found that the cyclists consumed an average of 12 g of carbohydrate/kg each day during the race.[15] A case study of two male cyclists during a 10-day, 2050-mile (3280-km) ride by Gabel and colleagues found that the cyclists consumed an average of 18 g of carbohydrate/kg/day.[16] Garcia-Roves and associates reported an average intake of 12.6 g of carbohydrate/ kg/day for male cyclists during the Tour de Spain.[17]

Lindeman reported that a male cyclist who competed in the RAAM consumed an average of 22.6 g of carbohydrate/kg/day.[20] The cyclist obtained the majority of his total energy intake from a high-carbohydrate liquid supplement (23% carbohydrate).[20] Knechtle and associates reported an average carbohydrate intake of 24.8 g of carbohydrate/kg/day for another male RAAM cyclist.[21] Eden and Abernathy reported that a male ultradistance runner competing in the Australian Sidney to Melbourne foot race consumed an average of 17 g of carbohydrate/ kg/day.[19] For a summary of these statistics, see Table 8.2.

Nutrient-dense carbohydrate foods and fluids should be emphasized during training as they contain other nutrients such as vitamins and minerals that are important for the overall diet as well as recovery from exercise.[5] Adequate energy intake is also important to promote glycogen restoration. Consumption of a reduced-energy diet can impair endurance performance due to suboptimal muscle and liver glycogen stores.[5]

Training for endurance events involves hours of prolonged exercise that may include multiple daily training sessions. The stress of such rigorous training can decrease appetite, resulting in reduced consumption of energy and carbohydrate.[5,27]

Brouns and colleagues evaluated the effect of a simulated Tour de France study on food and fluid intake, energy balance, and substrate oxidation.[27] Although the

TABLE 8.2
Carbohydrate Intake

Event	Gender	Carbohydrate intake
Elite ultra-endurance triathletes[7]	M	9 g/kg/day
Marathon runners[7]	M	8 g/kg/day
Elite Kenyan distance runners[8]	M	9 g/kg/day
Elite road cyclists[9]	M	11 g/kg/day training 12 g/kg/day racing
Elite road cyclists[10]	F	9 g/kg/day training 9.9 g/kg/day racing
Tour de France cyclists[15]	M	12 g/kg/day
Pony Express Trail cyclists[16]	M	18 g/kg/day
Tour de Spain cyclists[17]	M	12.6 g/kg/day
RAAM Cyclist[20]	M	22.6 g/kg/day
RAAM Cyclist[21] 4th place finish	M	24.8 g/kg/day
Sidney to Melbourne run[19]	M	17 g/kg/day

cyclists consumed 630 g of carbohydrate (8.6 g/kg per day), they oxidized 850 g of carbohydrate per day (11.6 g/kg per day).[27] In spite of *ad libitum* intake of conventional foods, the cyclists were unable to ingest sufficient carbohydrate and calories to compensate for their increased energy expenditure.[27] When the diet was supplemented with a 20% carbohydrate beverage, carbohydrate intake increased to 16 g/kg per day and carbohydrate oxidation rose to 13 g/kg per day.[27]

Athletes who have extremely high carbohydrate requirements and suppressed appetites due to heavy endurance training should include compact, low-fiber forms of carbohydrate, such as pasta, white rice, and sugar-rich foods. Carbohydrate-rich fluids such as sports drinks, juices, high-carbohydrate liquid supplements, commercial liquid meals, milk shakes, and fruit smoothies may also be appealing to athletes who are very tired and dehydrated.[5]

B. Protein

While acute endurance exercise results in the oxidation of several amino acids, the total amount of amino acid oxidation amounts to only 1–6% of the total energy cost of exercise.[28,29] The branched chain amino acid leucine has been most frequently studied in relation to endurance exercise.[28,29] A low-energy or -carbohydrate intake will increase amino acid oxidation and total protein requirements.[28,29]

During low- to moderate-intensity endurance activity, 1.2 g of protein/kg/day is sufficient when energy and carbohydrate intake are adequate.[28] Elite endurance athletes may require 1.6 g/kg/day or twice the recommended dietary allowance of protein for sedentary people.[29–32] In a simulated Tour de France cycling study, Brouns and colleagues found that well-trained male cyclists required 1.5 to 1.8 g of protein/kg/day to maintain nitrogen balance.[30] Tarnopolsky and associates found that elite male endurance athletes required 1.6 g of protein/kg/day to maintain nitrogen balance.[31] Friedman and Lemon found that well-trained endurance runners required 1.5 g of protein/kg/day to maintain nitrogen balance.[32]

Endurance athletes can meet their higher protein requirements by consuming a mixed diet that provides adequate energy and 15% of the calories from protein.[28] Although most endurance athletes get enough protein, those with low-energy or -carbohydrate intakes may require nutritional advice to optimize dietary protein intake.[28,29]

Studies of male endurance athletes suggest they are consuming an appropriate amount of protein. The data on female endurance athletes is extremely limited. Burke and colleagues found that male ultra-endurance triathletes consumed 2 g of protein/kg/day during training.[7] They also reported that male marathon runners consumed 2 g of carbohydrate/kg/day during training.[7] Garcia-Roves and associates reported that elite male cyclists consumed 2.9 g of protein/kg/day during heavy training and 2.6 g/kg/day g of protein/kg/day during racing.[9] Martin and associates reported that elite female cyclists consumed 2.6 g of protein/kg/day during heavy training and 2.2 g/kg/day g of protein/kg/day during racing.[10]

A study of Tour de France male cyclists found that they consumed an average of 3.1 g of protein/kg/day during the race.[15] A study of Tour de Spain male cyclists found they consumed 3.0 g of protein/kg/day during the race.[17]

TABLE 8.3
Protein Intake

Event	Gender	Protein intake
Elite ultra-endurance triathletes[7]	M	2 g/kg/day
Marathon runners[7]	M	2 g/kg/day
Elite Kenyan distance runners[8]	M	2.1 g/kg/day
Elite road cyclists[9]	M	2.9 g/kg/day training 2.6 g/kg/day racing
Elite road cyclists[10]	F	2.6 g/kg/day training 2.2 g/kg/day racing
Tour de France cyclists[15]	M	3.1 g/kg/day
Pony Express Trail cyclists[16]	M	2.7 g/kg/day
Tour de Spain cyclists[17]	M	3.0 g/kg/day
RAAM Cyclist[20]	M	3.6 g/kg/day
RAAM Cyclist[21] 4th place finish	M	2.8 g/kg/day
Sidney to Melbourne run[19]	M	2.9 g/kg/day

A case study of two male cyclists during a 10-day, 2050-mile (3280-km) ride found that the cyclists consumed an average of 2.7 g of protein/kg/day.[16] The two male cyclists who competed in the RAAM consumed an average of 3.6 g of protein/kg/day[20] and 2.8 g of protein/kg/day.[21] A male ultradistance runner competing in the Australian Sidney to Melbourne foot race consumed an average of 2.9 g of protein/kg/day.[19] Fudge and colleagues reported that elite endurance Kenyan distance runners consumed 2.1g of protein/kg/day during heavy training (see Table 8.3).[8]

Gender may affect protein metabolism. During endurance exercise, women oxidize more lipids and less carbohydrate and protein compared to equally trained and nourished men. Tarnopolsky suggests that female endurance athletes may have a 10 to 20% lower protein requirement than male endurance athletes.[33]

C. Fat

The Food and Nutrition Board of the Institute of Medicine established an Acceptable Macronutrient Distribution Range (AMDR) for fat at 20 to 35 percent of total calories.[34] Fat is an essential nutrient and provides energy, fat soluble vitamins, and essential fatty acids.[34] Endurance athletes should consume at least 1 g of fat per kg of body weight.

Individuals who consume high-fat diets (greater than 35% of calories) also consume more total energy and saturated fatty acids. Low-fat diets (less than 20% of calories) increase the risk of inadequate intakes of vitamin E and essential fatty acids, and may contribute to unfavorable changes in high-density lipoprotein cholesterol and triglycerides.[35]

Studies of male endurance athletes suggest they are consuming an appropriate amount of fat. Data on female endurance athletes is extremely limited. Burke

TABLE 8.4
Fat Intake

Event	Gender	Fat intake
Elite ultra-endurance triathletes[7]	M	1.8 g/kg/day (27% of calories)
Marathon runners[7]	M	2 g/kg/day (17% of calories)
Elite Kenyan distance runners[8]	M	1 g/kg/day (32% of calories)
Elite road cyclists[9]	M	2.8 g/kg/day training (29.9% of calories)
		2.2 g/kg/day racing (25.3% of calories)
Elite road cyclists[10]	F	1 g/kg/day training and racing (17% of calories)
Tour de France cyclists[15]	M	2.1 g/kg/day (23% of calories)
Pony Express Trail cyclists[16]	M	3.5 g/kg/day (27% of calories)
Tour de Spain cyclists[17]	M	2.3 g/kg/day (25.5% of calories)
RAAM Cyclist[20]	M	1 g/kg/day (9% of calories)
RAAM Cyclist[21] 4th place finish	M	2.3 g/kg/day (16.2 % of calories)
Sidney to Melbourne run[19]	M	3.2 g/kg/day (27% of energy intake)

and colleagues found that male ultra-endurance triathletes consumed 1.8 g of fat/kg/day (27% of energy intake) during training.[7] They also reported that male marathon runners consumed 2 g of protein/kg/day (32% of energy intake) during training.[7] Garcia-Roves and associates reported that elite male cyclists consumed 2.8 g of fat/kg/day (29.9% of energy) during training and 2.2 g/kg/day (25.3% of energy intake) during racing.[9] Martin and associates reported that elite female cyclists consumed 1 g of fat per kg/day (17% of energy intake) during both training and racing.[10]

Saris and colleagues found that male Tour de France male cyclists consumed 2.1 g of fat/kg/day (23% of energy intake) during the race.[15] A study of Tour de Spain male cyclists found they consumed 2.3 g of fat/kg/day (25.5% of energy intake) during the race.[17]

Gabel and colleagues found that two male cyclists consumed an average of 3.5 g of fat/kg (27% of energy intake) during a 10 day, 2,050 mile (3280 km) ride.[16] The two male cyclists who competed in the RAAM consumed an average of 1 g of fat/kg/day[20] (9% of energy intake) and 2.3 g/kg/day[21] (16.2% of energy intake). The male ultradistance runner competing in the Australian Sidney to Melbourne foot race consumed an average of 3.2 g of fat/kg (27% of energy intake).[19] Fudge and colleagues reported that elite endurance Kenyan distance runners consumed 1 g of fat/kg/day (17% of energy intake) during heavy training (see Table 8.4).[8]

V. MICRONUTRIENTS

Endurance athletes who consume adequate total energy usually meet or exceed population reference values such as the Dietary References Intakes (DRI) for vitamins and minerals.[36] Consuming a nutrient-dense diet containing fruits, vegetables, whole grains, legumes, lean meat, and dairy foods during training also helps to ensure adequate micronutrient intake.[37]

Endurance athletes who regularly restrict energy intake or eat a limited variety of foods may be at risk for suboptimal micronutrient intakes. Some endurance and ultra-endurance athletes may have increased requirements due to excessive losses in sweat and or urine.[36,37]

Supplementation may be necessary when intake is inadequate. However, athletes should not exceed the upper limit (UL) for any nutrient to prevent possible adverse effects on health and performance. Supplementation with single micronutrients is not recommended unless there is a medical necessity (e.g., iron to treat iron deficiency anemia).[37,38]

The antioxidant vitamins C and E play an important role in protecting cell membranes from oxidative damage. Although endurance exercise is associated with increased oxidative stress, it also increases the body's enzymatic and non-enzymatic antioxidant defenses as an adaptation to training. Supplemental vitamin C may reduce oxidative stress and help prevent upper respiratory tract infections in endurance and ultra-endurance athletes. Supplemental vitamin E may reduce oxidative stress and protect against muscle damage, but does not improve endurance performance.[36,37]

Until research suggests otherwise, it is prudent to recommend that endurance and ultra-endurance athletes consume an antioxidant-rich diet, rather than supplements, to protect against oxidative damage.[37,39,40]

Endurance training can increase iron requirements (due to increases in hemoglobin, myoglobin and iron-containing proteins involved in aerobic metabolism) and iron losses (through sweating, gastrointestinal bleeding, and mechanical trauma such as foot strike hemolysis). Endurance and ultra-endurance athletes, especially female athletes and runners, are at risk for depleting their iron stores.[36,41,42] If untreated, iron depletion can progress to iron deficiency anemia, which reduces VO_{2max}, aerobic efficiency, and endurance performance.[42] Athletes at risk for iron deficiency should have routine checks of their iron status and counseling on dietary strategies to increase iron intake.[42] Iron supplements are recommended for documented iron deficiency anemia.[42]

Calcium is important for the building and repair of bone tissue and the maintenance of blood calcium levels. Inadequate dietary calcium increases the risk of low bone mineral density and stress fractures. Female endurance and ultra-endurance athletes who have low energy intakes, eliminate dairy products, or have menstrual dysfunction are at high risk for low bone mineral density. Situations where medical referral is indicated include: (1) being amenorrheic for longer than six months; (2) a history of anorexia nervosa; (3) occurrence of stress fractures; (4) being postmenopausal; and (5) having a strong family history of osteoporosis.[43]

There is limited data on the micronutrient intake of endurance athletes. Data on the micronutrient intake of female endurance athletes is virtually nonexistent. Burke and colleagues found that male ultra-endurance triathletes and marathoners had adequate intakes of the major micronutrients during training.[7] Singh and colleagues reported that ultramarathoners had adequate pre-race intakes of vitamin and minerals from both food and supplements.[44] The biochemical indices of the ultramarathoners' vitamin and mineral status were also normal.[44] Lindeman noted that a male cyclist had an adequate intake of micronutrients during training for the RAAM.[20] Garcia-Roves and associates reported that all of the vitamin and mineral intakes for elite male cyclists during training and competition were above the recommended daily allowances.[9]

O'Connor reported that the male ultradistance runner who completed the run around Australia consumed two to three times the recommended dietary allowances (RDA) for micronutrients.[11] Eden and Abernathy found that all of the micronutrients except riboflavin were met in the diet of a male ultradistance runner competing in the Australian Sidney to Melbourne foot race.[19]

Gabel and colleagues found that vitamin and mineral intakes were two to three times the RDA for most vitamins and minerals for two male cyclists during a 10-day, 2050-mile (3280-km) ride.[16] Saris and associates found that Tour de France cyclists had low intakes of thiamin (in spite of very high energy intakes) due to their high consumption of refined carbohydrate foods such as sweet cakes and soft drinks.[15] The researchers conceded that any questions and concerns about food quality and nutrient density became immaterial after the consideration of micronutrients from pills and injections.[15]

A balanced diet is the ideal source of micronutrients.[37] In addition to providing a variety of nutrients, foods contain a large number of bioactive compounds that have health benefits such as phytochemicals.[37,45] And, endurance athletes eat foods, not single nutrients. The influence of diet on health occurs not only from the subtle effects of numerous individual food components, but from whole foods and the associated interactions that occur among these components.[45] Messina and colleagues refer to this concept as "food synergy" and recommend emphasizing healthy dietary patterns rather than individual foods or nutrients.[45]

Some endurance athletes may jeopardize their micronutrient status during training by emphasizing convenient, familiar high-carbohydrate foods (e.g., bagels and pasta made from refined flour, commercial sports drinks, high-carbohydrate liquid supplements) that are low in fiber and lack nutrient density.[22] The following additions can help improve the quality of the training diet: (1) emphasize whole grains (oatmeal, whole wheat bread, popcorn); (2) add vegetables in pasta dishes, pizza, stir fry, and soups; (3) try tropical fruits, berries, and fruit smoothies; and (4) use foods fortified with calcium (e.g. orange juice) and iron (e.g., hot cereal).[37]

VI. WATER AND SODIUM

Drinking during endurance exercise is necessary to prevent the detrimental effects of excessive dehydration (> 2% body weight loss) and electrolyte loss on exercise performance and health.[46] Dehydration increases physiologic stress as measured by core temperature, heart rate, and perceived exertion and these effects are accentuated during exercise in warm to hot weather.[46] The greater the body-water shortage, the greater the physiologic strain and impairment of endurance performance.[47]

Physiologic factors that contribute to reduced endurance performance when dehydrated include increased core temperature, increased cardiovascular strain, increased glycogen utilization, altered metabolic function, and possibly altered central nervous system function.[46]

The amount and rate of fluid replacement depends on the athlete's individual sweating rate, exercise duration, and opportunities to drink. It is not possible to propose a one-size-fits-all fluid and electrolyte replacement schedule due to the multiple factors that influence sweating rate and sweat electrolyte concentration.[46]

Sodium is the principal electrolyte lost in sweat. The concentration of sodium in sweat averages about 35 mEq/L or 805 mg/L (range 10 to 70 mEq/L).[46] As sweating rate increases, the concentration of sweat sodium and chloride also increases.[46] Dehydration can also increase the sweat concentrations of sodium and chloride.[46] Heat acclimatization generally reduces sweat sodium concentrations.[46] Endurance and ultra-endurance athletes who have high sweat rates and a high sweat-sodium concentration ("salty sweat") can sustain substantial losses of sodium.[48]

Symptomatic exercise-associated hyponatremia (plasma sodium concentration < 135 mmol/L) can occur in prolonged endurance exercise lasting > 4 hours. The lower the plasma sodium falls, the faster it falls, and the longer it remains low, the greater the risk of dilutional encephalopathy and pulmonary edema.[46]

Contributing factors to exercise-associated hyponatremia include drinking an amount of fluid that exceeds sweat and urinary water losses and excessive loss of total body sodium.[46] In events that last < 4 hours, hyponatremia is primarily caused by overdrinking before, during, and after the event.[48,49] During a marathon, symptomatic hyponatremia is more likely to occur in smaller and less lean individuals who run slowly, sweat less, and drink excessively before, during, and after the race.[48,49]

During prolonged ultra-endurance exercise such as an Ironman triathlon, total sodium losses can induce symptomatic hyponatremia whether the athlete is over- or under-drinking, so replacing some of the sodium losses is warranted.[46] High sweat rates and a high sweat-sodium concentration can also contribute to hyponatremia.[48] Large sweat-sodium losses confer a greater risk of developing hyponatremia because less fluid intake is required to produce dangerously low blood sodium levels.[48]

Endurance athletes can experience health problems from either dehydration or overdrinking. Dehydration is more common and can impair exercise performance and contribute to serious heat illness. Symptomatic hyponatremia, however, is more dangerous and can produce grave illness or death.[46]

There is limited data on fluid and sodium intakes and body-weight changes during endurance events. Mean intake during the Tour de France was 6.7 L but varied considerably throughout the race.[15] Fudge and colleagues reported that elite endurance Kenyan distance runners consumed 4.2 L per day during heavy training.[8] The Tour de Spain researchers recorded an intake of only 3.29 L per day during the April race.[17] The runner in the Sidney to Melbourne foot race consumed an average of 11 L per day.[50] The male ultradistance runner who completed the run around Australia had an average daily water turnover of about 6 L over a 14-day period on the temperate eastern coast.[50] A male cyclist consumed 13.5 L of fluid and 12.3 g of sodium during a 24-hour mountain bike race on an all-terrain course.[11]

Several studies have reported hourly fluid intake during exercise. The two male cyclists drank an average of (approximately 620 mL per hour of exercise) during their 10-day, 2050-mile (3280-km) ride.[16] The male RAAM cyclist drank an average of 15.7 L per day (approximately 677 mL per hour of exercise).[20] The Iroman triathletes drank 889 mL per hour on the bike and 632 mL per hour on the run.[51] The authors calculated average fluid losses of 808 mL per hour on the bike and 1021 mL per hour on the run.[51] The triathletes lost an average of 2.5 kg—about 3% of body weight for the males and 4% of body weight for the females.[51]

Two studies by Glace and colleagues evaluated fluid and sodium intakes and body-weight changes during two 100-mile (160-km) trail runs.[13,14] Male ultrarunners consumed 18 L of fluid (0.7 L/hour) and 12 g (0.5 g/hour) of sodium during a 160-km trail run. The ultrarunners lost 1.6 kg—about 2% of body weight.[13] The authors estimated that body fat accounted for about 1.13 kg of the weight loss according to skinfold measurements.[13]

In a second study, male and female ultrarunners consumed 19.4 L of fluid (0.7 L/hour) and 16.4 g of sodium (0.6 g/hour) during a 160 km trail run in the heat.[14] Despite extreme energy expenditure and thermal stress, body mass was very well maintained throughout the race—the runners lost only 0.5 kg.[14] High fluid intakes were associated with decreased serum sodium levels and increased risk of mental status change, suggesting possible fluid overload.[14] However, finishers consumed more fluids than non-finishers and also were better at meeting their energy requirements (see Table 8.5).[14]

Endurance exercise can cause substantial water and electrolyte losses, particularly in warm to hot weather. If not appropriately replaced, water and electrolyte imbalances (dehydration and hyponatremia) can develop and impair the athlete's exercise performance and health. Athletes should customize their fluid replacement plans due to the considerable variability in sweating rates and sweat electrolyte content between individuals.[46]

TABLE 8.5
Fluid and Sodium Intake

Event	Gender	Fluid Intake	Sodium Intake
Tour de France cyclists[15]	M	6.7 L/day	
Elite Kenyan distance runners[8]	M	4.2 L/day	
Tour de Spain cyclists[17]	M	3.29 L/day	
Sidney to Melbourne run[19]	M	11 L/day	
Run around Australia[50]	M	6 L/day	
24-hour mountain bike race[11]	M	13.5 L/day	12.3 g
Pony Express Trail cyclists[16]	M	10.5 L/day ~620 mL/hour of exercise	
RAAM Cyclist[20]	M	15.7 L/day 677 mL/hour of exercise	
New Zealand Ironman triathlon[12]	M and F	Bike: 889 mL/hour Run: 632 mL/hour	
Ultrarunners[13]	M	18 L/24.3 hours 700 mL/hour	12 g/24.3 hours 500 mg/hour
Ultrarunners[14]	M and F	19.4 L/26.2 hours 700 mL/hour	16.4 g/26.2 hours 600 mg/hour

VII. FUELING AND FLUID REPLACEMENT

A. Carbohydrate Loading for Competition

Muscle glycogen depletion is a well-recognized limitation to endurance performance.[1] Carbohydrate loading (glycogen supercompensation) can elevate muscle glycogen stores from resting levels of 100–120 mmol/kg to about 150–250 mmol/kg and improve performance in endurance events exceeding 90 minutes.[52,53] For endurance athletes, carbohydrate loading could be viewed as an extended period of "fueling up" to prepare for competition.[4] The regimen can postpone fatigue and extend the duration of steady-state exercise by about 20%.[54] Carbohydrate loading may also improve endurance performance by about 2 to 3%, in which a set distance is covered as quickly as possible.[54]

The "classical" 7-day model of carbohydrate loading involved a 3- to 4-day "depletion" phase of hard training and a low carbohydrate intake. The athlete finished with a 3- to 4-day "loading" phase of tapered training and a high carbohydrate intake before the event.[4]

Sherman and colleagues demonstrated that endurance athletes were able to supercompensate muscle glycogen stores without a depletion phase. Muscle glycogen stores were elevated to the same extent after 3 days of tapered training and a high carbohydrate intake (10 g/kg/day), whether preceded by a 3-day "depletion" phase or a more typical diet and training regimen.[55] The modified carbohydrate loading protocol is more practical and avoids the fatigue and extreme diet and training requirements associated with the depletion phase of the classical regimen.[4]

Several studies have suggested that endurance athletes can carbohydrate load in as little as 1 day.[56,57] Bussau and colleagues found that muscle glycogen increased significantly from pre-loading levels of ~90 mmol/kg to ~180 mmol/kg after 1 day and remained stable despite another 2 days of rest and a high-carbohydrate diet of 10 g/kg/day.[56] Fairchild and associates found that a high-carbohydrate intake of 10.3g/kg following a 3-minute bout of high-intensity exercise enabled athletes to increase muscle glycogen levels from preloading levels of ~109 mmol/kg to 198 mmol/kg in 24 hours.[57] Burke notes that muscle glycogen supercompensation is probably achieved within 36 and 48 hours of the last exercise session, provided the athlete rests and consumes adequate carbohydrate (10 to 12 g carbohydrate/kg/day).[4]

For most athletes, a carbohydrate loading regimen will involve 3 days of a high-carbohydrate intake (8–12 g of carbohydrate/kg).[4] Some athletes may have difficulty tolerating the higher fiber content of a high-carbohydrate diet.[4] To avoid gastrointestinal distress, the athlete may benefit from consuming low-fiber foods such as white bread, plain cereal, pasta, peeled fruit, and liquid sources of carbohydrate.[4] Athletes who struggle to consume enough carbohydrate can add liquid meals, high-carbohydrate supplements, and fat-free sweets (jam, honey, hard candy). As with other nutritional strategies, athletes should test their carbohydrate loading regimen prior to a prolonged workout or a low-priority race.[4]

The performance benefits of carbohydrate loading may add to the benefits of consuming carbohydrate during exercise.[5] The combination of carbohydrate loading with other dietary strategies that are used to improve endurance performance (e.g., pre-exercise meal, consuming carbohydrate during exercise, caffeine ingestion) should be thoroughly studied.[5]

B. Pre-Exercise Meal and Hydration

Consuming foods and fluids in the 4 hours before exercise helps to: (1) restore liver glycogen, especially for morning exercise when liver glycogen is depleted from an overnight fast; (2) increase muscle glycogen stores if they are not fully restored from the previous exercise session; (3) ensure the athlete is hydrated; (4) prevent hunger, which may in itself impair performance and (5) give the athlete a psychological boost.[4]

The pre-exercise meal should emphasize carbohydrate-rich foods and fluids.[4] Consuming carbohydrate on the morning of an endurance event may help to maintain blood glucose levels during prolonged exercise. Compared with an overnight fast, consuming a pre-event meal 2 to 4 hours before exercise containing 200 to 300 g of carbohydrate improves endurance performance.[58–60]

The performance benefits of a pre-exercise meal appear to add to those of consuming carbohydrate during endurance exercise. However, the improvement in performance from a pre-exercise meal is less than when smaller quantities of carbohydrate are consumed throughout endurance exercise.[59]

Research suggests that the pre-exercise meal contain ~1.0 to 4.5 g of carbohydrate/kg, consumed 1 to 4 hours prior to exercise (see Table 8.7).[60,61] To avoid potential gastrointestinal distress, the carbohydrate and calorie content of the meal should be reduced the closer to exercise the meal is consumed.[60,61] Foods that are low in fat, low–moderate in protein, and low in fiber are recommended, as they are less likely to cause gastrointestinal upset.[4] Commercial liquid meal supplements or home-made smoothies are beneficial when an athlete is nervous and unable to tolerate solid foods before competition (see Table 8.6).[4]

Endurance athletes may want to experiment with low-glycemic index foods (e.g., pasta, oatmeal, apples, oranges, beans, yogurt) before exercise to promote a more sustained release of carbohydrate during prolonged exercise.[4] While there is no clear evidence of a performance benefit, a low-glycemic pre-exercise meal may be helpful when consuming carbohydrate during exercise is not practical or possible.[4]

A small number of endurance athletes experience symptoms of hypoglycemia and a rapid onset of fatigue after consuming carbohydrate in the hour before exercise.

TABLE 8.6
Pre-Exercise Meal Recommendations[60,61]

Time before Exercise	Amount of Carbohydrate
1 hour	1 g/kg
2 hours	2 g/kg
3 hours	3 g/kg
4 hours	4 g/kg

The reason for this is not known. In most cases, the blood glucose lowering that may occur during the first 20 minutes of exercise following carbohydrate ingestion is self-correcting during exercise and not associated with performance decrements.[4]

Endurance athletes who react negatively to consuming carbohydrate before exercise can choose from several strategies: consume a low-glycemic index carbohydrate before exercise; take in carbohydrate a few minutes before exercise; or wait until exercising to consume carbohydrate. The exercise-induced rise in the hormones epinephrine, norepinephrine, and growth hormone inhibit the release of insulin and thus counter insulin's effect in lowering blood glucose.[4]

Endurance athletes should begin exercise with normal hydration and plasma electrolyte levels.[46] Athletes will generally be normally hydrated when they have consumed ample beverages with meals and had adequate time (8 to 12 hours) to recover from their last exercise session.[46] If the athlete has experienced extensive sweat losses and hasn't had enough time to reestablish normal hydration, an aggressive prehydration program may be warranted.[46] This will help ensure that fluid and electrolyte deficits are rectified prior to exercising.

Prior to exercise, the athlete should slowly drink fluid (about 5 to 7 mL/kg per body weight) at least 4 hours before activity.[46] (Note: 7 mL/kg is equivalent to about 1 oz or 30 mL for every 10 lb or 4.5 kg of body weight). If the athlete does not produce urine, or the urine is dark or highly concentrated, he or she should slowly drink more fluid (an additional 3 to 5 mL/kg or about one-half oz for every 10 lb) about 2 hours before exercise (see Table 8.7).[46]

Drinking several hours before exercise allows adequate time for the urine output to return toward normal.[46] Drinking beverages that contain sodium (20 to 50 mEq/L, or 460 to 1150 mg/L) such as sports drinks or eating small amounts of salted snacks or sodium-containing foods at meals helps to stimulate thirst and promote fluid retention.[46]

Athletes should experiment with different pre-exercise foods and fluids in training. Before competition, the athlete should choose familiar, well-tolerated, and palatable foods and fluids.[4]

C. Glycerol Hyperhydration

Hyperhydration can be achieved by over-drinking combined with an agent such as glycerol that "binds" water within the body. In theory, glycerol hyperhydration improves heat dissipation and decreases cardiovascular stress, thereby improving

TABLE 8.7
Pre-Exercise Hydration Recommendations[46]

Time before Exercise	Amount of Fluid (drink slowly)
4 hours	5 to 7 mL/kg 7 mL/kg = ~1 oz for every 10 lb
2 hours (if athlete has not produced urine)	3 to 5 mL/kg 5 mL/kg = ~ ½ oz for every 10 lb

endurance performance. Studies have evaluated consumption of 1 to 1.2 g of glycerol per kg along with a large fluid bolus of 25 to 35 mL per kg in the hours before exercise. This typically allows a fluid expansion or retention of about 600 mL (above consuming fluid alone) by reducing urinary volume.[4]

Glycerol hyperhydration may aid high-intensity endurance exercise in hot and humid environments where sweat losses are high and the opportunities to replace fluid are significantly lower than the rates of fluid loss.[62–63] However, glycerol hyperhydration has not improved performance in all studies of this type.[4] In addition, the underlying mechanism is not clear because the purported improvements in heat dissipation and decreases in cardiovascular stress have not been observed.[4]

Side effects reported with glycerol hyperhydration include nausea, gastrointestinal distress, and headaches resulting from increased intracranial pressure.[4] Glycerol hyperhydration can also substantially dilute and lower plasma sodium prior to starting exercise[64] and may thus increase the risk of dilutional hyponatremia if the individual drinks too much during exercise.[48]

Endurance athletes who want to hyperhydrate with glycerol should be supervised and monitored by appropriate sports medicine professionals. Athletes should use it in competition only after adequate experimentation and fine-tuning.[4]

D. Exercise Fueling and Hydration

It is well established that consuming 30 to 60 g of carbohydrate per hour during endurance exercise can delay the onset of fatigue and improve endurance capacity by maintaining blood glucose levels and carbohydrate oxidation in the latter stages of exercise.[65–69] Carbohydrate feedings supplement the body's limited endogenous stores of carbohydrate.[6] During prolonged exercise, ingested carbohydrate can account for up to 30% of the total amount of carbohydrate oxidized.[70]

The maximum amount of carbohydrate that can be oxidized during exercise from a single carbohydrate source (e.g., glucose) is about 1 g per minute or 60 g per hour because the transporter responsible for carbohydrate absorption in the intestine becomes saturated.[71] Consuming more than 1 g per minute from one source does not raise the rate of carbohydrate oxidation and increases the risk of gastrointestinal distress.

By consuming multiple carbohydrates that use different intestinal transporters, the total amount of carbohydrate that can be absorbed and oxidized is increased. When glucose and fructose or glucose, fructose, and sucrose are ingested together during exercise at a rate of 2.4 g per minute (144 g per hour), the rate of exogenous carbohydrate oxidation can reach 1.7 g per minute or about 105 g per hour.[72,73] Drinks containing multiple transportable carbohydrates are also less likely to cause gastrointestinal distress.[74,75]

Water absorption is also enhanced when sports drinks include two to three different carbohydrate sources (glucose, sucrose, fructose, or maltodextrins) compared with solutions containing only one carbohydrate source.[76] The addition of a second or third carbohydrate activates additional mechanisms for intestinal transport and involves transport by separate pathways that are noncompetitive.[76]

In theory, consuming multiple transportable carbohydrates should enhance endurance performance by increasing exogenous carbohydrate oxidation and reducing the reliance on endogenous carbohydrate stores. Compared with an isocaloric amount of glucose, the ingestion of glucose and fructose (1.5 per g minute) increased peak exogenous carbohydrate oxidation, reduced ratings of perceived exertion, and increased self-selected cadence in the latter stages of 5 hours of cycling at 50% of maximal work rate.[77] While these findings suggested a reduction in fatigue with the ingestion of glucose and fructose compared with glucose, direct measures of performance were not obtained.[77]

Currell and Jeukendrup found that ingestion of glucose and fructose (1.8 g per minute) improved cycling time trial performance by 8% compared with an isocaloric amount of glucose following 2 hours of cycling at 55% of maximal work rate.[78] The glucose and fructose may have promoted better ATP resynthesis than glucose, thus allowing the maintenance of a higher power output.[78] This was the first study to provide evidence that increased exogenous carbohydrate oxidation improves endurance performance.

The series of studies conducted by researchers at the University of Birmingham have shown that consuming between 1.8 to 2.4 g of carbohydrate per minute (108 to 144 g per hour) from a mixture of carbohydrates increases carbohydrate oxidation up to 75 to 104 g of carbohydrate per hour.[72–75,77,78] When providing recommendations for carbohydrate intake during exercise, it is reasonable to take into account the athlete's body weight. To maximize carbohydrate oxidation and improve performance, endurance athletes should consume ~1 g of carbohydrate per kg per hour from either carbohydrate-rich fluids or foods providing a mixture of carbohydrates. Athletes should individually determine the optimum amount of carbohydrate to enhance their performance.[6]

Kimber and colleagues found that male Ironman triathletes consumed 1.1 g of carbohydrate/kg/hr.[12] The female triathletes consumed 1.0 g/kg/hr. All athletes consumed significantly more energy during the bike (2233 calories for women; 2896 calories for men) than during the run (883 calories for women; 1049 calories for men).[12] Calorie intake during cycling provided 73% of the total energy intake.[12] This is not surprising, as cycling composed about 54% of the total race time for these athletes, and foods and fluid are easier to consume and digest while on the bike.[12] The bike portion of an Ironman also gives athletes the opportunity to obtain energy and fluid in preparation for the marathon run.[12]

A study of Tour de France male cyclists by Saris and colleagues found that the cyclists consumed nearly half of the daily calories that were consumed during the race, resulting in a carbohydrate intake of 94 g per hour (1.3g/kg/hr).[15] About 30% of the total carbohydrate consumed came from high-carbohydrate beverages (e.g. high-carbohydrate drink, sports drink, soft drinks, and liquid meal).[15]

A case study of two male cyclists during a 10-day, 2050-mile (3280 km) ride by Gabel and colleagues found that the cyclists consumed about 60 to 75 g of carbohydrate per hour of cycling and obtained about 24% of their total energy intake from high carbohydrate beverages (e.g. sports drinks, fruit juices).[16] Garcia-Roves and associates reported that male cyclists in the Tour de Spain consumed only 14% of the daily calories during the race, resulting in a carbohydrate intake of 25 g per hour.[17]

Eden and Abernathy reported that a male ultradistance runner competing in the Australian Sidney to Melbourne foot race consumed approximately 39 g of carbohydrate per hour.[19] The runner utilized a combination of high-carbohydrate solid foods and a sports drink during running to meet his energy requirements.[19] Glace

TABLE 8.8
Carbohydrate Intake

Event	Gender	Carbohydrate Intake
New Zealand Ironman triathlon[12]	M	1.1 g/kg/hour
New Zealand Ironman triathlon[12]	F	1.0 g/kg/hour
Tour de France cyclists[15]	M	1.3g/kg/hour
Pony Express Trail cyclists[16]	M	60 to 75 g/hour
Tour de Spain cyclists[17]	M	25 g/hour
Run around Australia[50]	M	39 g/hour
Ultrarunners[13]	M	44 g/hour
Ultrarunners[14]	M and F	54 g/hour

and associates found that male ultrarunners consumed 44 g of carbohydrate per hour during a 160-km trail run.[13] In another study, Glace and colleagues found that male and female ultrarunners consumed 54 g of carbohydrate per hour during a 160-km trail run in the heat (see Table 8.8).[14]

The athlete should develop and refine a fueling plan weeks and months ahead of the priority race by experimenting in workouts and in lower-priority races. The athlete should test this fueling plan while exercising at race pace and in environmental conditions that simulate race conditions. Athletes should not consume untested foods or fluids during the race as the result may be severe indigestion and poor performance (see Table 8.9).[6]

Endurance athletes should monitor body weight changes during training and competition in different environmental conditions to estimate their sweat losses.[46] This allows them to develop customized fluid replacement programs for their particular needs.[46] To determine sweat rate, the athlete should weigh before and after a specified time of exercise (e.g., 1 hour). Nude weights should be used when possible to avoid corrections for sweat trapped in the clothing. The post-workout weight and

TABLE 8.9
Carbohydrate Content of Typical Items Consumed during Endurance Exercise

1 quart of Gatorade® = 60 gm
1 PowerBar® = 47 gm
2 Gu® gels = 50 gm
1 banana = 30 gm
3 large graham crackers = 66 gm
4 Fig Newtons = 42 gm

TABLE 8.10
Determining Sweat Rate

Weigh before and after activity (e.g., 1 hour run)
(Pre-Weight – Post Weight)
+ Fluid Intake During Activity
= Athlete's Individual Sweat Rate

any urinary fluid losses should be subtracted from the pre-workout weight. Then, the amount of fluid consumed during the workout should be added (see Table 8.10).[46]

Endurance athletes should drink only enough during exercise to closely match fluid loss from sweating.[46] The athlete should monitor weight losses during training and competition and drink sufficient fluid to limit weight loss to 1–2% of initial body weight.[6,79] A weight loss of up to 3% may be tolerable and not impair performance in cool weather.[46]

During training, athletes should experiment with different fluid replacement drinks and practice adjusting their drinking strategies based on the workout intensity, duration, and environmental conditions.[6] Drinking appropriately in workouts enables the athlete to maintain a desirable training pace (and so maximize training adaptations), protects against heat illness, and allows the athlete to practice proper drinking strategies for competition.[6]

To prevent hyponatremia, endurance athletes should avoid overconsumption of fluids and associated weight gain.[46] Athletes should determine their hourly sweat rate and drink only enough to closely match fluid loss from sweating.[46] During endurance exercise, a loss of 1 to 2% of body weight is likely to occur from factors unrelated to sweat losses (substrate oxidation) and is acceptable.[6] Consuming a sodium-containing sports drink helps to maintain plasma sodium levels and may reduce the risk of hyponatremia during prolonged exercise.[80,81]

Athletes participating in endurance exercise lasting over 3 hours should be particularly meticulous in establishing their fluid replacement schedule. As the exercise duration increases, the cumulative effects of slight disparities between fluid intake and loss can cause extreme dehydration or hyponatremia.[46]

Endurance athletes use a variety of fluids, foods, and gels during training and competition. Liquid and solid carbohydrates are equally effective in increasing blood glucose and improving performance, though each has certain advantages.[82,83]

Sports drinks and other fluids containing carbohydrate encourage the consumption of water needed to maintain normal hydration during exercise. Carbohydrate ingestion and fluid replacement independently improve performance and their beneficial effects are additive.[84] The sodium in sports drinks helps to replace sweat sodium losses and stimulate thirst.[46] Sports drinks are a practical way to obtain water, carbohydrate, and sodium during endurance events lasting up to 3 hours and offer the benefit of simplifying the athlete's race nutrition plan.[6]

If both fluid replacement and carbohydrate delivery are going to be met with a single beverage, the carbohydrate concentration should not exceed 8% (or even be slightly less), as highly concentrated carbohydrate beverages reduce gastric emptying.[46]

TABLE 8.11
Exercise Fueling and Hydration

1 g of carbohydrate/kg/hour[72] (multiple transportable carbohydrates)
Drink to closely match sweat rate[46]
Ingest sodium: ~ 800 mg lost in 2 lb (907.1 g) of sweat[46] (sports drinks, gels, other items)

High-carbohydrate liquid supplements containing 18 to 24% carbohydrate may be utilized during ultra-endurance events to help increase carbohydrate and energy intake. However, they are too concentrated in carbohydrate to double for use as fluid replacement beverages and may cause gastrointestinal distress when consumed in large volumes.[20] Lindeman noted that a male RAAM cyclist's reliance on a 23% carbohydrate solution to meet the majority of his energy needs contributed to gastrointestinal distress during the race despite consistent dilution.[20]

Carbohydrate and electrolytes can also be obtained by non-fluid sources such as carbohydrate gels, energy bars, and other foods.[46] These items are compact, can be easily carried, and provide variety (different flavors and textures) to prevent a boredom-related decline in energy intake and help relieve hunger.[6,11,16,19]

Koopman and colleagues found that the combined ingestion of protein (0.25 g/kg/hour and carbohydrate (0.7 g/kg/hour) before, during, and after prolonged moderate intensity exercise (6 hours at 50% of VO_{2max}) improved net protein balance at rest, during exercise, and during subsequent recovery in endurance athletes.[85] Foods or fluids that contain small amounts of protein and fat may also help to provide satiety and maintain energy levels during prolonged exercise (see Table 8.11).

Gabel and colleagues reported that the two ultra-endurance cyclists who cycled 2050 (3280 km) miles in 10 days achieved an optimal intake due to the variety and palatability of foods that were available during the event.[16] Eden and Abernathy noted that the foods eaten during the Sidney to Melbourne race were based on what the male ultra-distance runner had enjoyed eating during training and what he could tolerate while competing.[19]

High-fiber foods should be limited during competition to avoid gastrointestinal distress (e.g., abdominal bloating, cramping, bathroom breaks).[6] Lindeman noted that a male RAAM cyclist's high fiber intake (57 g per day from consuming fiber-rich sports bars and fruit) may have contributed to his gastrointestional distress during the race.[20]

When the athlete's gut blood flow is low (e.g., during intense cycling or running) the athlete should emphasize carbohydrate-rich fluids (sports drinks, liquid meals, high-carbohydrate liquid supplements, fruit juices, and carbohydrate gels) to promote rapid gastric emptying and intestinal absorption. When the athlete's gut blood flow is moderate (e.g., during moderate-paced cycling or slow running) the athlete may be able to consume easily digested carbohydrate-rich foods such as sports bars, fruit, and grain products (fig bars, bagels, graham crackers) in addition to liquid foods and fluids.[86]

Athletes can generally consume more calories per hour cycling than running.[6] Ironman triathlon competitors often decrease their calorie intake toward the end of the bike segment to start the run with a fairly empty gut. During the run segment of

TABLE 8.12
Pace and Fueling

Intense Exercise = Low Gut Blood Flow:
liquid food
sports drinks
carbohydrate gels
Moderate Exercise = Moderate Gut Blood Flow:
fruits
grain products
sports bars

a triathlon, the athletes usually consume only sports drinks, gels, and water to reduce the risk of gut distress (see Table 8.12).

Endurance athletes should consume liquid or solid fuel before feeling hungry or tired, usually within the first hour of exercise. Consuming small amounts at frequent intervals (every 15 to 20 minutes) helps to prevent gastrointestinal upset, maintain blood glucose levels, and promote hydration. The athlete's foods and fluids should be easily digestible, familiar (tested in training), and enjoyable (to encourage eating and drinking).[6]

E. Recovery Nutrition and Hydration

Restoring muscle and liver glycogen stores, replacing fluid and electrolyte losses, and promoting muscle repair are important for recovery following strenuous endurance training.[5]

Endurance athletes commonly engage in prolonged high-intensity workouts once or twice a day with a limited amount of time (6 to 24 hours) to recover before the next exercise session. Utilizing effective refueling strategies following daily training sessions helps to optimize recovery and promote the desired adaptations to training. During competition, especially multiday events such as bicycle stage races, there may be less control over the exercise–recovery ratio. In this case, the goal is to recover as much as possible for the next day's event.[5]

The most important factor affecting muscle glycogen storage is the total amount of carbohydrate consumed.[26] An adequate intake of carbohydrate and energy will optimize muscle glycogen repletion during consecutive days of hard workouts.[87–89] During the early period of recovery (0 to 4 hours), the endurance athlete should consume 1 to 1.2 g of carbohydrate per kg each hour. Recovery meals and snacks contribute toward the athlete's daily carbohydrate requirements of 7 to 12 g of carbohydrate/kg/day.[5]

When there is less than 8 hours between workouts or competitions that deplete muscle glycogen stores, the endurance athlete should start consuming carbohydrate immediately after the first exercise session to maximize the effective recovery time. The athlete may be more comfortable eating small amounts more frequently (e.g., every 30 minutes). During longer periods of recovery (24 hours), it doesn't appear to matter how intake is spaced throughout the day as long as the athlete consumes adequate carbohydrate and energy.[5]

There is no difference in glycogen synthesis whether liquid or solid forms of carbohydrate are consumed.[89] However, as noted in the "Carbohydrate" section earlier in the chapter, liquid forms of carbohydrate may be appealing when athletes have decreased appetites due to fatigue or dehydration.[5] Carbohydrate-rich foods with a moderate to high glycemic index should be emphasized in recovery meals or snacks to supply a readily available source of carbohydrate for muscle glycogen synthesis.[90]

The addition of protein to the recovery feeding does not enhance muscle glycogen storage when the amount of carbohydrate is at or above the threshold for maximum glycogen synthesis (1 to 1.2 g/kg/hr).[91–93] However, consuming protein with recovery snacks and meals may help to increase net muscle protein balance, promote muscle tissue repair, and enhance adaptations involving synthesis of new proteins.[5,28] The endurance athlete's initial recovery snack or meal should include 10 to 20 g of high quality protein (about 6 to 12 g of essential amino acids) in addition to carbohydrate.[5] Recovery meals and snacks count toward the athlete's daily protein requirements of ~1.6 g of protein/kg/day.[5]

The foods consumed during recovery meals and snacks should contribute to the athlete's overall nutrient intake. Nutritious carbohydrate-rich foods and lean sources of protein and dairy also contain vitamins and minerals that are essential for health and performance. These micronutrients may be important for post-exercise recovery processes.[5]

Endurance athletes should avoid consuming large amounts of foods high in fat or protein when total energy requirements or gastrointestinal distress limits food intake during recovery. These foods can displace carbohydrate-rich foods and reduce muscle glycogen storage.[5]

Ideally, the endurance athlete should fully restore fluid and electrolyte losses between exercise sessions.[46] Consuming regular meals and beverages will restore normal hydration over 24 hours, provided the food contains enough sodium to replace sweat losses.[46] If the individual is significantly dehydrated and has a short period (less than 12 hours) in which to recover before exercise, an aggressive rehydration program may be necessary.[46,94,95]

Inadequate replacement of sodium losses prevents the return of normal hydration and stimulates excessive urine production.[96] Consuming sodium during recovery promotes fluid retention and stimulates thirst.[96] Sodium losses are harder to determine than water losses because athletes have vastly different rates of sweat electrolyte losses.[46] Although drinks containing sodium (e.g., sports drinks) may be beneficial, many foods can supply the needed electrolytes.[46] Extra salt (one-half teaspoon or 2.5 g of salt supplies 1000 mg of sodium) can be added to meals and recovery fluids when sweat sodium losses are high.[46]

Endurance athletes should drink 1.5 L of fluid for each kg lost (24 oz or 720 mL for each pound or 0.5 kg lost) to achieve rapid and total recovery from dehydration.[94] The additional volume (150% of sweat losses) is required to compensate for the increased urine production that goes along with the rapid intake of large volumes of fluid.[46] When possible, fluids should be consumed over time and with ample electrolytes to maximize fluid retention (see Table 8.13).[97]

TABLE 8.13
Recovery Nutrition

0 to 4 hours: 1 to 1.2 g of carbohydrate/kg/hour[5]
10 to 20 g of high quality protein in initial feeding[5]
24 oz for each lb lost (150% of sweat lost)[94]
Ample electrolytes to maximize fluid retention[97]

VIII. STRATEGIES TO ENHANCE FAT OXIDATION

A. CAFFEINE

There is substantial evidence that caffeine enhances endurance performance.[98] Caffeine was removed from the World Anti-Doping Association's list of prohibited substances in January 2004. While caffeine's mechanism of action is unknown, it is unlikely that it improves endurance by increasing fat oxidation and sparing muscle glycogen utilization (the popular so-called "metabolic theory").[98,99] As a central nervous system stimulant, caffeine may reduce the perception of effort by lowering the neuron activation threshold and making it easier to recruit muscles for exercise.[98,99] Caffeine may also increase the force of muscle contractions by positively influencing calcium kinetics and sodium–potassium pump activity.[98,99]

A commonly recommended dose to improve endurance is 3 to 6 mg of caffeine/kg, consumed 1 hour before exercise.[100] However, recent evidence suggests that the beneficial effects of caffeine occur at lower levels of intake—1 to 3 mg of caffeine per kg—when it is consumed before or during exercise.[101] Cox and colleagues found a similar 3% improvement in time trail performance with (1) six doses of 1 mg caffeine/kg spread throughout 2 hours of submaximal cycling prior to the time trial; (2) 6 mg caffeine/kg consumed 1 hour prior to the cycling bout; or (3) 1.5 mg caffeine/kg consumed over the last third of the exercise protocol.[101] Further research is needed to identify the dose and timing of caffeine intake to improve endurance performance.[98]

Caffeine is unlikely to elevate urine output or cause dehydration if consumed in moderation before or during exercise.[102] In fact, Kovacs and associates found that the addition of caffeine to a 7% carbohydrate-electrolyte solution improved 1 hour cycling time-trial performance at all caffeine doses compared with the carbohydrate-electrolyte drink alone.[103] The performance improvement was the same with caffeine doses of 3.2 mg/kg and 4.5 mg/kg and greater than with 2.1 mg/kg.[103] The addition of caffeine to a sports drink may enhance performance by increasing carbohydrate oxidation. Yeo and colleagues found that ingesting 5 mg of caffeine/kg/hr with a 5.8% glucose solution during endurance exercise increased exogenous carbohydrate oxidation compared with glucose ingestion alone, possibly due to enhanced intestinal absorption.[104]

Coffee is not an ideal source of caffeine due to the variability of caffeine content and the possible presence of chemicals that may impair exercise performance.[98] The majority of research studies have used pure caffeine rather than caffeinated drinks or sports products.[98] Further research is required on the effectiveness of caffeinated products (energy drinks, caffeinated beverages and gels) commonly used by athletes.

Some athletes do not respond to caffeine and others experience adverse effects such as tremors, increased heart rate, headaches, and disrupted sleep.[98] These side effects are more common at caffeine doses exceeding 6 mg/kg.[98] Endurance athletes who want to use caffeine should experiment with pure caffeine in training before and during exercise to determine the dose that elicits the greatest benefits and least adverse effects.[98]

B. Short-Term Fat Adaptation

Several studies have evaluated the effects of a 5-day fat adaptation period (60 to 70% energy from fat) followed by 1 day of carbohydrate restoration (10 g carbohydrate/kg) on exercise metabolism and performance in endurance-trained athletes.[105–107] A 5-day time frame represents a more manageable period for extreme dietary change and minimizes the potential health and training disadvantages caused by longer periods of fat adaptation.

Short-term fat adaptation significantly increases fat oxidation and reduces muscle glycogen utilization during submaximal exercise (< 70% of $V0_{2max}$) compared with an isocaloric high-carbohydrate diet.[105–107] These higher rates of fat oxidation persist even under conditions in which carbohydrate availability is increased by having athletes consume a high-carbohydrate meal before exercise or ingest carbohydrate during exercise.[106,107] Despite a dramatic increase in fat oxidation, however, fat-adaptation and carbohydrate restoration strategies do not enhance endurance or ultra-endurance performance.[105–107]

The metabolic changes that occur with dietary fat adaptation suggest an upregulation of fat metabolism. Burke and Kiens propose that what was initially viewed as "glycogen sparing" following fat adaptation may actually represent a downregulation of carbohydrate metabolism or "glycogen impairment."[108]

Stellingwerff and colleagues found that fat adaptation and carbohydrate restoration were associated with reduced activity of pyruvate dehydrogenase at rest and during exercise.[109] This would impair rates of glycogenolysis at a time when muscle carbohydrate requirements are high.[108,109] Havemann and colleagues found that fat adaptation/carbohydrate restoration had no effect on overall performance during a 100 km time-trial but compromised the ability of well-trained cyclists to perform 1 km sprints during the time-trial.[110]

Competitive success in endurance and ultra-endurance sports requires more than the ability to exercise for hours at a moderate intensity.[108] The strategic moves that occur during these sports—breaking away, surging during an uphill stage, and sprinting to the finish line—all depend on the athlete's ability to work at high intensities, which are in turn fueled by carbohydrate.[108] Since fat adaptation appears to impair this critical ability[110] and does not enhance prolonged endurance exercise,[105–107] there appears to be no scientific support to recommend this dietary strategy.[108]

IX. ULTRA-ENDURANCE AND MULTI-DAY EVENTS

The importance of proper refueling and rehydrating during ultra-endurance events cannot be overemphasized.[11,111,112] The primary nutritional needs are water, carbohydrate, and sodium.[11] During the event, athletes should limit foods that are high in fat, protein, and fiber to decrease the risk of gastrointestinal distress.[113] The following pointers are also helpful:

- The food plan should be built around the athlete's food preferences and include a variety of foods rather than a limited number of items.[11,16,19,22]
- Food and fluid intake should be closely monitored.[11,16,19,20] The crew should be prepared to enforce an eating and drinking schedule during multiple day events. If necessary, separate timers can be set for both liquid and solid feedings.[22]
- Weighed food records are recommended to assess dietary intake.[16] Ideally, body weight should be assessed daily during multiple-day events.[16] By tracking the athlete's food and fluid intake and body weight, the crew can take immediate corrective action if the athlete starts to fall behind on fluid or energy intake.[16,22]
- Solid food should be easy to handle, chew, and digest. Beverages should promote rapid gastric emptying so that fluids and nutrients are quickly absorbed.[46,113] Concentrated nutrition such as high-carbohydrate supplements or liquid meals may be offered immediately before scheduled rest.[20,22,86]

In an ultra-endurance event, the athlete's fueling and fluid replacement strategies can mean the difference between successfully completing the event or dropping out of it. The advice of a registered dietitian with expertise in sports nutrition is recommended to determine the ultra-endurance athlete's nutritional requirements and develop an individualized dietary plan. The sports dietitian can also help to monitor the athlete's nutrition during multiple-day events and help enforce programmed food and fluid intake when necessary.[11,16,19,20]

X. FUTURE RESEARCH NEEDS

Limited data exists on the macronutrient and energy intake of female endurance athletes during training and competition. Further research is recommended to determine the adequacy of female endurance athletes' macronutrient and energy intakes, especially during training.

There is insufficient data on the micronutrient intake and status of endurance athletes,[114] especially for female endurance athletes. Further research is recommended to determine the adequacy of endurance athletes' micronutrient intakes.

Muscle glycogen supercompensation may add to the benefits of other dietary strategies that are used to improve endurance performance. These combined strategies should be systematically researched.

Recent research suggests that low doses of caffeine—1 to 3 mg of caffeine per kg—improve performance when consumed before or during exercise. Further research is warranted to identify the dose and timing of caffeine intake to improve endurance performance as well as the effectiveness of caffeinated products commonly used by athletes.

XI. CONCLUSIONS

Consuming adequate carbohydrate (5 to 12 g/kg/day) and energy on a daily basis is necessary to meet the fuel requirements of the athlete's training program as well as replenish muscle and liver glycogen between training sessions and competitive events. These athletes can meet their higher protein requirements (~1.2 to 1.6 g/kg/day) by consuming a mixed diet that provides adequate energy and 15% of the calories from protein. Endurance athletes should consume at least 1 g of fat per kg of body weight (~20 to 35% of calories from fat).

Endurance athletes who consume adequate total energy usually meet or exceed population reference values such as the DRI for vitamins and minerals. Consuming a nutrient-dense diet containing fruits, vegetables, whole grains, legumes, lean meat, and dairy foods during training and competition also helps to ensure adequate micronutrient intake. Endurance training can increase iron requirements as well as iron losses.

Drinking during endurance exercise is necessary to prevent the detrimental effects of excessive dehydration (> 2% body weight loss) and electrolyte loss on exercise performance and health. Athletes should customize their fluid replacement plans due to the considerable variability in sweating rates and sweat electrolyte content between individuals.

Carbohydrate loading can improve performance in endurance events exceeding 90 minutes. For most athletes, a carbohydrate loading regimen will involve 3 days of a high-carbohydrate intake (8 to 12 g of carbohydrate/kg) and tapered training. Fat adaptation impairs the athlete's ability to work at high intensities and does not enhance prolonged endurance exercise.

Consuming carbohydrate prior to exercise can help performance by "topping off" muscle and liver glycogen stores. The pre-exercise meal should contain ~1.0 to 4.5 g of carbohydrate/kg, consumed 1 to 4 hours prior to exercise. To avoid potential gastrointestinal distress, the carbohydrate and calorie content of the meal should be reduced the closer to exercise the meal is consumed. Prior to exercise, the athlete should slowly drink about 5 to 7 mL/kg at least 4 hours before activity. When sweat losses are high and the opportunities to replace fluid are low, glycerol hyperhydration may help intense endurance exercise in hot and humid environments. Athletes using glycerol to hyperhydrate should be supervised and monitored by appropriate sports medicine professionals.

Consuming carbohydrate during exercise can improve performance by maintaining blood glucose levels and carbohydrate oxidation. Endurance athletes should consume ~1 g of carbohydrate per kg each hour from either carbohydrate-rich fluids or foods providing a mixture of carbohydrates. To prevent dehydration and hyponatremia, endurance athletes should drink only enough during exercise to closely match fluid loss from sweating. The athlete should monitor weight losses during training and competition and drink sufficient fluid to limit weight loss to 1 to 2% of initial body weight. Low doses of caffeine—1 to 3 mg of caffeine per kg—may improve performance when consumed before or during exercise.

Consuming carbohydrate following exercise facilitates rapid refilling of carbohydrate stores. During the early period of recovery (0 to 4 hours), the endurance athlete should consume 1 to 1.2 g of carbohydrate per kg each hour. Consuming 10 to 20 g of high-quality protein with recovery snacks and meals may help to increase net muscle protein balance, promote muscle tissue repair, and enhance adaptations involving synthesis of new proteins. Endurance athletes should drink 1.5 L of fluid for each kg lost (24 oz or 720 mL for each pound or 0.5 kg lost) and consume adequate sodium to achieve rapid and total recovery from dehydration.

Endurance athletes should practice adjusting their fueling strategies based on workout intensity, duration, and environmental conditions. Testing specific foods and fluids before, during, and after training sessions also allows the athlete to determine effective fueling strategies for competition.

REFERENCES

1. Hargreaves, M., Exercise physiology and metabolism, in *Clinical Sports Nutrition*, 3rd ed., Burke, L. and Deakin, V. Eds. McGraw-Hill, Australia, 2006, chap. 1.
2. Coyle, E.F., Substrate utilization during exercise in active people, *Am. J. Clin. Nutr.* 61 suppl, 968S–979S, 1995.
3. Manore, M.M., and Thompson, J.L., Energy requirements of the athlete: Assessment and evidence of energy efficiency, in *Clinical Sports Nutrition*, 3rd ed., Burke, L. and Deakin, V. Eds. Australia, 2006, chap. 5.
4. Burke, L., Preparation for competition, in *Clinical Sports Nutrition*, 3rd ed., Burke, L. and Deakin, V. Eds. McGraw-Hill, Australia, 2006, chap. 12.
5. Burke, L., Nutrition for recovery after training and competition, in *Clinical Sports Nutrition*, 3rd ed., Burke, L. and Deakin, V. Eds. McGraw-Hill, Australia, 2006, chap. 14.
6. Maughan, R., Fluid and carbohydrate intake during exercise, in *Clinical Sports Nutrition*, 3rd ed., Burke, L. and Deakin, V. Eds. McGraw-Hill, Australia, 2006, chap. 13.
7. Burke, L.M., Gollan, R.A., and Reed, R.S.D., Dietary intakes and food use of groups of elite Australian male athletes. *Int. J. Sport Nutr.* 1, 378–94, 1991.
8. Fudge, B.W., Westerterp, K.R., Kiplamai, F.K., Onywera, V.O., Boit, M.K., Kayser, B., and Pitsiladis, Y.P. Evidence of negative energy balance using doubly labelled water in elite Kenyan endurance runners prior to competition. *Br. J. Nutr.*. 95, 59–66, 2006.
9. García-Rovés, P.M., Terrados, N., Fernández, S., and Patterson, A.M., Comparison of dietary intake and eating behavior of professional road cyclists during training and competition, *Int. J. Sport Nutr. Exerc. Metab.* 10, 82–98, 2000.
10. Martin, M.K., Martin, D.T., Collier, G.R., and Burke, L.M., Voluntary food intake by elite female cyclists during training and racing: Influence of daily energy expenditure and body composition, *Int. J. Sport Nutr. Exerc. Metab.* 12, 249–67, 2002.
11. O'Connor, H., Cox, G. Feeding ultra-endurance athletes: An interview with Dr. Helen O'Connor and Gregory Cox, Interview by Louise M Burke, *Int. J. Sport Nutr. Exerc. Metab.* 12, 490–494, 2002.
12. Kimber, N.E., Ross, J.J., Mason, S.L., and Speedy D.B., Energy balance during an ironman triathlon in male and female triathletes, *Int. J. Sport Nutr. Exerc. Metab.* 12, 47–62, 2002.
13. Glace, B., Murphy, C., and McHugh, M., Food and fluid intake and disturbances in gastrointestinal and mental function during an ultramarathon, *Int. J. Sport Nutr. Exerc. Metab.* 12,414–13, 2002.
14. Glace, B.W., Murphy, C.A, and McHugh, M.P., Food intake and electrolyte status of ultramarathoners competing in extreme heat, *J. Am. Coll. Nutr.* 21, 553–9, 2002.

15. Saris, W.H.M., van Erp-Baart, M.A., Brouns, F., Westerterp, K.R., and ten Hoor, F., Study of food intake and energy expenditure during extreme sustained exercise: The Tour de France, *Int. J. Sport Med.* 10 suppl, 26–31, 1989.
16. Gabel K.A., Aldous, A., Edgington, C., Dietary intake of two elite male cyclists during a 10 day, 2,050 mile ride, *Int. J. Sport Nutr.* 5, 56–61, 1995.
17. García-Rovés P.M., Terrados, N., Fernández, S., and Patterson, A.M., Macronutrients intake of top level cyclists during continuous competition—change in the feeding pattern, *Int. J. Sports Med.* 19, 61–7, 1998.
18. Hill, R.J., and Davies, P.S., Energy expenditure during 2 wk of an ultra-endurance run around Australia, *Med. Sci. Sports Exerc.* 33, 148–51, 2001.
19. Eden, B.D., and Abernathy, P.J., Nutritional intake during an ultra-endurance running race, *Int. J. Sport Nutr.* 4, 166–174, 1994.
20. Lindeman, A.K., Nutrient intake of an ultra-endurance cyclist, *Int. J. Sport Nutr.* 1, 79–85, 1991.
21. Knechtle, B., Enggist, A, and Jehle T., Energy turnover at the Race Across America (RAAM)—A case report, *Int. J. Sports Med.* 26, 499–503, 2005.
22. Clark, N., Tobin, J., Ellis, C., Feeding the ultra-endurance athlete: Practical tips and a case study, *J. Am. Diet. Assoc.* 92, 1258–62, 1992.
23. Fallowfield, J.L., and Williams C., Carbohydrate intake and recovery from prolonged exercise, *Int. J. Sport Nutr.* 3, 150–164, 1993.
24. Achten, J., Halson, S.L., Moseley, L., Rayson, M.P., Casey, A., and Jeukendrup, A.E., Higher dietary carbohydrate content during intensified running training results in better maintenance of performance and mood state, *J. Appl. Physiol.* 6, 1331–40, 2004.
25. Simonsen, J.C., Sherman, W.M., Lamb, D.R., Dernbach, A.R., Doyle, J.A., and Strauss R., Dietary carbohydrate, muscle glycogen, and power output during rowing training, *J. App.l Physiol.* 70, 1500–5, 1991.
26. Burke, L.M., Kiens, B., and Ivy, J.L., Carbohydrates and fat for training and recovery, *J Sports Sci.* 22, 15–30, 2004.
27. Brouns, F., Saris, W.H.M., Stroecken, J., Beckers, E., Thijssen, R., Rehrer, N.J., and ten Hoor, F., Eating, drinking, and cycling: A controlled Tour de France simulation study, Part II. Effect of diet manipulation, *Int. J. Sport. Med.* 10 suppl, S41–S48, 1989.
28. Tarnopolsky M., Protein and amino acid needs for bulking up, in *Clinical Sports Nutrition*, 3rd ed., Burke, L. and Deakin, V. Eds. McGraw-Hill, Australia, 2006, chap. 4.
29. Tarnopolsky, M., Protein requirements for endurance athletes, *Nutrition.* 20, 662–8, 2004.
30. Brouns, F., Saris, W.H., Stroecken, J., Beckers, E., Thijssen, R., Rehrer, N.J., and ten Hoor, F., Eating, drinking, and cycling. A controlled Tour de France simulation study, Part I, *Int. J. Sports Med.* 10 Suppl 1, S32–40, 1989.
31. Tarnopolsky, M.A., MacDougall, J.D., and Atkinson, S.A., Influence of protein intake and training status on nitrogen balance and lean body mass, *J. Appl. Physiol.* 64, 187–93, 1988.
32. Friedman, J.E., and Lemon, P.W., Effect of chronic endurance exercise on retention of dietary protein, *Int. J. Sports Med.* 10, 118–23, 1989.
33. Tarnopolsky, L.J., MacDougall, J.D., Atkinson, S.A., and Tarnopolsky M.A., and Sutton JR., Gender differences in substrate for endurance exercise, *J. Appl. Physiol.* 68, 302–8, 1990.
34. Food and Nutrition Board, Institute of Medicine, *Dietary Reference Intakes for Energy, Carbohydrate, Fiber, Fat, Fatty Acids, Cholesterol, Protein, and Amino acids.* National Academy Press, Washington, DC, 2002.
35. Jonnalagadda, S., Dietary fat and exercise, in *Sports Nutrition: A Practice Manual for Professionals*, 4th ed., Dunford, M. Ed. American Dietetic Association, 2006, chap. 4.

36. Volpe, S., Vitamins, minerals, and exercise, in *Sports Nutrition: A Practice Manual for Professionals*, 4th ed., Dunford, M. Ed. American Dietetic Association, 2006, chap. 5.
37. Fogelholm, M. Vitamin, mineral, and antioxidant needs of athletes. in *Clinical Sports Nutrition*, 3rd ed., Burke, L. and Deakin, V. Eds. McGraw-Hill, Australia, 2006, chap. 11.
38. Position of the American Dietetic Association, Dietitians of Canada, and the American College of Sports Medicine: Nutrition and athletic performance, *J. Am. Diet. Assoc.* 100, 1543–56, 2000.
39. Bjelakovic, G., Nikolova, D., Gluud, L.L., Simonetti, R.G., and Gluud, C., Mortality in randomized trials of antioxidant supplements for primary and secondary prevention: Systematic review and meta-analysis, *JAMA*. 297, 842–57, 2007.
40. Watson, T. The science of anti-oxidants and exercise performance, in *Clinical Sports Nutrition*, 3rd ed., Burke, L. and Deakin, V. Eds. McGraw-Hill, Australia, 2006, commentary B.
41. Schumacher Y.O., Schmid, A., Grathwohl, D., Bültermann, D., and Berg, A., Hematological indices and iron status in athletes of various sports and performances, *Med. Sci. Sports Exerc.* 34, 869–75, 2002.
42. Deakin V., Iron depletion in athletes. in *Clinical Sports Nutrition*, 3rd ed., Burke, L. and Deakin, V. Eds. McGraw-Hill, Australia, 2006, chap. 10.
43. Kerr, D., Kahn, K., and Bennell, K. Bone, exercise, and nutrition. in *Clinical Sports Nutrition*, 3rd ed., Burke, L. and Deakin, V. Eds. McGraw-Hill, Australia, 2006, chap. 9.
44. Singh, A., Evans, P., Gallagher, K.L., and Deuster PA., Dietary intakes and biochemical profiles of nutritional status of ultramarathoners, *Med. Sci. Sports Exerc.* 25, 328–34, 1993.
45. Messina, M., Lampe, J.W., Birt, D.F., Appel, L.J., Pivonka, E., Berry, B., and Jacobs, D.R. Jr., Reductionism and the narrowing nutrition perspective: time for reevaluation and emphasis on food synergy, *J. Am. Diet. Assoc.* 101, 1416–9, 2001.
46. Sawka, M.N., Burke, L.M., Eichner, E.R., Maughan, R.J., Montain, S.J., and Stachenfeld, N.S., American College of Sports Medicine. Position stand: Exercise and fluid replacement, *Med. Sci. Sports Exerc.* 39, 377–390, 2007.
47. Montain, S.J., and Coyle, E.F., Influence of graded dehydration on hyperthermia and cardiovascular drift during exercise, *J. Appl. Physiol.* 73, 1340–50, 1992.
48. Montain, S.J., Cheuvront, S.N., and Sawka, N.M., Exercise associated hyponatremia: Quantitative analysis for understanding the aetiology, *Br. J. Sports Med.* 40, 98–106, 2006.
49. Hew, T.D., Chorley J.N., Cianca J.C., Divine J.G. The incidence, risk factors, and clinical manifestations of hyponatremia in marathon runners, *Clin. J. Sports Med.* 13, 41–47, 2003.
50. Hill, R.J., and Davies, P.S., Energy expenditure during 2 wk of an ultra-endurance run around Australia, *Med. Sci. Sports Exerc.* 33, 148–51, 2001.
51. Speedy, D.B., Noakes, T.D., Kimber, N.E., Rogers, I.R., Thompson, J.M., Boswell, D.R., et al., Fluid balance during and after an ironman triathlon, *Clin. J. Sport Med.* 11, 44–50, 2001.
52. Bergstrom, J., Hermansen, L., and Saltin, B., Diet, muscle glycogen, and physical performance, *Acta Physiol. Scand.* 71, 140–150, 1967.
53. Karlsson, J., and Saltin, B., Diet, muscle glycogen, and endurance performance, *J. Appl. Physiol.* 31, 203–206, 1971.
54. Hawley, J.A, Schabort, E.J., Noakes, T.D., and Dennis SC., Carbohydrate-loading and exercise performance: An update, *Sports Med.* 24,73–81, 1997.
55. Sherman, W.M., Costill, D.L., Fink, W.J., and Miller, J.M., The effect of exercise and diet manipulation on muscle glycogen and its subsequent use during performance, *Int. J. Sport. Med.* 2, 114–118, 1981.
56. Bussau, V.A., Fairchild, T.J., Rao, A., Steele, P., and Fournier, P.A., Carbohydrate loading in human muscle: An improved 1 day protocol, *Eur. J. Appl. Physiol.* 87, 290–5, 2002.

57. Fairchild, T.J., Fletcher, S., Steele, P., Goodman, C., Dawson, B., and Fournier, P.A., Rapid carbohydrate loading after a short bout of near maximal-intensity exercise, *Med. Sci. Sport Exerc.* 34, 980–986, 2002.
58. Nueffer, P.D., Costill, D.L., Flynn, M.G., Kirwan, J.P., Mitchell, J.B., and Houmard, J., Improvements in exercise performance: Effects of carbohydrate feedings and diet, *J. Appl. Physiol.* 62, 983–988, 1987.
59. Wright, D.A., Sherman, W.M., and Dernbach, A.R., Carbohydrate feedings before, during, or in combination improves cycling performance, *J. Appl. Physiol.* 71, 1082–1088, 1991.
60. Sherman, W.M, Brodowicz, G., Wright, D.A, Allen, W.K., Simonsen, J., and Dernbach, A., Effects of 4 hr preexercise carbohydrate feedings on cycling performance, *Med. Sci. Sport Exerc.* 12, 598–604, 1989.
61. Sherman, W.M., Peden, M.C., and Wright, D.A. Carbohydrate feedings 1 hr before exercise improves cycling performance, *Am. J. Clin. Nutr.* 54, 866–870, 1991.
62. Hitchins, S., Martin, D.T., Burke, L., Yates, K., Fallon, K., Hahn, A., and Dobson, G.P., Glycerol hyperhydration improves cycle time trial performance in hot humid conditions, *Eur. J. Appl. Physiol. Occup. Physiol.* 80, 494–501, 1999.
63. Anderson, M.J., Cotter, J.D., Garnham, A.P., Casley, D.J., and Febbraio, M.A., Effect of glycerol-induced hyperhydration on thermoregulation and metabolism during exercise in heat, *Int. J. Sport Nutr. Exerc. Metab.* 11, 315–33, 2001.
64. Kavouras, S.A., Armstrong, L.E., and Maresh, C.M. et al. Rehydration with glycerol: Endocrine, cardiovascular and thermoregulatory responses during exercise in heat. *J. Appl. Physiol.* 100, 442–50. 2006.
65. Coyle, E.F., Hagberg, J.M., Hurley, B.F., Martin, W.H., Ehsani, A.A., and Holloszy, J.O., Carbohydrate feeding during prolonged strenuous exercise can delay fatigue. *J. Appl. Physiol.* 55, 230–235, 1983.
66. Coyle, E.F., Coggan, A.R., Hemmert, W.K., and Ivy, J.L., Muscle glycogen utilization during prolonged strenuous exercise when fed carbohydrate, *J. Appl. Physiol.* 61, 165–172, 1986.
67. Millard-Stafford, M.L., Sparling, P.B., Rosskopf, L.B., Hinson, B.T., and Dicarlo, L.J., Carbohydrate-electrolyte replacement improves distance running performance in the heat, *Med. Sci. Sports Exerc.* 24, 934–940, 1992.
68. Wilber, R.L., and Moffatt, R.J., Influence of carbohydrate ingestion on blood glucose and performance in runners, *Int. J. Sport Nutr.* 2, 317–327, 1992.
69. Coyle, E.F., Fluid and fuel intake during exercise, *J. Sports Sci.* 22, 39–55, 2004.
70. Hawley, J.A., Dennis, S.C., and Noakes, T.D., Oxidation of carbohydrate ingested during prolonged endurance exercise. *Sports Med.* 14, 27–42, 1992.
71. Wagenmakers, A.J., Brouns, F., Saris, W.H., and Halliday, D., Oxidation rates of orally ingested carbohydrates during prolonged exercise in men. *J. Appl. Physiol.* 75, 2774–80, 1993.
72. Jentjens, R.L., Achten, J., and Jeukendrup, A.E. High oxidation rates from combined carbohydrates ingested during exercise, *Med. Sci. Sports Exerc.* 36, 1551–8, 2004.
73. Jentjens, R.L., and Jeukendrup, A.E., High rates of exogenous carbohydrate oxidation from a mixture of glucose and fructose ingested during prolonged cycling exercise, *Br. J. Nutr.* 93, 485–92, 2005.
74. Jentjens, R.L., Moseley, L., Waring, R.H., Harding, L.K., and Jeukendrup, A.E., Oxidation of combined ingestion of glucose and fructose during exercise. *J. Appl. Physiol.* 96, 1277–1284, 2004.
75. Jentjens, R.L., Underwood, K., Achten, J., Currell, K., Mann, C.H., and Jeukendrup, A.E., Exogenous carbohydrate oxidation rates are elevated after combined ingestion of glucose and fructose during exercise in the heat. *J. Appl. Physiol.* 100, 807–16, 2006.

76. Shi, X., Summers, R.W., Schedl, H.P., Flanagan, S.W., Chang, R., and Gisofi, C.V., Effects of carbohydrate type and concentration and solution osmolality on water absorption, *Med. Sci. Sports Exerc*. 27, 1607–1615, 1995.
77. Jeukendrup, A.E., Moseley, L., Mainwaring, G.I., Samuels, S., Perry, S., and Mann, C.H., Exogenous carbohydrate oxidation during ultra–endurance exercise, *J. Appl. Physiol*. 100, 1134–41, 2006.
78. Currell, K. and Jeukendrup, A.E., Superior endurance performance with ingestion of multiple transportable carbohydrates, *Med. Sci. Sports Exerc*. 40, 275–81, 2008.
79. Coyle, E.F., Fluid and fuel intake during exercise, *J Sports Sci*. 22, 39–55, 2004.
80. Vrijens, D.M. and Rehrer, N.J. Sodium–free fluid ingestion decreases plasma sodium during exercise in the heat, *J. Appl. Physiol*. 86, 1847–51, 1999.
81. Twerenbold, R., Knechtle, B., Kakebeeke, T.H., Eser, P., Müller, G., von Arx P., and Knecht H., Effects of different sodium concentrations in replacement fluids during prolonged exercise in women, *Br. J. Sports Med*. 37, 300–3, 2004.
82. Lugo, M., Sherman, W.M., Wimer, G.S., and Garleb, K. Metabolic responses when different forms of carbohydrate energy are consumed during cycling, *Int J Sport Nutr*. 3, 398–407, 1993.
83. Robergs, R.A., McMinn, S.B., Mermier, C., Leabetter, G., Ruby, B., and Quinn, C., Blood glucose and glucoregulatory hormone responses to solid and liquid carbohydrate ingestion during exercise, *Int. J. Sport Nutr*. 8, 70–83, 1998.
84. Below, P.R., Mora-Rodriguez, R., Gonzalez-Alonso, J., and Coyle, E.F., Fluid and carbohydrate ingestion independently improve performance during 1 hour of intense exercise, *Med. Sci. Sports Exerc*. 27, 200–210, 1995.
85. Koopman, R., Pannemans, D.L., Jeukendrup, A.E., Gijsen, A.P., Senden, J.M., Halliday D., et al., Combined ingestion of protein and carbohydrate improves protein balance during ultra-endurance exercise, *Am. J. Physiol. Endocrinol. Metab*. 87, E712–20, 2004.
86. Laursen, P.B., and Rhodes, E.C., Physiological analysis of a high-intensity ultra-endurance event, *J. Strength Cond. Res*. 21, 26–38, 1999.
87. Ivy, J.L., Katz, A.L., Cutler, C.L., Sherman, W.M,, and Coyle, E.F., Muscle glycogen synthesis after exercise: Effect of time of carbohydrate ingestion, *J. Appl. Physiol*. 6, 1480–85, 1988.
88. Ivy, J.L., Lee, M.C., Broznick, J.T., and Reed, M.J., Muscle glycogen storage after different amounts of carbohydrate ingestion, *J. Appl. Physiol*. 65, 2018–23, 1988.
89. Reed, M.J., Broznick, J.T., Lee, M.C., and Ivy, J.L., Muscle glycogen storage postexercise: Effect of mode of carbohydrate administration, *J. Appl. Physiol*. 75, 1019–1023, 1989.
90. Burke, L.M., Collier, G.R., and Hargreaves, M., Muscle glycogen storage after prolonged exercise: Effect of glycemic index, *J. Appl. Physiol*. 75, 1019–23, 1993.
91. Jentjens, R., van Loon, L., Mann, C., Wagenmakers, A.J., and Jeukendrup, A.E., Additional protein and amino acids to carbohydrates does not enhance postexercise muscle glycogen synthesis, *J. Appl. Physiol*. 91, 839–846, 2001.
92. Van Hall, G., Shirreffs, S., and Calbet, J., Muscle glycogen resynthesis during recovery from cycle exercise: No effect of additional protein ingestion, *J. Appl. Physiol*. 88, 1631–36, 2000.
93. Carrithers, J., Williamson, D., Gallagher, P., Godard, M.P., Schulze, K.E., and Trappe S.W., Effects of postexercise carbohydrate-protein feedings on muscle glycogen restoration, *J. Appl. Physiol*. 88, 1976–1982, 2000.
94. Shirreffs, S.M., and Maughan, R.J., Volume repletion after exercise-induced volume depletion in humans: Replacement of water and sodium losses, *Am. J. Physiol*. 274, F868–75, 1998.

95. Maughan, R.J., Leiper, J.B., and Shirreffs, S.M., Restoration of fluid balance after exercise-induced dehydration: Effects of food and fluid intake, *Eur. J. Appl Physiol.* 73, 317–25, 1996.
96. Nose, H.G., Mack, W., Shi, X.R., and Nadel, E.R., Involvement of sodium retention hormones during rehydration in humans, *J. Appl. Physiol.* 65, 332–336, 1988.
97. Kovacs, E.M., Schmahl, R.M., Senden, J.M., Brouns, F., Effect of high and low rates of fluid intake on post–exercise rehydration, *Int. J. Sport Nutr. Exerc. Metab.* 12, 14–23, 2002.
98. Burke, L., Cort, M., Cox, G., Crawford, R., Desbrow, B., Farthing, L., Minehan, M., Shaw, N., and Warnes, O. Supplements and sports foods, in *Clinical Sports Nutrition*, 3rd ed., Burke, L. and Deakin, V. Eds. McGraw-Hill, Australia, 2006, chap. 16.
99. Spriet, L., Caffeine, in *Performance Enhancing Substances in Sport and Exercise*, Bahrke, M. and Yesalis, C. Eds. Human Kinetics. Champaign, IL, 2002, chap. 22.
100. Graham, T.E., Spriet, L.L., Metabolic, catecholamine, and exercise performance responses to various doses of caffeine, *J. Appl. Physiol.* 78, 867–74, 1995.
101. Cox, G.R., Desbrow, B., Montgomery, P.G., Anderson, M.E., Bruce, C.R., Macrides T.A., et al. Effect of different protocols of caffeine intake on metabolism and endurance performance, *J. Appl. Physiol.* 93(3), 990–9, 2002.
102. Armstrong, L.E., Pumerantz, A.C., Roti, M.W., Judelson, D.A., Watson, G., Dias, J.C., et al., Fluid, electrolyte, and renal indices of hydration during 11 days of controlled caffeine consumption, *Int. J. Sport Nutr. Exerc. Metab.* 15, 252–65, 2005.
103. Kovacs, E.M., Stegen, J.H.C.H., and Brouns, F., Effect of caffeinated drinks on substrate metabolism, caffeine excretion, and performance, *J. Appl. Physiol.* 85, 709–15, 1998.
104. Yeo, S.E., Jentjens, R.L., Wallis, G.A, and Jeukendrup, A.E. Caffeine increases exogenous carbohydrate oxidation during exercise, *J. Appl. Physiol.* 99, 844–50, 2005.
105. Burke, L.M., Angus, D.J., Cox, G.R., Cummings, N.K., Febbraio, M.A., Gawthorn, K., et al., Effect of fat adaptation and carbohydrate restoration on metabolism and performance during prolonged cycling, *J. Appl. Phys.* 89, 2413–2421, 2000.
106. Burke, L.M., Hawley, J.A., Angus, D.J., Cox, G.R., Clark, S.A., Cummings, N.K., et al., Adaptations to short-term high-fat diet persist during exercise despite high carbohydrate availability, *Med. Sci. Sports Exerc.* 34, 83–91, 2002.
107. Carey, A.L., Staudacher, H.M., Cummings, N.K., Stepto, N.K., Nikolopoulos, V., Burke, L.M., and Hawley, J.A., Effects of fat adaptation and carbohydrate restoration on prolonged endurance exercise, *J. Appl. Physiol.* 91, 115–122, 2001.
108. Burke, L.M., and Kiens, B. Fat adaptation for athletic performance: The nail in the coffin? *J. Appl. Physiol.* 100, 7–8, 2006.
109. Stellingwerff, T., Spriet, L.L., Watt, M.J., Kimber, N.E., Hargreaves, M., Hawley, J.A., and Burke, L.M., Decreased PDH activation and glycogenolysis during exercise following fat adaptation with carbohydrate restoration, *Am. J. Physiol. Endocrinol. Metab.* 290, E380–8, 2006.
110. Havemann, L., West, S., Goedecke, J.H., Macdonald, I.A., St Clair Gibson, A., Noakes, T.D., and Lambert, E.V., Fat adaptation followed by carbohydrate-loading compromises high intensity sprint performance, *J. Appl. Physiol.* 100, 194–202, 2006.
111. Kreider, R.B, Physiological considerations of ultra-endurance performance, *Int. J. Sport Nutr.* 1, 3–27, 1991.
112. Applegate, L., Nutritional considerations for ultra-endurance performance, *Int. J. Sport Nutr.* 1, 118–26, 1991.
113. Jeukendrup, A.E., Jentjens, R.L., and Moseley, L., Nutritional considerations in triathlon, *Sports Med.* 35, 163–81, 2005.
114. Nogueira, J.A., and Da Costa, T.H., Nutritional status of endurance athletes: What is the available information? *Arch. Latinoam Nutr.* 55, 15–22, 2005.

9 Purported Ergogenic Aids

Abbie E. Smith, Sarah E. Tobkin, Jeffrey R. Stout, and Christopher M. Lockwood

CONTENTS

I. INTRODUCTION

The ultimate goal of athletics is to maximize potential and deliver peak performance, whether the competitor is one's opponent or oneself. When these entrenched goals relate to performance, a true athlete's drive toward reaching them is unmatched. It is this profound incentive that triggered the advent of the use of ergogenic aids and continues to propel the further development of this emerging science.

The term "ergogenic" has its etymologic origin in ancient Greece, a culture that was captivated by human athletic achievement. From the Greek, *ergon* meaning "work" and *gennan* meaning "to produce," evident in this definition is the potential of some of these substances to provide the highly sought missing pieces in one's path toward enhanced performance. The variety of ergogenic aids available allow different athletes to approach diverse goals, including those that are sport-specific and those that relate to achieving general improvements in endurance, strength, or power performance. However, many of these supplements, some highly marketed, lack research-based evidence of their efficacy in humans, while others are backed by concrete support for their veritable ineffectiveness in improving human performance.

This chapter is designed to serve as a reference for sound, applicable information on 35 of the most prominent purported ergogenic aids. Herein, we explore the present state of the highly dynamic field of ergogenic aids through a concise presentation of the current substances of interest and the sum of the relevant human-based evidence.

II. ERGOGENIC AIDS AND HUMAN USE

A. Strong Human Research to Support Use

1. β-Alanine

As the only beta amino acid that exists in nature, beta-alanine has gained recent attention in the world of sports nutrition. Beta-alanine is a naturally occurring nonessential amino acid that is typically found in a carnivorous diet (chicken and turkey). The performance-enhancing effects as a result of beta-alanine alone are minimal. However, beta-alanine has been identified as the rate-limiting substrate necessary for the synthesis of a dipeptide protein called carnosine.[1,2] While, initially, carnosine may appear to be the substrate of interest, this dipeptide cannot be taken up into the muscle intact and is readily hydrolyzed into histidine and beta-alanine. It is the presence of beta-alanine that promotes a rise in carnosine levels. In fact, scientists reported an average increase of 64% in muscle carnosine after 4 weeks of supplementing with 4–6 g per day of beta-alanine.[3,4]

Carnosine (β-alanyl-L-histidine) is primarily found in fast-twitch skeletal muscle, where it acts as a physiochemical hydrogen ion (H^+) buffer and is essential in delaying the drop in pH associated with anaerobic metabolism. Carnosine appears to buffer as much as 40% of the H^+ that cause the acidic conditions in skeletal muscle.[2,3] In theory, increasing the muscle carnosine levels through chronic training or beta-alanine supplementation would improve the muscle's buffering capabilities and further lead to an improvement in anaerobic performance. However, methods to increase muscle carnosine concentration have been somewhat disputed. While carnosine has been suggested to be elevated in chronically trained athletes, the effects of acute training are less clear. Earlier research suggested that 10 days to 8 weeks of intensive training could increase intramuscular carnosine content.[5,6] However, more recently, studies have shown that intense training, utilized as an acute method to induce intramuscular acidosis, has been unable to promote a rise in skeletal muscle carnosine levels.[7–9] Harris et al. reported that 5 weeks of intense interval training (1- and 3-minute intervals) had no significant effect on muscle carnosine levels in women.[7] In addition, using a 4-week single-leg training program for the *vastus lateralis* resulted in no change in skeletal muscle carnosine content in either the trained or untrained legs.[9]

Sports scientists have investigated the relationship between skeletal muscle carnosine levels and high-intensity exercise performance in trained cyclists.[10] They reported a significant and positive relationship between carnosine concentration and the average power from a 30-second maximal sprint on a cycle ergometer. These results offer support for the theory that an increase in skeletal muscle carnosine concentration is positively associated with improved anaerobic performance due to the muscle's enhanced buffering ability.

The role of beta-alanine supplementation in augmenting intramuscular carnosine levels has been the topic of several recent studies. Supplementing with beta-alanine has been shown to significantly increase skeletal muscle carnosine content by 60% or more.[2] More interestingly, a study published by Derave et al.[11] contested the idea of a "ceiling effect" with respect to carnosine levels in highly trained sprint athletes, reporting 37–47% and 57–67% increases after 4 and 6 weeks of beta-alanine supplementation, respectively. Furthermore, the combination of training and supplementation appears to stimulate a greater increase in carnosine concentration than supplementation alone.[9] Harris et al. reported that beta-alanine supplementation combined with intense training may double the increase in carnosine content.[7,9] Kim et al. also showed an enhanced effect of combining supplementation and training. In a group of elite cyclists, muscle carnosine was not altered after 12 weeks of training in the absence of beta-alanine, but increased 46% with beta-alanine supplementation.[12]

Elevated intramuscular carnosine levels have also been positively related to improvements in performance. Hill and colleagues[2] examined the effect of beta-alanine supplementation on muscle carnosine levels and exercise performance in untrained individuals. In a double-blind fashion, 25 men, ages 19–31, supplemented either 4.0 g beta-alanine or sugar placebo for the first week, followed by a dose of 6.4 g for an additional 9 weeks. Muscle carnosine levels (via muscle biopsy) and total work done (kJ) were measured at weeks 0, 4, and 10 during cycling to exhaustion

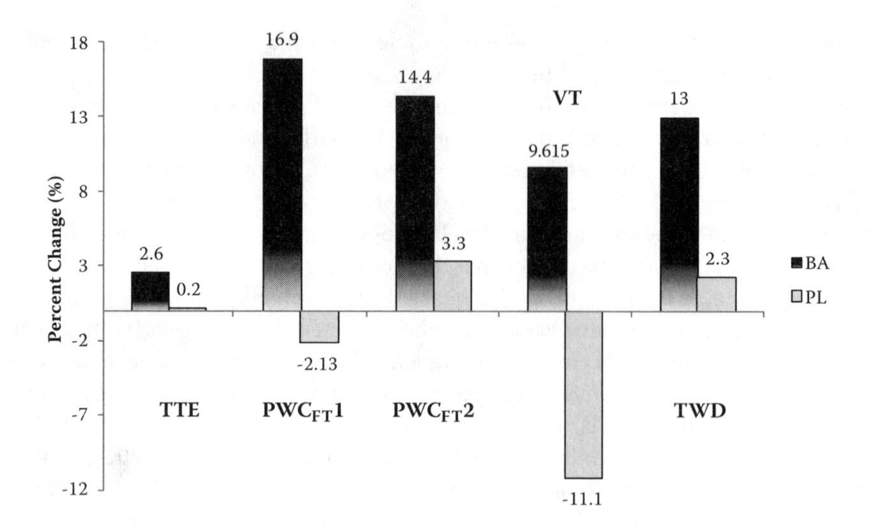

FIGURE 9.1 The influence of beta-alanine supplementation vs. placebo on time to exhaustion (TTE; Stout, *Amino Acids* 2006),[257] physical working capacity at fatigue threshold (PWCFT1; Stout, *JSCR* 2006; PWCFT2; Stout, *Amino Acids* 2006),[13,257] ventilatory threshold (VT; Zoeller 2006)[258] and total work done (TWD; Hill 2007).[2]

at 110% of max power established from a graded exercise cycle ergometry test. Average carnosine levels increased by 58% at week 4 and an additional 15% at week 10. Furthermore, there was a 13% and 16% increase in total work done during cycle ergometry at weeks 4 and 10, respectively (Figure 9.1). Another study examined the influence of beta-alanine on neuromuscular fatigue in a group of untrained men.[13] In a double-blind approach, participants consumed either 1.6 g of beta-alanine or sugar placebo four times per day for 6 days, followed by a 3.2 g per day period for 22 days. Prior to and following supplementation, the men performed an incremental cycle ergometry test to assess neuromuscular fatigue using the physical working capacity at fatigue threshold (PWC_{FT}) method. In theory, the PWC_{FT} represents the highest exercise intensity a person can maintain without signs of fatigue and is highly related to anaerobic threshold measurements. This technique offers insight into peripheral fatigue by utilizing surface electromyography to quantify electrical activity of the *vastus lateralis*. The results revealed a significantly greater increase in PWC_{FT} (9%) in the beta-alanine group compared with no change in the placebo group. In a follow-up study, Stout and colleagues[14] examined the effects of beta-alanine supplementation in untrained college-age women and reported similar significant increases in PWC_{FT} (12.6%), ventilatory threshold (13.9%), and time to exhaustion (2.5%) during a graded exercise cycle ergometry test (Figure 9.1). These findings suggest that 28-day beta-alanine supplementation appears to increase the level of intensity at which men and women can train or compete without signs of rapid fatigue. Essentially, performance and quality of training would be enhanced by elevating the onset of fatigue threshold due to a delay in metabolite accumulation.

In conclusion, beta-alanine supplementation (3.2 g–6.4 g per day) appears to significantly elevate intramuscular carnosine levels and further enhance performance in both trained and untrained individuals by maintaining the homeostatic pH environment of the muscle cell. Additionally, improvements in performance have been reported in both men and women and have been centered on anaerobic activities.

2. β-Hydroxy-β-Methylbutyrate (HMB)

HMB is a natural metabolite of the essential amino acid leucine.[15] Scientists at Iowa State University generated the theory that HMB may play an important role in protein metabolism, particularly in stressful situations. Specifically, HMB may regulate enzymes responsible for muscle tissue breakdown.[15] A meta-analysis substantiated the use of HMB as an effective sports supplement, detailing its effect on improved strength and lean mass gains in anaerobic and aerobic training. It was further reported to spare muscle protein catabolism and speed recovery.[15]

Researchers at Iowa State conducted the first HMB supplementation study in humans, in which untrained male subjects participated in a resistance-training program and were assigned to one of three groups: a control group, a group that consumed 1.5 g HMB per day, or a group that consumed 3 g HMB per day.[15] Following 1 week of resistance training, the 3 g HMB-supplementing group demonstrated a 44% reduction in muscle protein catabolism compared with the control group. The HMB group also continued to maintain a lower degree of muscle protein breakdown for the entire 3-week study. Furthermore, the subjects in both HMB-supplemented groups experienced significant gains in strength: +23% for the 1.5 g per day group and +29% for the 3 g per day group. In support, a study conducted at East Tennessee University examined the effects of resistance training plus HMB supplementation in untrained men and women.[16] All subjects trained three times per week for 4 weeks while supplementing 3 g per day of HMB or a placebo. The HMB group demonstrated greater gains in strength and lean body mass over the placebo group. In a more recent study, recreationally active college students underwent five weeks' high-intensity interval training on a treadmill, while supplementing with 3 g per day of HMB or placebo. Only the HMB-supplementing group resulted in a significant increase (13.4%) in aerobic performance (VO_{2max}).[17]

While HMB has been shown to be an effective anti-catabolic supplement, its use in trained individuals has yet to demonstrate any benefits. Kreider et al.,[18] in a double-blind fashion, provided 3 or 6 g per day of HMB to a group of experienced resistance trained athletes for 28 days. No improvements were reported for protein synthesis, 1RM strength, or body composition. It has been proposed that trained individuals may need a higher dose to demonstrate the anti-catabolic effect, but more research with this population is necessary.

In summary, HMB supplementation appears to work best for those who are untrained or in the process of altering their training program and want to lessen the associated muscle soreness and damage. Based on the available evidence, 3.0 g per day is recommended for 3 to 5 weeks when starting a new program.

3. Caffeine

The stimulatory effects of caffeine have been known for centuries, and it continues to be one of the most widely used supplements in the world (Figure 9.2). Caffeine is a central nervous system and metabolic stimulant utilized to reduce feelings of fatigue and to restore mental acuity. Caffeine readily crosses the blood–brain barrier, where it acts as an adenosine antagonist. While adenosine typically has an inhibitory effect on the central nervous system, causing feelings of fatigue and drowsiness, caffeine's structure allows it to mimic the shape of adenosine and bind to adenosine receptors, causing the opposite effect, accelerating neural cell activity. Many studies have demonstrated the exercise performance-enhancing effects of caffeine.[19,20] The traditional hypothesis is that caffeine increases the levels of our "fight or flight" chemical messengers, including epinephrine and norepinephrine, that promote fat utilization and result in the sparing of intramuscular glycogen.

Caffeine supplementation prior to exercise has been shown to increase fat oxidation (using fat for energy)[21] and to spare muscle glycogen utilization by up to 55%.[22,23] The decrease in glycogenolysis during exercise would prove to be essential for endurance and prolonged athletic activities during which carbohydrate stores deplete before finishing the activity. In support, performance data suggest that an elevation in fat oxidation, as well as a reduction in muscle glycogen utilization, leads to an increase in time to exhaustion. In support, Schneiker and colleagues demonstrated significant improvements in intermittent sprint ability (two 36-minute tests consisting of 18 4-second sprints on a cycle ergometer) after 7 days of caffeine supplementation (6 mg per kg of body weight per day).[24] In addition, caffeine may help endurance athletes by positively influencing psychological state and altering pain perception.

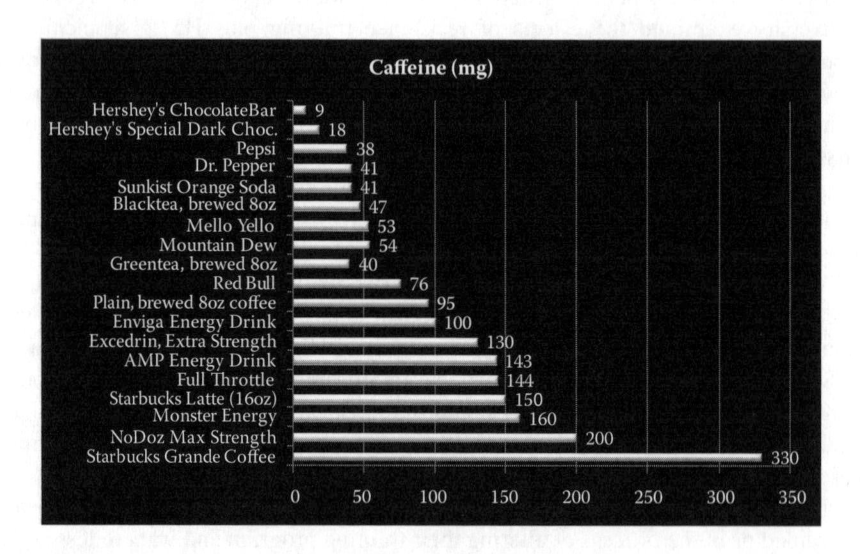

FIGURE 9.2 Caffeine content in commonly consumed food and beverages. 8 oz. is equivalent to 237 mL; 16 oz. is equivalent to 473 mL. All other items listed are prepackaged or recommended doses.

In a meta-analysis, caffeine supplementation subsequently resulted in a reduced rating of perceived exertion during constant load exercise.[19]

While caffeine has been primarily used in improving endurance-related activities, its effect in strength and power-type exercises may be attributed to an enhanced ability to maximally activate skeletal muscle.[25] The research supporting use in anaerobic activities is equivocal. Anaerobic power, assessed with a 30-second cycle ergometer sprint, after a range of caffeine doses (3.2–7 mg/lb), demonstrated no improvements[26,27] with one study resulting in a 7% increase in anaerobic power for the caffeine group only.[28] In addition, a report by Wiles et al. demonstrated improved performance time during a bout of short-duration, high-intensity exercise and an improvement in mean power, following 5 mg per kg body weight of caffeine per day.[29] Furthermore, another study provided support for an improvement in bench press 1RM following caffeine supplementation.[30] While the use of caffeine as an ergogenic aid in anaerobic activities is not conclusive, the mild stimulant effect of caffeine on the central nervous system may make it a worthwhile preworkout supplement.

Studies seem to suggest that an ergogenic benefit from caffeine can be achieved with a dose of 3 mg per kg (1.4 mg per lb) body weight, while a dose of 5 to 6 mg per kg (2.3–2.7 mg per lb) body weight may be more effective at increasing free fatty acid levels. The most common effective dosing recommendation would be to supplement with 3–6 mg per kg (1.4–2.7 mg per lb) of body weight 30–60 minutes before exercise.[19,20]

4. Creatine

Creatine (Cr) is an organic compound that is synthesized in small amounts (2%) in the liver, pancreas, and kidneys from the amino acids arginine, methionine, and glycine.[31] Creatine can also be obtained through exogenous sources, from foods that are high in protein, such as fish and beef.[31,32] Approximately 95% of all Cr stores in the body are found in skeletal muscle, and over 500 studies have demonstrated an increase in intramuscular Cr stores through supplementation.[31] The rationale for augmenting Cr levels is based on initial energy substrate use during the onset of exercise. The adenosine triphosphate (ATP)-phosphocreatine (PCr) system is always the first to supply energy during exercise, yet PCr and creatine phosphate (CP) are depleted at an extremely rapid rate.

Creatine supplementation of 20 to 30 g per day for 3 days has been suggested to enhance exercise performance in two ways. Through supplementation, Cr may first provide a greater primary source of energy by increasing the initial amount of available PCr in the muscle, and, second, it may increase the amount of free Cr, which aids the rate of PCr regeneration during recovery.[33] Further physiological explanations for the ergogenic effects have been demonstrated by an increase in muscle growth and muscle strength, measured by bench press and leg press, due to enhanced Cr levels (Figure 9.3),[34–37] and an increase in lean body mass as a result of an increase in training volume.[35,38] In addition, Cr supplementation has been demonstrated to increase muscle cross-sectional area (Type I, IIA, IIB)[35,38] and augment myosin heavy chain expression,[39] and may result in intramyocellular swelling, which, in turn, may affect protein and carbohydrate/glycogen storage.[40–42]

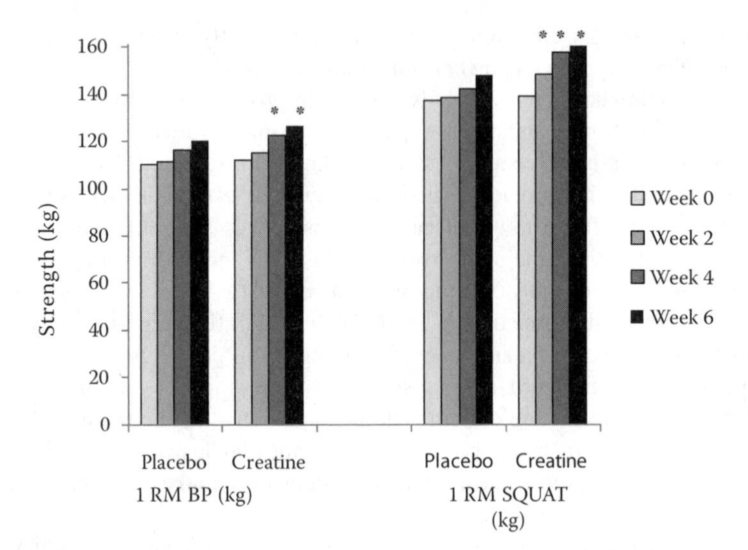

FIGURE 9.3 Strength adaptations from a six-week creatine supplementation and resistance training intervention. * Adapted from Volek et al. *Eur J Appl Physio.* 2004.[36]

In summary, the International Society of Sports Nutrition's (ISSN) published position stand states that Cr monohydrate is the most effective ergogenic nutritional supplement currently available in terms of increasing high-intensity exercise capacity and lean body mass during training. The ISSN states that Cr supplementation is not only safe, but possibly beneficial in regard to preventing injury. There is also no evidence of detrimental short- or long-term effects of Cr supplementation. The quickest method of increasing muscle Cr stores appears to be to consume approximately 0.3 g per kg of body weight per day of Cr monohydrate for at least 3 days followed by 3–5 g per day thereafter to maintain elevated stores. Ingesting smaller amounts of Cr monohydrate (e.g. 2–3 g per day) will increase muscle Cr stores over a 3- to 4-week period; however, the performance effects of this method are less supported. The addition of carbohydrate or carbohydrate and protein to a Cr supplement appears to increase muscular retention of Cr, although the effect on performance measures may not be greater than using Cr monohydrate alone.[32]

5. Essential Amino Acids (EAAs)

EAAs are amino acids that the body cannot manufacture and must be consumed in the diet. There are nine EAAs, which include histidine, isoleucine, leucine, lysine, methionine, phenylalanine, threonine, tryptophan, and valine (Table 9.1). When combining the use of EAAs, formulations vary considerably. In general, however, the literature supporting the use of EAAs suggests a dose-dependent effect on protein synthesis and supports use in recovery, not as a means for "energy" (calories).

Research has demonstrated that consuming EAAs pre- and post-exercise augments amino acid uptake and availability for protein synthesis.[43] In support, Tipton

TABLE 9.1
Essential Amino Acids

	Essential Amino Acids	Minimum Daily (mg)	Augments	Food Sources
1	Histidine	9	Tissue repair, muscle growth	Pork, poultry, rice, wheat, cheese
2	Isoleucine*	10	Mucle development/repair, energy	Eggs, fish, lentils, poultry, beef, soy, wheat, almonds, dairy
3	Leucine*	14	Protein synthesis, gluconeogenisis	Cottage cheese, sesame seeds, peanuts, lentils, chicken, fish
4	Lysine	12	Triglycerides	Green beans, lentils, soybeans, spinach
5	Methionine	13	Metabolism	Fish, whole grains, dairy
6	Phenylalanine	14	Catecholamine response	Dairy, almonds, avocados, lima beans, peanuts, seeds
7	Threonine	7	Collagen, tooth enamel	Dairy, beef, poultry, eggs, beans, nuts
8	Tryptophan	3.5	Serotonin, melatonin	Chocolate, oats, bananas, milk, cottage cheese, fish, turkey, peanuts
9	Valine*	10	Muscle metabolism, tissue repair	Whole grain, meat, mushrooms, peanuts, soy protein

* = Branched Chain Amino Acids

and colleagues[44] demonstrated a significant additive effect of combining EAA supplementation with a resistance training bout, compared with resistance training alone. Fifteen grams of an EAA beverage was given immediately before and another 15 g of EAAs 1 hour after resistance training, for a total of 30 g of EAAs, resulting in an improved muscle protein balance over a 24-hour period. These findings confirm that supplementing EAAs before and after training can have a powerful anabolic effect on skeletal muscle that persists for more than just a few hours post-exercise.[44] Other studies have shown that consuming EAAs pre-exercise may be more important than consuming them post-exercise for boosting the anabolic effect of resistance training and building muscle more rapidly. Furthermore, combining EAAs with carbohydrates (CHO) before an exercise training session has been shown to improve protein synthesis to a greater extent than when consumed after exercise.[45–48] A recent study by Bird et al.[49,50] demonstrated anti-catabolic effects of combining EAA and CHO (6% CHO; 6 g EAA) during a short-term resistance training bout, which resulted in decreased cortisol and attenuated myofibrillar protein degradation.

In addition, there may be a threshold for EAA intake of approximately 20 g, above which greater doses may not further improve the protein synthesis response.[45–47,51–53] In light of the sum of reviewed studies, specifically those confirming that EAA concentrations directly stimulate protein synthesis, it would be recommended for any athlete desiring to increase the benefits of training to consume EAAs before and after exercise. Based on the available evidence, to enhance the effects of training and to improve recovery, 3–20 g per day is recommended consumed in combination with carbohydrate 30 minutes pre-exercise and within 1 hour post-exercise.

6. Sodium Bicarbonate

As a result of muscular contraction, ATP is reduced to supply energy, resulting in an increase in H^+. During intense exercise, the accumulation of H^+ surpasses physiological buffering capabilities, decreasing the intracellular pH and, therefore, reducing the muscles' ability to contract (metabolic acidosis), which can result in fatigue, increased use of protein for energy, and loss of muscle mass.[54] Sodium bicarbonate, however, is extremely alkaline (low acidity/high pH) and has generally been shown to be effective for increasing intra- and extracellular pH of muscle cells, further corresponding to a delay in the onset of muscle fatigue and improving recovery from high-intensity events.[54–63] For example, McNaughton and Thompson[58] reported a 12% and 10% improvement in total work capacity and power, respectively, after 5 days of sodium bicarbonate supplementation (500 mg per kg body weight). In addition, Coombes and McNaughton[64] investigated the effects of 300 mg per kg body weight sodium bicarbonate ingestion on isokinetic strength and endurance, demonstrating an improved ability to perform work. Their results further support the use for sodium bicarbonate in anaerobic activities. However, with respect to endurance events, no performance-enhancing benefits have been demonstrated following sodium bicarbonate supplementation prior to the activity.[65–69]

While sodium bicarbonate is favored as an effective supplement, several factors must be considered for recommended dosing. Based on supporting research, positive results are demonstrated from consuming 300 to 500 mg per kg body weight. However, such dosages have been associated with side effects of diarrhea, cramping, nausea, and vomiting. These side effects are reduced when using doses of 100 to 200 mg per kg body weight, yet these doses may not be as useful for enhancing performance.[61,70,71] Side effects may also be reduced when supplementation is accompanied by copious water intake. Additionally, the timing of sodium bicarbonate supplementation can affect its ability to influence performance. Most studies have utilized a 90-minute pre-exercise consumption to allow for absorption into the bloodstream and greater buffering capacity. In summary, the recommendation for delaying fatigue from intense exercise is 300 mg per kg body weight per day as sodium bicarbonate diluted in 1L of water, consumed 1–2 hours prior to exercise or competition.

7. Sodium Citrate

Like sodium bicarbonate, sodium citrate can reduce blood acidity and increase the body's capacity to buffer the H^+ responsible for causing fatigue during high-intensity exercise. During high-intensity exercise, anaerobic glycolysis continually produces H^+ ions, decreasing intramuscular pH. Absorption of sodium citrate into the bloodstream after oral ingestion produces an increase in blood pH. The dissonance between the intramuscular and blood pH concentration accelerates the movement of H^+ from the working muscle into extracellular spaces. This movement consequently reduces the negative effects of metabolic acidosis. Thus, sodium citrate acts to balance the pH and further delay the onset of fatigue.

According to existing research, sodium citrate's performance-enhancing effects appear to be dependent on exercise duration. Short-duration exercise, even at very high intensities, does not allow enough time for a maximal rise in H^+; therefore, sodium citrate's buffering capabilities are not fully utilized and have not demonstrated a contribution to improved exercise performance in events lasting less than 60 seconds.[72–75] However, more studies have shown enhanced exercise performance when maximal intensity exercise lasted between 2 and 15 minutes.[76–80] Hausswirth and colleagues[76] reported a 20% improvement in maximal isometric knee extension endurance. Later, sodium citrate, given 90 minutes prior to exercise, was demonstrated to improve 3000-meter running performance in a group of Olympic caliber athletes.[81]

When given 60–90 minutes before high-intensity events lasting more than 2 minutes, a single dose of 0.4–0.5 g sodium citrate per kg body mass may elicit the greatest benefits. In addition, sodium citrate is well tolerated by most users, with few accounts of gastrointestinal distress.

B. Equivocal Human Research to Support Use

1. Alpha-Ketoglutarate (AKG)

As an intermediate in the Krebs cycle, AKG is naturally involved energy metabolism. It is also a precursor for glutamine synthesis and pyridoxal-5-phosphate (vitamin B_6), one of two critical co-factors used in transamination, a reaction by which the body forms non-essential amino acids or new amino acids from other amino acids.

AKG is most often recognized as an anticatabolic, or protein-sparing, agent, which works by sparing endogenous glutamine pools and increasing glutamine synthesis and availability. The evidence to support AKG supplementation comes primarily from clinical human studies. In a group of hip replacement patients, Blomqvist and colleagues[82] demonstrated that AKG (administered at 0.28 g per kg body weight) was effective in preventing protein catabolism and sparing free glutamine at 24 hours post-surgery. Wernerman et al.[83] also reported reduced losses of muscle mass following surgery when high doses of AKG were orally administered.

Few studies have used AKG supplementation in healthy individuals. One study, however, using trained but noncompetitive men, supplemented a combination of AKG (14 mg per kg body weight) and vitamin B_6 (16 mg per kg body weight), resulting in a 6% increase in maximal aerobic exercise performance and significantly reduced peak levels of blood lactate following supramaximal running workloads lasting less than 140 seconds.[84]

To gain a sports performance benefit, an average person (70 kg) would need to consume 980 mg of AKG, whereas a much larger dose of 20 g would be needed to reduce protein breakdown and spare muscle glutamine.

2. Alpha-Ketoisocaproate (KIC)

KIC is the branched-chain keto acid derived from the amino acid leucine, and, when ingested, about 50% of the consumed dose is converted into leucine.[85] KIC is also a direct precursor to the production of beta-hydroxy-beta-methylbutyrate (HMB) and has demonstrated anabolic and anticatabolic characteristics.[86] In particular, a recent study investigated the effects of supplementing with HMB (3 g) and KIC (0.3 g) daily on a muscle damaging protocol. The supplementing group demonstrated significantly reduced measures of delayed onset muscle soreness, an attenuated creatine kinase response, and a reduced decrement in 1RM.[87] KIC supplementation has demonstrated a protein-sparing effect, meaning that, under certain conditions, supplementing with KIC may help offset the loss of muscle mass. Theoretically, KIC may improve performance by increasing energy,[88] delaying the build-up of metabolites that cause fatigue,[89] and decreasing muscle damage caused by intense exercise.[87] Despite some positive results, a recent study suggested that a dose of 9 g of KIC per day, given immediately prior to an exercise test, did not result in improved performance.[90] Although various studies have tested the effects of KIC doses ranging from 1.5–20 g, more research is necessary before a verified recommendation for the effective dose can be given. It should be noted, however, that high doses, greater than 10 g, may cause gastrointestinal problems in some individuals.

3. Alpha-Lipoic Acid (ALA)

ALA is associated with an array of biological functions. While it is found in abundance in red meat in a carnivorous diet, it is also produced endogenously, and, therefore, is considered a nonessential nutrient. As it relates to athletic performance, ALA primarily functions as a potent antioxidant, assists in energy-producing reactions, and mimics the actions of the hormone insulin.

ALA's antioxidant effects were demonstrated in healthy adults, in which a dose of 600 mg per day for 8 weeks significantly reduced LDL-cholesterol oxidation, a process involved in initiating atherosclerosis. ALA was also found to be superior to vitamin E at decreasing plasma protein carbonyls, high levels of which may be linked to an increased risk for cancer.[91] Furthermore, ALA may increase the availability of glutathione, a powerful antioxidant that fights the free radicals that cause fatigue. By sparing glutathione, ALA may delay fatigue and improve performance during vigorous, long-duration aerobic exercise, supporting ALA's role as a "metabolic antioxidant."[92] While ALA is primarily reputed as a metabolic agent, athletes commonly ingest ALA in combination with glucose to promote an augmented post-exercise insulin response, potentially speeding recovery. In a randomized controlled study, healthy untrained men consumed 1 g of ALA in combination with 20 g of creatine monohydrate and 100 g of sucrose each day for 5 days. The supplementing group demonstrated significantly greater increases in muscle phosphocreatine levels than men who consumed creatine plus sucrose or creatine alone.[93] To achieve an antioxidant effect, an ALA supplement of 300–600 mg per day is recommended. To benefit from ALA's insulin-like action, the recommended supplemental dose is 1 g per day with glucose immediately after exercise.

4. Branched-Chain Amino Acids (BCAAs)

The essential amino acids leucine, isoleucine, and valine collectively form a group referred to as branched-chain amino acids, composing approximately 30% of the total muscle protein content. BCAAs are essential amino acids that the body cannot synthesize and, thus, must be obtained through the diet. BCAAs are found in high concentration in whey protein (26% BCAA), milk (21%), meats, fish, eggs, and other quality protein sources. Although they are readily available in dietary sources, BCAAs are in high demand as the primary amino acids oxidized during exercise (especially endurance exercise) and oxidative stress and are fundamental for protein synthesis. Research investigating BCAA supplementation pre-, during-, and post-exercise has demonstrated augmented protein synthesis and a reduction in protein degradation, ultimately enhancing recovery time.[94,95] For example, the effect of supplementing approximately 4–15 g of BCAAs per day or about 35 mg per pound (77 mg per kg) of body weight during resistance exercise resulted in a decrease in muscle protein breakdown and an increase in muscle building. Shimomura et al.[96] have also reported BCAA supplementation to be effective in reducing delayed-onset muscle soreness (DOMS) and fatigue for a few days following a fatiguing squat protocol. Bloomstrand and colleagues also provided support for BCAA supplementation in delaying central fatigue during and after prolonged exercise, by competing with tryptophan (an amino acid precursor to serotonin) and reducing its uptake into the brain.[97]

Furthermore, an investigation of the effects of BCAAs in a group of marathon runners revealed that, when mixed into a glucose rehydration drink, 7.5 g of BCAAs improved mental performance, and 16 g of BCAAs improved physical performance.[97] BCAAs may conceivably enhance performance in runners by enabling them to run harder and maintain mental focus. In addition, in a study from Rutgers University, 14 men and women ingested either a placebo or BCAA (5 mL per kg body weight) drink every 30 minutes during cycling at 40% of maximal exercise capacity. The BCAA-consumption groups demonstrated a 11.7% increase in time to exhaustion.[98]

Although the positive research supporting the use of BCAA supplementation is vast, some studies have failed to show any ergogenic effects.[99–101] However, BCAA research clearly supports improved recovery from exercise and enhanced protein synthesis and it could be argued that BCAAs indirectly improve performance. Thus far, however, BCAAs have not been shown to be *directly* ergogenic during exercise. In summary, these results indicate that supplementing with BCAAs during endurance or resistance training may spare valuable muscle by performing an anticatabolic function, while simultaneously increasing muscle protein building,[94,95,102] which would assist in recovery, training adaptations, and performance. The recommended dosages range between 9 and 15 g for the total dose consumed during exercise lasting approximately 2 hours. Also, some evidence indicates that supplementing 12 g daily for 2 weeks may assist in alleviating exercise-induced skeletal muscle damage.

5. Colostrum

Colostrum is a form of milk produced by the mammary glands for the nourishment of newborns. Its release occurs just before the onset of genuine lactation (milk secretion). While milk has many bioactive compounds that may be beneficial for active individuals, colostrum is even more complex. Along with nutrients and antibodies, colostrum contains multiple bioactive components, with growth factor fraction (IGF-1) and immunoglobulin fraction having gained the most attention for future ergogenic potential.[103] A third remaining fraction contains enzymes, proteins, and various peptides that are of less interest to athletes.[103] Research suggests that IGF-1 and the high-quality protein found in colostrum may stimulate muscle growth and promote protein synthesis.[104,105] In a double-blind, placebo-controlled study, 39 men completed an 8-week running program (45 minutes, 3 times per week) with supplementation (60 g colostrum per day or placebo). After 4 weeks, both groups improved comparably in treadmill running performance. However, at 8 weeks, the colostrum group ran 10% farther than the placebo group. In addition, the colostrum group demonstrated reduced levels of creatine kinase (an indicator of muscle damage) and an associated reduction in muscle trauma. Furthermore, a group of 51 males, combining 8 weeks of resistance and plyometric training and colostrum supplementation (60 g per day), resulted in improvements in peak vertical jump power and peak cycle power, with no change in 1RM of anaerobic work capacity, compared with placebo.[106]

Additionally, a few studies have demonstrated enhanced endurance performance due to the influence of IGF-1 on lipoprotein lipase (fat breakdown for energy utilization) and the inhibition of insulin activity in fat cells.[107] Coombes and colleagues[108] reported significant improvements in cycling time trial performance after a 2-hour ride at 65% VO_{2max} after 8 weeks of 20 g or 60 g of colostrum per day. Buckley et al.[109] also demonstrated that 8 weeks of colostrum supplementation (60 g per day) may enhance recovery between two bouts of incremental treadmill running to exhaustion by 5.2%. Colostrum supplementation may also positively influence body composition by augmenting the loss of body fat and reducing muscle breakdown (increase in or maintenance of lean body mass).[106,110–112]

The recommended dose of colostrum is 20–60 g per day. However, research presented by Antonio and colleagues[110] demonstrated that 20 g per day over an 8-week period in regular exercisers resulted in significant gains in lean body mass but no change in performance. Furthermore, combining a lower dose (20 g) with a high-quality protein (such as whey) may offer less expensive and additional benefits.

6. Dehydroepiandrosterone (DHEA)

DHEA, a steroid that is produced naturally by the adrenal glands, serves as a precursor to the sex hormones testosterone and estradiol. The conversion of DHEA to estradiol would not be advantageous for athletes in light of its anabolic effect on fat cells. However, the conversion of DHEA to testosterone may have potential performance-enhancing effects.

Testosterone is a potent anabolic hormone that promotes skeletal muscle protein accrual, and more muscle mass should translate into improved strength-power performance. However, the ergogenic effects of DHEA supplementation have been questioned. Wallace et al.[113] investigated the effects of a 12-week resistance training program and DHEA supplementation (100 mg per day) in a group of healthy middle-aged men and reported no significant changes in the DHEA group for upper- and lower-body strength. In addition, another study, employing 3 weeks of DHEA supplementation and resistance training in healthy adults, reported no significant changes in lean mass or strength gains.[15] However, several studies employing DHEA supplementation in elderly men and women have demonstrated significant improvements in immune function, muscle strength, muscle mass, and quality of life.[114,115]

While the effects of DHEA on athletic performance are uncertain, a dose of 100 mg per day might offer health-related benefits. Furthermore, DHEA may have a role in enhancing quality of life and improving strength and lean body mass in aging men and women. Caution should be used surrounding the ergogenic use of DHEA, as it is listed as a banned substance on the International Olympic Committee's list.

7. Gamma-Aminobutyric Acid (GABA)

GABA is an inhibitory neurotransmitter present in high concentrations throughout the central nervous system. Although it is an amino acid, it is not found in proteins, rather, it is synthesized by converting the principal excitatory neurotransmitter, glutamate, into the inhibitory form. GABA became popular among bodybuilders after a study revealed that acute supplementation (one single dose) resulted in an increase in growth hormone (GH) within 3 hours of consuming a 5 g oral dose.[116] Two follow-up studies confirmed the effectiveness of a 5 g oral dose in healthy adults, as well as revealing a dose-dependent increase when 10 g GABA was ingested.[117,118] One of these studies did, however, reveal a curvilinear response when 18 g of GABA was supplemented 4 days in a row and effectively resulted in a blunted GH response.[116] Consequently, ingesting too much GABA may actually have the opposite of the desired effect on GH release. Furthermore, recent data suggest that GABA may have inhibitory effects on the motor cortex after anaerobic exercise, thus reducing central fatigue.[119]

Additionally, while data are limited, some evidence suggests the potential use of GABA as an anti-anxiety aid that may also promote improved sleep. Based on the available data, in order to stimulate GH release, 5–10 g per day should be consumed on an empty stomach about 1 hour before bedtime.

8. Ginseng

While there are many species of ginseng, *Panax ginseng* (or Asian ginseng) and *Panax quinquefolius* (or American ginseng) are the two most commonly used forms and are believed to be the most effective due to the presence of biologically active ginsenosides (steroid-like compounds). In addition to historical use as aphrodisiacs and stimulants, both American and Asian ginseng are taken orally as adaptogens, substances believed to increase the body's resistance to stresses such as trauma, anxiety, and bodily fatigue. However, as with most herbs, there is considerable variation in chemical make-up and density of active ingredients between, and even within, ginseng species,[120] so all ginseng cannot be expected deliver analogous performance or physiological benefits.

In a comprehensive review of research data relevant to ginseng as performance enhancer, scientists have concluded that Asian ginseng extracts, standardized to not less than 4% total ginsenosides, produced some ergogenic effects in 74% of the studies that supplemented for more than 4 weeks, while Asian ginseng was suggested to be ineffective if used for less than 4 weeks.[121] In addition, evidence suggests that Asian ginseng, when consumed before exercise, can improve performance and act as a stimulant, and strong evidence supports the use of American ginseng in glucose disposal and recovery. For example, the use of Asian ginseng has been shown to improve endurance time to exhaustion and VO_2 during endurance exercise,[122] and to enhance recovery.[123] However, evidence suggests that Asian ginseng does not appear to enhance physical performance.[124,125] Furthermore, the use of American ginseng may reduce skeletal muscle damage following high-intensity exercise.[126] In addition, Vuksan et al. have provided evidence for reduced plasma glucose levels following 1, 2, or 3 g of American ginseng when taken 40 minutes before a glucose load.[127,128]

Based on the available science, for energy, performance enhancement, or for use as an adaptogen, 200 mg per day as *Panax ginseng* root (standardized to not less than 4% total ginsenosides) is recommended, consumed in divided doses: once in the morning and again 30–60 minutes prior to exercise. When taking ginseng as an aid to dispose glucose, 1–3 g per day is suggested as American ginseng (*Panax quinquefolius*) consumed in divided doses, 40 minutes before meals or under high glucose loads.

9. Glycerol

Also known as glycerin, glycerol is a colorless, odorless, sweet-tasting, syrupy liquid that is marketed as a sugar alcohol that does not affect blood sugar or increase insulin.[129] It is commonly used for added sweetness and palatability to high-protein or low-carbohydrate nutrition bars. In addition, glycerol has been suggested to serve as an ergogenic aid due to its hyperhydrating effects. Much of the data suggest that glycerol is an effective hyperhydrating agent,[130–132] yet its influence on performance is uncertain. Hitchins et al.[133] demonstrated an increase in power output without an increased perception of effort, after an acute dose (1 g per kg body weight) prior to exercise. Glycerol supplementation (1.0–1.2 g per kg body weight) has also been associated with an average 23% increase in time to exhaustion,[134] as well as maintaining normal body temperature and heart rate during exercise in the heat.[135,136] While some evidence is positive, not all studies have shown an ergogenic effect. For instance, Latzka and colleagues reported that glycerol ingestion was unable to lower oral or skin temperatures, improve sweating efficiency, or reduce heart rate while exercising in a hot environment.[137] Furthermore, other studies revealed that 1.0–1.2 g per kg body weight glycerol supplementation has no significant influence on cardiovascular, metabolic, or thermoregulatory function.[131,135]

While glycerol supplementation may not work for everyone,[138] individual responses vary, and one's personal reaction may be uncovered through experimentation. Sport scientist Dr. Wagner advises "as with any sport drink or nutritional aid, if an athlete decides to try glycerol-induced hyperhydration, he or she should experiment with it in training before using it in competition" (p. 210).[135] Based on the available data, a dose of 1 g of glycerol per kg (0.45 g per lb body weight) in about 1–2 cups (237–473 mL) of water or a favorite juice is suggested.

10. N-Acetylcysteine (NAC)

NAC supplementation has been shown to improve immune function and reduce the free radial stress that can cause muscle fatigue and damage. These benefits appear to result from an increase in glutathione (GSH) availability with NAC supplementation.[92,139,140] GSH is a potent antioxidant that protects the body from destructive free radicals that can cause fatigue or tissue damage. When the demand for GSH is high, as it is during exercise, there is a dramatic decrease in intramuscular GSH and increase in circulating GSH. However, if the demand for GSH continuously exceeds the available supply, muscle catabolism and contraction-induced fatigue increase.[141–143] In light of this, supplemental NAC may be needed to support GSH levels and could result in a sports performance benefit when administered before exercise.[144–147] For example, one study demonstrated that NAC supplementation prior to (15 minutes and 20 minutes) and during continuous exercise attenuated muscle fatigue and improved Na^+-K^+-pump kinetics.[148] Matuszczak and colleagues[149] also support a delay in fatigue during repetitive exercise following NAC supplementation. Furthermore, there are reports of a direct correlation between an improvement in aerobic fitness and NAC response, which may imply an improvement in aerobic performance following NAC supplementation.[145] Similarly, NAC supplementation more strongly influences slow-twitch fiber GSH kinetics and has been shown to delay muscle fatigue in prolonged aerobic activities with no direct ergogenic benefits in short-duration or maximal anaerobic exercise.[144,146,147] Moreover, some evidence suggests that the ergogenic benefits from NAC supplementation may be dependent upon training status.[145]

Based on the available research, for endurance performance benefits or to delay muscle fatigue, 600–1500 mg per day should be consumed with food approximately 60–120 minutes prior to aerobic exercise training or competition. For general and antioxidant use, 600 mg per day to 4 g per day is recommended in divided doses with meals.

11. Rhodiola

Rhodiola, like ginseng, is considered an adaptogen that optimizes serotonin and dopamine levels.[150] Rhodiola use may promote a wide variety of benefits, including neurostimulatory, antidepressant, antifatigue, antioxidant, immunostimulatory, sex hormone stimulatory, antistress, anti-inflammatory, and anticancer actions, among others.[151–157] For example, acute supplementation of *Rhodiola rosea* (200 mg per day for 2 days) resulted in improved time to exhaustion during a 30-minute endurance test, along with improvements in VO_{2peak}. In the same group of healthy men, chronic (4 weeks) rhodiola supplementation did not elicit any significant performance gains.[158] Furthermore, *Rhodiola rosea* has been suggested as an anti-inflammatory agent in healthy untrained individuals, which may indirectly lead to improved performance.[152]

Individuals should be aware that rhodiola consists of a variety of species, whereas the majority of the data employ supplementation with *Rhodiola rosea* root extract. For general chronic use and as a potential adaptogen, it is recommended that 100–600 mg per day as *Rhodiola rosea* root extract (standardized to provide 3.6–21.6 mg per day rosavin) be consumed on an empty stomach. For an acute performance effect, it is recommended that 300–1,800 mg as *Rhodiola rosea* root extract (standardized to provide 10.8–64.8 mg rosavin) be consumed on an empty stomach, approximately 30–60 minutes prior to exercise or competition.

12. Ribose

Ribose, a simple sugar naturally synthesized in the body, is used to make energy for skeletal and cardiac muscle and other tissues. While ribose is immediately absorbed intracellularly and converted to energy, the process is slow. As an essential component to the backbone of ATP,[159] ribose may play an important role in energy availability when mechanical energy demand is high. During intense activity, energy is depleted more rapidly than it can be replenished, ultimately leading to fatigue. Thus, it is believed that supplementing ribose may be useful in rebuilding ATP and therefore creating more available energy during and after exercise.[160] Although inconclusive, research suggests that ribose supplementation does accelerate ATP resynthesis, but this has seldom been associated with improved performance.[160–166] However, a few studies have demonstrated positive effects of ribose ingestion on performance. For example, Witter et al.[167] and Gallagher et al.[168] compared the effects of 10 g of ribose per day versus placebo on cycling performance in a group of college-aged men. They reported greater gains after ribose supplementation for mean power output over 5 days of training and greater peak power at the last training session than the placebo group. In another study, strength and endurance were measured in male bodybuilders supplementing with 10 g per day over a 4-week period. The ribose group experienced significant increases in the number of bench press repetitions to failure, in addition to improvements in maximal strength.[169]

Additional long-term studies are warranted before a more conclusive use of ribose in sport-specific activities is suggested. Therefore, based on the absence of exercise benefits indicated by the majority of studies, no recommend dose for ribose supplementation can be made to enhance performance.[169]

13. Taurine

Taurine is the most abundant free amino acid in excitable tissues, such as muscle, heart, and brain.[170] Although taurine is classified as a non-essential amino acid, it plays a fundamental role in several physiological functions within the body, in particular modulation of neurotransmission, cell-volume regulation, cell-membrane stabilization, adipose-tissue regulation, and calcium homeostasis.[171–176] In addition to regulating physiological phenomena, taurine has been proposed to improve time to exhaustion, reduce exercise-induced injury, decrease oxidative stress, and regulate core body temperature,[177–179] which may translate into augmented performance. Furthermore, it is considered a *conditionally* essential amino acid, meaning that under certain conditions, such as intense training, the body cannot synthesize adequate amounts, suggesting the importance of taurine supplementation.

Studies have reported that intramuscular taurine concentrations decrease as a result of exhaustive high-intensity exercise lasting 30, 60, or 100 minutes, and the deficit is particularly pronounced in fast-twitch muscle fibers.[178,180,181] Notably, Zhang and colleagues demonstrated an increase in performance following 1 week of taurine supplementation. When their healthy young subject population supplemented taurine for 1 week prior to an exhaustive exercise bout, taurine significantly improved exercise time to exhaustion, maximal oxygen consumption, and maximal workload achieved.[177] Also, due to the influence of taurine on regulation of core body temperature, its use may reduce athletes' risk of heat stress and heat stroke.[179] Based on the current research, recommendations consist of 100–500 mg per kg body weight per day consumed prior to meals and/or glucose-containing solutions.

C. Limited to No Human Research to Support Use

1. Adenosine Triphosphate (ATP)

ATP, an essential source of energy for numerous cellular processes, is fundamental for the transfer of energy. ATP is hydrolyzed to adenosine diphosphate (ADP) and inorganic phosphate (P_i), where the P_i bond is split, releasing chemical energy, and initiating physiological processes.[182] During physical activity, energy from ATP is released during muscle contraction but is limited by the body's capabilities for resynthesis.[183] Furthermore, supplementing with ATP may influence available concentrations for energy, resulting in an improvement in performance. However, the influence of ATP supplementation on performance is limited and uncertain. One study investigated the effects of 150 or 225 mg ATP supplementation over a 14-day period on aerobic and anaerobic performance.[184] There were no reported changes in whole blood concentrations of ATP immediately after supplementation or at 14 days post-supplementation. Furthermore, ATP supplementation did not alter bench press strength or endurance, or peak power or total work during repeated Wingate tests. The researchers did, however, note improvements in the number of repetitions to fatigue at 1RM and total lifting volume after 14 days of 225 mg ATP supplementation. Herda and colleagues[185] examined the acute effects of a supplement intended to improve ATP concentrations on performance in college-aged men. Following 7 days of supplementation, there were no observed improvements in vertical jump height, leg strength, leg endurance, or forearm endurance. Due to the lack of research, more data are required before any recommendation can be made for the use of ATP as an efficacious sports supplement.

2. Betaine

A metabolite of choline, and the trimethylated form of glycine, betaine is present in the diet in large concentrations in wheat germ and bran, as well as in sources such as spinach, shrimp, beets, and some wheat products.[186] Betaine's two primary functions in the body are as a methyl donor and an osmolyte, a compound that maintains normal cell volume. As an osmolyte, betaine protects cells, proteins, and enzymes from heat, dehydration, and other environmental and physiological stresses. As a methyl donor, betaine is used to convert homocysteine to L-methionine and is, therefore, also a precursor to creatine and S-adenosylmethionine (SAMe), which has been used as a dietary supplement for bone and joint health, as well as mood regulation. In healthy adults, 6 weeks of betaine supplementation at 1.5, 3, and 6 g per day was shown to decrease levels of homocysteine, an indicator of heart and blood vessel disease, in a dose-dependent manner.[187] In another study, 6 g per day of betaine for 12 weeks provided to 42 obese men and women resulted in a significant reduction in homocysteine levels; however, no changes in body composition, body weight, or resting energy expenditure occurred.[188]

Data to substantiate a sports enhancing effect is limited; two studies, currently available only as abstracts, provide evidence that when betaine was co-ingested with a carbohydrate and electrolyte beverage during and after exercise in hot climates, sprint time to exhaustion, as well as anaerobic and aerobic metabolism, improved.[189,190] Based on available science, the recommendation is to supplement 600 mg–6 g per day consumed with meals or immediately post-exercise with recovery drink.

3. Choline

Choline is considered an essential nutrient and is required for the synthesis of cell membrane phospholipids, betaine, and the neurotransmitter acetylcholine. Choline plays a key role in neuromuscular function, as well as in cell structure integrity and fat metabolism. It can be found in high concentrations in a variety of foods, the two most common of which are eggs and soy lecithin.[191,192] While choline is essential for many biological functions, studies have demonstrated that choline levels can decrease significantly as a result of strenuous exercise and that supplementation with choline may significantly increase choline availability; however, supplementation has shown no effect on endurance performance.[193–196] Although there have been no reports of improvements in performance following choline supplementation, all available studies have used only an acute dose immediately before or no more than 1 day before competition, in highly trained indvidiuals. Thus, we cannot completely dismiss its use. Based on available science, 300 mg–1.2 g per day of choline supplementation is recommended, in the form of choline bitartrate or choline citrate, consumed in divided doses, with meals or pre-exercise.

4. Chromium

Chromium is an essential trace mineral found in small amounts in the typical American diet. As a cofactor for insulin, chromium may amplify insulin's effects on the transport of glucose, amino acids, and fatty acids into the cell. This enhanced transport could possibly boost the anabolic effects of insulin by increasing protein and glycogen synthesis in the muscle cell.[197] While chromium is essential, it would appear that most, if not all, Americans consuming a sufficient number of calories obtain enough chromium from diet alone.[198,199] However, athletes who are on a low-calorie diet and in intense training for an extended period may consider adding supplemental chromium to their diet. It is also important to note that chromium supplementation serves as a preventive method for chromium depletion. In such cases, the data suggest improvements in strength and glycogen synthesis are limited, however, more research is needed. The current recommended intake of chromium is 50–200 mcg per day.

5. Citrulline Malate

Citrulline is a non-essential amino acid that is vital for the synthesis of arginine and nitric oxide. Research suggests that citrulline may increase lactate reabsorption, and more importantly, ATP resynthesis.[200] The potential result of citrulline's action is enhanced exercise performance as a consequence of delayed fatigue. In the majority of the existing research, citrulline was administered in the form of citrulline malate (L-citrulline-DL-malate). Moreover, researchers noted that the combination of citrulline malate was significantly more effective for increasing ATP resynthesis than either compound given independently.[200] In a later "exercise"-specific study of the effects of 6 g per day for 15 days on finger flexion, orally consumed citrulline malate was given to 18 men. The results showed that ATP production during exercise increased by 34%, and phosphocreatine resynthesis after exercise improved by 20%.[4] Concerning the synergistic effect of the combination of citrulline and malate, scientists have proposed that citrulline preferentially increases lactate re-absorption, while DL-malate facilitates ATP resynthesis via its role in the TCA cycle, a part of the aerobic metabolic pathway. Based on limited research, in order to delay muscle fatigue by increasing ATP resynthesis and lactate re-absorption, 6 g per day as citrulline malate (53.9% L-citrulline; 46.1% DL-malate) is suggested.

6. Conjugated Linoleic Acid (CLA)

CLA is a naturally occurring free fatty acid that is found in meat and dairy products such as beef, turkey, milk, and cheese. The use of CLA is widely promoted as an aid to reduce body fat. However, in humans, the effects of CLA supplementation on body composition and exercise performance have been highly inconclusive. For example, Lambert et al.[201] demonstrated no effect of 3.9 g CLA per day for 12 weeks on body composition, resting metabolic rate, resting energy expenditure, or appetite in 62 healthy women. However, the effects of chronic CLA supplementation (3.4 g per day for 6 and 24 months) in overweight and obese participants have been more notable, resulting in improvements in total and regional decreases in body fat.[202–204] Due to the minimally available data in healthy, normal-weight individuals, no recommended dose can be suggested.

7. D-Pinitol

D-pinitol is found in rich concentrations in various legumes, fruits, pine tree components, and other botanicals. Chemically similar to the sugar-like compound inositol, it appears to stimulate glucose uptake and, thus, may reduce blood glucose. D-pinitol is most effective at decreasing blood glucose when consumed either in the absence of glucose or prior to a glucose-containing drink.[205–207] For this reason, D-pinitol has become popular with bodybuilders, fitness enthusiasts, and athletes attempting to promote muscle cell loading and recovery. It is quite expensive, and its value in exercise performance enhancement is still inconclusive. However, the available data involving supplementation and D-pinitol's insulin-mimetic effects in the absence of glucose do present a host of sports-specific applications if validated. The current data suggest that consuming 600 mg immediately before a high-carbohydrate recovery drink after an intense, high-volume workout, may allow the recovery process, namely the rebuilding of glycogen stores, to proceed more rapidly and to a greater extent. However, no data supports this hypothesis.

8. Ecdysterone

Ecdysterone is an ecdysteroid, or insect hormone, that is also present in most plant species. In 1976, Russian researchers reported that ecdysterone significantly increased body weight and protein content in muscle and other organs in rats that had received 0.5 mg per 100 g of body weight per day for 7 days. The effect appeared to be present in younger, growing rats, and it was noted that the increased anabolism was not due to the same pathway as the male hormone testosterone.[208] The results of several Eastern European studies support the beneficial effects of ecdysterone consumption when combined with protein in endurance and strength-trained athletes. After 3 weeks of supplementation, they reported an increase in muscle mass and total work performance during exercise testing, as well as a reduction in body fat. However, most of these studies are in Russian, and English translations of the full texts are not available.[209–215] Despite these limitations in translation, pure ecdysterone may have enough supporting data to justify its use in sports. Based on the available data, 0.5–10 mg per kg body weight per day of ecdysterone (as 20-hydroxyecdysone) consumed in equally divided doses, with protein, or immediately post-workout with protein has been recommended.

9. Glutamine

Glutamine is the most prevalent free amino acid in plasma and among the most prevalent in muscle. It acts as a substrate for gluconeogenesis, an oxidative energy source in growing or regenerating tissue, and is involved in the regulation of muscle protein synthesis, protein degradation in skeletal muscle and liver glycogen synthesis.[216] It is considered to be a *conditionally essential* nutrient needed in the diet under certain catabolic conditions. Glutamine was reclassified as such when patients receiving standard parenteral nutrition consistently became glutamine depleted.[217] Decreases in glutamine concentrations have also been commonly associated with overtraining syndrome or very high-intensity training regimens in generally healthy populations.[218]

Most studies of glutamine supplementation have demonstrated little to no benefit on exercise performance or body composition. However, some research has reported success in using glutamine as an energy recovery aid to boost glycogen resynthesis after exhaustive exercise.[219,220] Interestingly, data also demonstrated that glutamine plus a carbohydrate beverage provided no additional effect on muscle glycogen over glutamine alone, but did increase whole body glycogen resynthesis in the liver. In addition, glutamine alone did not raise insulin, whereas insulin increased significantly with the ingestion of the carbohydrate-containing drink.[220] This effect may be of value to athletes who seek recovery between workouts but are trying to lose weight and avoid extra calories. However, this theory needs to be examined more closely. It should be stressed that claims that glutamine reduces protein breakdown and supports immune function, which originated largely from research conducted in ill or injured people, are somewhat misleading. Several independent reviews of the literature have all come to much the same conclusion:

glutamine supplementation is required to be very high (at least 20 g per day) and in sustained doses (consumed immediately upon injury and continuously thereafter) to be effective in influencing net protein balance and immune function.[221–224] Based on the available science, to augment glycogen resynthesis a recommended dose of 8 g of glutamine should be consumed immediately post-exercise. For anti-catabolic and general use, 20 g per day or more should be consumed immediately post-exercise or in divided doses.

10. Hydroxycitric Acid (HCA)

HCA is extracted from the dried fruit rind of *Garcinia cambogia*, which grows in west and central Africa and Southeast Asia. HCA has a chemical structure similar to that of citric acid and has been suggested to potentially promote the utilization of fat for energy and contribute to the inhibition of lipogenesis by competing with the enzyme ATP-citratelyase. Anecdotal reports suggest that HCA supplementation may cause weight loss in humans without the central nervous system stimulatory effect that occurs with most weight reduction supplements. However, the majority of studies across athletic and non-athletic populations have found that supplementing HCA alone was not significantly better than ingesting a placebo in terms of fat oxidation, satiety, energy expenditure, or weight loss.[225–227] In one study, although not significant, a greater number of the people in the HCA group lost weight compared with the placebo group. The authors suggest that this could have resulted from a decrease in appetite due to a potential satiety effect of HCA.[228–232] Several Japanese studies also offer support for HCA's role in glycogen sparing and fat oxidation.[233–235] Perhaps in conjunction with exercise and diet, HCA may help control appetite and allow people to lose a significant amount of weight. Based on available data, the recommended dosages range from 750–2800 mg per day.

11. Octacosanol

A waxy plant extract found in wheat germ oil and sugar cane, octacosanol is a nutraceutical that has received attention for its potential role in muscle and strength development by acting on nervous tissue. Theoretically, if supplementation of octocosanol exerts a positive influence on the efficiency of the nervous system, it may facilitate speed and strength production, as well as influence the growth response in skeletal muscle by activating more muscle fibers during athletic movements. In one study, when 16 subjects were supplemented with 1 mg of octacosanol for 8 weeks, they experienced improved reaction time to visual stimuli, as well as a significant increase in grip strength.[236] To date, other human studies involving octacosanol as an ergogenic aid have exhibited severe design flaws and cannot provide conclusive evidence for its use. Limited data suggest that 1 mg per day may improve exercise performance; however, more recent, controlled research is needed to validate these results.

12. Pyruvate

Pyruvate is a three-carbon ketoacid product of glucose metabolism. During longer-duration, lower-intensity exercise, pyruvate is primarily utilized aerobically to make copious amounts of energy; whereas, during higher-intensity exercise, pyruvate is used mostly anaerobically to make energy very rapidly but is accompanied by the accumulation of lactic acid and hydrogen ions and subsequent fatigue after as little as 15 seconds. Researchers hypothesize that supplementing pyruvate may help the aerobic system operate more efficiently, improve endurance capacity, and reduce premature fatigue.[237] Two studies reported an 80% improvement in endurance capacity in trained men, reflected in their ability to run longer, when they supplemented 25 g per day of pyruvate for a week.[238,239] These studies were criticized on the basis that the tremendously high dose of pyruvate supplemented would not be affordable and may not be safe over the long term. As a result, other investigators tested the effect of 7–8 g per day in trained and untrained men for 1 to 2 weeks, yet they found no effect on endurance performance.[240,241] Two other studies examining the ergogenic potential of lower doses of pyruvate also found pyruvate supplementation to have no significant effect on exercise performance or body composition in untrained adults or football players, respectively.[242,243] In general, unless athletes supplement with a very costly 25 g per day of pyruvate, endurance performance benefits are unlikely.

13. Tribulus

Supplemental tribulus is derived from *Tribulus terrestris*, a groundcover plant widespread throughout many of the world's warm temperate and tropical climates. Bodybuilders have long used tribulus with the goal of increasing testosterone, strength, and muscularity, but thus far, the clinical data in humans is limited and not positive. Research in humans has demonstrated tribulus to be ineffective for resistance-trained males who consumed a daily dose 3.21 mg per kg of body weight or 450 mg for 5 to 8 weeks. Tribulus was found to offer no performance-enhancing or physique-altering benefit compared with placebo.[244,245] However, research in rats suggests that, to observe any benefits, the amount and purity of tribulus's active component, protodioscin, is critical.[246] While no research in humans has substantiated the benefits seen in rat studies, data in rats suggest that a much higher dose of 5–10 mg per kg body weight per day of active protodioscin (from *Tribulus terrestris*) be consumed in divided doses with meals or as a single dose immediately prior to exercise to potentially see any hormonal or performance benefits. However, based on available science, Tribulus is not recommended at this time.

14. Tyrosine

Tyrosine is a conditionally essential amino acid that is naturally produced in the body under normal conditions but may not be synthesized in adequate quantities under stressful conditions, such as disease states or intense exercise training. Tyrosine is a well-documented precursor to the thyroid hormone thyramine, and plays a critical role in the production of the skin pigment melanin and in the release of luteinizing hormone, which is instrumental to reproductive system function.[247] Tyrosine's primary function in the body is to serve as the direct precursor to the synthesis of catecholamines, including dopamine (DA), epinephrine (E), and norepinephrine (NE). Considering its direct involvement in the sympathetic nervous system's stimulation of the "fight or flight" response and hormone release from the adrenal glands, tyrosine supplementation may improve both endurance and anaerobic performance by increasing NE and DA release. However, recent studies have demonstrated no performance enhancement from tyrosine supplementation prior to high-intensity exercise.[248,249] Interestingly, in sleep-deprived subjects, 150 mg per kg body weight of tyrosine improved memory, reasoning ability, mathematical processing, tracking, and visual vigilance in comparison with the known stimulants, D-amphetamine, phentermine, and high-dose caffeine (approximately 300 mg).[250] Researchers also reported that a dose of 150 mg per kg body weight of tyrosine, when provided to sleep-deprived subjects, reduced the typical psychomotor performance declines associated with mental fatigue.[251] Along these lines, tyrosine supplementation could potentially improve performance in sleep-deprived athletes. Data have also supported the ergogenic potential of tyrosine for use in extreme temperature conditions. Mahoney et al.[252] exposed human subjects to water immersion testing at various temperatures and found that tyrosine supplementation helped to alleviate memory decrements associated with acute cold exposure. While data is limited in humans, the recommendation consists of 50–150 mg of tyrosine per kg body weight consumed on an empty stomach, approximately 60–90 minutes prior to exercise.

15. Yohimbine

Yohimbe, an herbal extract from the bark of the African evergreen tree *Pausinystalia yohimbe*, contains the active ingredient yohimbine, an alpha-antagonist, or a substance capable of blocking alpha-adrenergic receptors. Adipocytes, or fat cells, have both alpha- and beta-adrenergic receptors, which trigger different functions. Stimulation of the alpha-receptors signals the cells to start storing more fat. However, when these receptors are blocked (i.e., by alpha-antagonists such as yohimbine), the fat storage process is averted. Some researchers suggest that supplementing yohimbine, in combination with exercise, can maximize fat loss by increasing lipolysis.[253] Exercise stimulates beta-receptors on fat cells, resulting in fat being released and used for energy, and supplemental yohimbine, through its actions on alpha-receptors, may block the normal resynthesis of fat during recovery. Research has demonstrated that supplementation of yohimbine in adults significantly elevated blood markers of fat metabolism and was further enhanced with the addition of exercise.[254] In one study, highly trained men who supplemented 10 mg of yohimbine twice a day for 3 weeks experienced significantly greater fat loss than the placebo group.[255] However, because alpha-receptors are present in the heart, arteries, and lungs, in addition to fat tissue, many side effects of yohimbine use may occur. Some of the most common side effects are feelings of panic, clumsiness, and confusion.[256] Based on the available research, the current recommendations are 0.2 mg per kg of body weight per day in two equally divided doses.

III. SUMMARY AND CONCLUSIONS

The field of sports nutrition is rapidly advancing, with new research providing evidence in support of, or contesting the use of, supplements to augment performance (see Table 9.2). Concomitantly, the use of supplements in athletics and performance has increased considerably in efforts to enhance training, strength adaptations, recovery, metabolism, and hydration, as well as to reduce fatigue and deter injury. While many advantageous supplements exist, an equal number of ineffective aids persist, many of which are highly marketed, leaving consumers with uncertainty and a cause for possible harm. This chapter outlines the more widely used supplements, evaluating the available human-related evidence and the true performance and physiological effects that may be observed. Guidelines for rational use are profiled throughout the chapter and illustrated in Table 9.3.

TABLE 9.2
National Collegiate Athletic Association—List of Banned Substances—2007–2008

Stimulants	
Amiphenazole	Diethylpropion
Amphetamine	Dimethylamphetamine
Bemigride	Doxapram
Benzphetamine	Ephedrine (ephedra, mahuang)
Bromantan	Ethamivan
Caffeine (>15 μl mL concentration in urine)	Ethylamphetamine
Chlorphentermine	Fencamfamine
Cocaine	Meclofenoxate
Cropropamide	Methamphetamine
Crothetamide	Methylenedioxymethamphetamine
Diethylpropion	Methylphenidate
Dimethylamphetamine	Nikethamide
Anabolic Agents	
Androstenediol	Dehydrocholrmethyl-testosterone
Androstenedione	Dehydroep oxymesterone
Boldenone	Dihydrotestosterone (DIH)
Colstebol	

(Continued)

TABLE 9.2 (CONTINUED)
National Collegiate Athletic Association—List of Banned Substances—2007–2008

Anabolic Agents	
Dromostanolone	Norethandrolone
Epitrenbolone	Oxandrolone
Fluoxymesterone	Oxymetholone
Gestrinone	Stanozolol
Mesterolone	Testosterone
Methandienone	Tetrahydrogestrinone (THG)
Methyltestosterone	Trenbolone
Nandrolone	
Norandrostenediol	
Norandrostenedione	
Diuretics and Other Urine Manipulators	
Acetazolamide	Furosemide
Bendroflumethiazide	Hydrochlorothiazide
Benzhiazide	Hydroflumethiazide
Bumetanide	Methylclothiazide
Chlorothiazide	Metolazone
Chlorthalidone	Polythiazide
Ethacrynic acid	Probenecid
Finasteride	Triamterene
Flumethiazide	Trichlormethiazide
Street Drugs	
Heroin	
Marijuana (concentration in urine in THC metabolite >15 ng/mL)	
Tetrahydrocannabinol (THC; concentration in urine of THC metabolite >15 mg/mL)	
Peptide Hormones and Analogs	
Corticotrophin (ACTH)	
Growth hormone (HGH, somatotrophin)	
Human chorionic gonadotrophin (HCG)	
Insulin-like growth factor (IGF-1)	
Luteinizing hormone (LH)	
Releasing factors that are also banned: darbepoetin, erythropoietin (EPO) & sermorelin.	
Anti-Estrogens	
Anastrozole	
Clomiphene	
Tamoxifen	

TABLE 9.3
Guidelines for Use

Common Name	Recommended Use(s)	Recommended Dose(s)	Pre-Exercise	During Exercise	Post-Exercise	Other	Special Notes
Adenosine triphosphate	n/a	n/a					Insufficient data
Alpha-ketoglutarate	Anti-catabolic	13.905 mg/kg b.w. –0.28 g/kg/d b.w.	✓		✓	✓-with meals	Consume with glucose and vitamin B6
Alpha-ketoisocaproate	Exercise recovery muscle buffer	1.5 g/d–20 g/d			✓	✓-with meals	>10 g/d may cause gastrointestinal stress
Alpha-lipoic acid	Anti-oxidant insulin mimetic	300 mg/d–1 g/d as R-ALA			✓	✓-between or with meals	Consume with or in the absense of glucose
Beta-alanine	Proton buffering anti-oxidant	3.2 g/d–6.4 g/d	✓				Consume on an empty stomach
Betaine	Protein utilization cell maintenance	600 mg/serving–6 g/d			✓	✓-with meals	Consume with meals and protein
Beta-hydroxy-beta-methylbutyrate	Anti-catabolic increased muscle strenqth	3 g/d–6 g/d	✓		✓		Only applies to previously untrained and/or elderly athletes
Branched chain amino acids	Anabolic anti-catabolic glycogen resynthesis recovery	9 g/d–20 g/d	✓	✓	✓	✓-with meals	Consume as 45%:25%:30% ratio of Leu:Iso:Val
Caffeine	Simulant glycogen sparing	3 mg/kg b.w.–6 mg/kg b.w.	✓				

Choline	Cell structure neuromuscular function	300 mg/d–1.2 g/d as Choline Bitartrate or Choline Citrate	✓			✓-with meals	May be substituted with 3 g/d–9 g/d Phosphotidylcholine (PC)
Chromium	Glucose transport	50 mcg/d–200 mcg/d	✓				
Citrulline	Delay muscle fatigue increase ATP resynthesis	6 g/d as Citrulline Malate	✓	✓		✓-between or with meals	Consume as 53.9% L-Citrulline and 46.1% DL-Malate
Colostrum	Protein synthesis anti-catabolic	20 g/d–60 g/d	✓	✓	✓	✓-with high quality protein	Consume with protein
Conjugated linoleic acid	n/a	n/a					Insufficient data
Creatine	Increase energy increase strength	0.3 g/kg b.w. for 3 days followed by 3–5 g/d	✓				
D-pinitol	Glucose disposal glycogen resynthesis	200 mg/dose–600 mg/dose	✓		✓	✓-prior to meals	
Dehydroepiandrosterone (DHEA)	Increase testosterone increase strength	100 mg/d	✓				Applies primarily to elderly men and women
Ecdysterone	Protein synthesis	0.5 mg/kg/d b.w.–10 mg/kg/d b.w. as 20-Hydroxyecdysone			✓	✓-with meals	Consume with protein
Essential amino acids	Protein synthesis exercise recovery	3 g/d–40 g/d	✓		✓	✓-between or with meals	Consume on an empty stomach or in combination with CHO
Gamma-aminobutyric acid	Increase GH blood pressure reduction reduce feelings of fatigue	5/g–10 g/d				✓-1 hr prior to bedtime	Consume on an empty stomach

(*Continued*)

TABLE 9.3 (CONTINUED)
Guidelines for Use

Common Name	Recommended Use(s)	Recommended Dose(s)	Pre-Exercise	During Exercise	Post-Exercise	Other	Special Notes
Ginseng	Stimulant Increase Energy Glucose Disposal Reduce Muscle Damage	200 mg/d as *Panax ginseng* root (standardized to ≥4% total ginsenosides, and ≥1.5% total ginsenosides as Rg1) 1 g/d–3 g/d as *Panax quinquefolius* root (standardized to ≥3.21% total ginsenosides, and ≥1.5% total ginsenosides as Rb1)	✓		✓	✓-prior to meals and/or glucose	
Glutamine	Anti-Catabolic Glycogen Resynthesis	8 g/dose ≥20 g/d			✓	✓-between meals	>20 g/d for anti-catabolic effect
Glycerol	Endurance Performance Hydration Heat Tolerance	1 g:20 mL–1.2 g:25 mL, per kg b.w. (as Glycerol:6% CHO-containing fluid)	✓	✓	✓		Consume slowly
Hydroxycitrate	Fat Oxidation	750 mg–2800 mg/d	✓				
Ipriflavone	Bone Support	600 mg/d			✓	✓-with meals	Consume with food
N-acetylcysteine	Endurance Performance Delay Muscle Fatigue Vasodilation Anti-Oxidant General Use	600 mg/d–4 g/d	✓		✓	✓-with meals	Consume with food

Octacosanol	n/a	n/a					Insufficient data
Pyruvate	Endurance performance	7 g/d–25 g/d					
Rhodiola	Neurostimulant adaptogen anti-Inflammatory	100 mg/d–1,800 mg/d as *Rhodiola rosea* root (standardized to ≥3.6 mg/d-64.8 mg/d rosavin, respectively)	✓			✓-between meals	Consume on an empty stomach
Ribose	n/a	n/a					Insufficient data
Sodium bicarbonate	Delay anaerobic muscle fatigue	300 mg/kg/d b.w.	✓				Dilute in 1 L of water
Sodium citrate	Delay anaerobic muscle fatigue	0.4 g/kg b.w–0.5 g/kg b.w.	✓				
Taurine	Glucose disposal anti-oxidant cellular function regulate body temperature	100 mg/kg/d b.w– 500 mg/kg/d b.w.	✓		✓	✓-prior to meals and/ or glucose	Consume on an empty stomach, prior to glucose
Tribulus	Increase strength increase testosterone	5 mg/kg/d b.w.–10 mg/ kg/d b.w. Protodioscin active (from *Tribulus terrestris* above ground parts)	✓			✓-with meals	
Tyrosine	Stimulant mental acuity energy	50 mg/kg/d b.w.– 150 mg/kg/d b.w.	✓			✓-immediately upon waking in the morning	Consume on an empty stomach w/ more potent catecholaminergic agonist(s); do not consume with BCAAs or glucosa
Yohimbine	Fat metabolism	0.2 mg/kg/d b.w.	✓				

REFERENCES

1. Dunnett M and Harris RC: Influence of oral beta-alanine and L-histidine supplementation on the carnosine content of the gluteus medius. *Equine Vet J Suppl* 30: 499–504, 1999.
2. Hill CA, Harris RC, Kim HJ, Harris BD, Sale C, Boobis LH, et al.: Influence of beta-alanine supplementation on skeletal muscle carnosine concentrations and high intensity cycling capacity. *Amino Acids* 32: 225–33, 2007.
3. Harris RC, Tallon MJ, Dunnett M, Boobis L, Coakley J, Kim HJ, et al: The absorption of orally supplied beta-alanine and its effect on muscle carnosine synthesis in human vastus lateralis. *Amino Acids* 30: 279–89, 2006.
4. Bendahan D, Mattei JP, Ghattas B, Confort-Gouny S, Le Guern ME and Cozzone PJ: Citrulline/malate promotes aerobic energy production in human exercising muscle. *Br J Sports Med* 36: 282–9, 2002.
5. Kim HJ, Cho J, Kim CK, Harris RC, Harris BD, Sale C and Wise JA: Effect on muscle fibre morphology and carnosine content after 12 days training of Korean speed skaters. *Med Sci Sports Exerc* 37: S192, 2005.
6. Suzuki Y, Ito O, Takahashi H and Takamatsu K: The effect of sprint training on skeletal muscle carnosine in humans. *Int J Sport Health Sci* 2: 105–110, 2004.
7. Harris RC, Edge J, Kendrick IP, Bishop D, Goodman C and Wise JA: The effect of very high interval training on the carnosine content and buffering capacity of V. lateralis from humans. In: *Experimental Biology*. Washington D.C., 2007.
8. Kim HJ, Kim CK, Lee YW, Harris RC, Sale C, Harris BD and Wise JA: The effect of a supplement containing B-alanine on muscle carnosine synthesis and exercise capacity, during 12 weeks combined endurance and weight training. *J Int Soc Sports Nutr* 3: S9, 2006.
9. Harris RC, Kendrick IP, Kim CK, Hyojeong K, Dang VH, Lam TQ, et al.: The effect of physical training on the carnosine content of V Lateralis using a one-leg training model. In: Abstract presented at the American College of Sports Medicine. Washington D.C., 2007.
10. Suzuki Y, Ito O, Mukai N, Takahashi H and Takamatsu K: High level of skeletal muscle carnosine contributes to the latter half of exercise performance during 30-s maximal cycle ergometer sprinting. *Jpn J Physiol* 52: 199–205, 2002.
11. Derave W, Ozdemir MS, Harris RC, Pottier A, Reyngoudt H, Koppo K, et al.: Beta-alanine supplementation augments muscle carnosine content and attenuates fatigue during repeated isokinetic contraction bouts in trained sprinters. *J Appl Physiol* 103: 1736–43, 2007.
12. Kim CK, Kim HJ, Lee YW, Harris RC, Sale C, Harris BD and Wise JA: Combined training and B-alanine supplementation: Muscle carnosine synthesis, ventilatory threshold and exercise capacity in cyclists. *Med Sci Sports Exerc* 39: 5364, 2007.
13. Stout JR, Cramer JT, Mielke M, O'Kroy J, Torok DJ and Zoeller RF: Effects of twenty-eight days of beta-alanine and creatine monohydrate supplementation on the physical working capacity at neuromuscular fatigue threshold. *J Strength Cond Res* 20: 928–31, 2006.
14. Stout JR, Cramer JT, Zoeller RF, Torok D, Costa P, Hoffman JR, et al.: Effects of beta-alanine supplementation on the onset of neuromuscular fatigue and ventilatory threshold in women. *Amino Acids* 32: 381–6, 2007.
15. Nissen SL, and Sharp RL: Effect of dietary supplements on lean mass and strength gains with resistance exercise: A meta-analysis. *J Appl Physiol* 94: 651–9, 2003.

16. Panton LB, Rathmacher JA, Baier S, Nissen S: Nutritional supplementation of the leucine metabolite beta-hydroxy-beta-methylbutyrate (hmb) during resistance training. *Nutrition* 16: 734–9, 2000.
17. Lamboley CR, Royer D, and Dionne IJ: Effects of beta-hydroxy-beta-methylbutyrate on aerobic-performance components and body composition in college students. *Int J Sport Nutr Exerc Metab* 17: 56–69, 2007.
18. Kreider RB, Ferreira M, Wilson M, and Almada AL: Effects of calcium beta-hydroxy-beta-methylbutyrate (HMB) supplementation during resistance-training on markers of catabolism, body composition and strength. *Int J Sports Med* 20: 503–9, 1999.
19. Doherty M, and Smith PM: Effects of caffeine ingestion on rating of perceived exertion during and after exercise: A meta-analysis. *Scand J Med Sci Sports* 15: 69–78, 2005.
20. Keisler BD, and Armsey TD, 2nd: Caffeine as an ergogenic aid. *Curr Sports Med Rep* 5: 215–9, 2006.
21. Costill DL, Dalsky GP, and Fink WJ: Effects of caffeine ingestion on metabolism and exercise performance. *Med Sci Sports* 10: 155–8, 1978.
22. Erickson MA, Schwarzkopf RJ, and McKenzie RD: Effects of caffeine, fructose, and glucose ingestion on muscle glycogen utilization during exercise. *Med Sci Sports Exerc* 19: 579–83, 1987.
23. Spriet LL, MacLean DA, Dyck DJ, Hultman E, Cederblad G, and Graham TE: Caffeine ingestion and muscle metabolism during prolonged exercise in humans. *Am J Physiol* 262: E891–8, 1992.
24. Schneiker KT, Bishop D, Dawson B, and Hackett LP: Effects of caffeine on prolonged intermittent-sprint ability in team-sport athletes. *Med Sci Sports Exerc* 38: 578–85, 2006.
25. Kalmar JM, and Cafarelli E: Effects of caffeine on neuromuscular function. *J Appl Physiol* 87: 801–8, 1999.
26. Collomp K, Ahmaidi S, Audran M, Chanal JL, and Prefaut C: Effects of caffeine ingestion on performance and anaerobic metabolism during the Wingate Test. *Int J Sports Med* 12: 439–43, 1991.
27. Greer F, McLean C, and Graham TE: Caffeine, performance, and metabolism during repeated Wingate exercise tests. *J Appl Physiol* 85: 1502–8, 1998.
28. Anselme F, Collomp K, Mercier B, Ahmaidi S, and Prefaut C: Caffeine increases maximal anaerobic power and blood lactate concentration. *Eur J Appl Physiol Occup Physiol* 65: 188–91, 1992.
29. Wiles JD, Coleman D, Tegerdine M, and Swaine IL: The effects of caffeine ingestion on performance time, speed and power during a laboratory-based 1 km cycling time-trial. *J Sports Sci* 24: 1165–71, 2006.
30. Beck TW, Housh TJ, Schmidt RJ, Johnson GO, Housh DJ, Coburn JW and Malek MH: The acute effects of a caffeine-containing supplement on strength, muscular endurance, and anaerobic capabilities. *J Strength Cond Res* 20: 506–10, 2006.
31. Stout JR, Antonio J, and Kalman D: *Essentials of Creatine in Sports and Health.* Humana Press, Totowa, NJ, 2007.
32. Buford TW, Kreider RB, Stout JR, Greenwood M, Campbell B, Spano M, et al.: International society of sports nutrition position stand: Creatine supplementation and exercise. *J Int Soc Sports Nutr* 4: 2007.
33. Demant TW and Rhodes EC: Effects of creatine supplementation on exercise performance. *Sports Med* 28: 49–60, 1999.
34. Arciero PJ, Hannibal NS, 3rd, Nindl BC, Gentile CL, Hamed J and Vukovich MD: Comparison of creatine ingestion and resistance training on energy expenditure and limb blood flow. *Metabolism* 50: 1429–34, 2001.

35. Volek JS, Kraemer WJ, Bush JA, Boetes M, Incledon T, Clark KL and Lynch JM: Creatine supplementation enhances muscular performance during high-intensity resistance exercise. *J Am Diet Assoc* 97: 765–70, 1997.
36. Volek JS, Ratamess NA, Rubin MR, Gomez AL, French DN, McGuigan MM, et al.: The effects of creatine supplementation on muscular performance and body composition responses to short-term resistance training overreaching. *Eur J Appl Physiol* 91: 628–37, 2004.
37. Volek JS, and Rawson ES: Scientific basis and practical aspects of creatine supplementation for athletes. *Nutrition* 20: 609–14, 2004.
38. Burke DG, Chilibeck PD, Parise G, Candow DG, Mahoney D and Tarnopolsky M: Effect of creatine and weight training on muscle creatine and performance in vegetarians. *Med Sci Sports Exerc* 35: 1946–55, 2003.
39. Willoughby DS, and Rosene J: Effects of oral creatine and resistance training on myosin heavy chain expression. *Med Sci Sports Exerc* 33: 1674–81, 2001.
40. Haussinger D, Roth E, Lang F, and Gerok W: Cellular hydration state: An important determinant of protein catabolism in health and disease. *Lancet* 341: 1330–2, 1993.
41. Nelson AG, Day R, Glickman-Weiss EL, Hegsted M, Kokkonen J and Sampson B: Creatine supplementation alters the response to a graded cycle ergometer test. *Eur J Appl Physiol* 83: 89–94, 2000.
42. Derave W, Eijnde BO, Verbessem P, Ramaekers M, Van Leemputte M, Richter EA and Hespel P: Combined creatine and protein supplementation in conjunction with resistance training promotes muscle GLUT-4 content and glucose tolerance in humans. *J Appl Physiol* 94: 1910–6, 2003.
43. Tipton KD, Elliott TA, Cree MG, Aarsland AA, Sanford AP, and Wolfe RR: Stimulation of net muscle protein synthesis by whey protein ingestion before and after exercise. *Am J Physiol Endocrinol Metab* 292: E71–6, 2007.
44. Tipton KD, Borsheim E, Wolf SE, Sanford AP, and Wolfe RR: Acute response of net muscle protein balance reflects 24-h balance after exercise and amino acid ingestion. *Am J Physiol Endocrinol Metab* 284: E76–89, 2003.
45. Levenhagen DK, Gresham JD, Carlson MG, Maron DJ, Borel MJ, and Flakoll PJ: Postexercise nutrient intake timing in humans is critical to recovery of leg glucose and protein homeostasis. *Am J Physiol Endocrinol Metab* 280: E982–93, 2001.
46. Miller SL, Tipton KD, Chinkes DL, Wolf SE, and Wolfe RR: Independent and combined effects of amino acids and glucose after resistance exercise. *Med Sci Sports Exerc* 35: 449–55, 2003.
47. Rasmussen BB, Tipton KD, Miller SL, Wolf SE, and Wolfe RR: An oral essential amino acid-carbohydrate supplement enhances muscle protein anabolism after resistance exercise. *J Appl Physiol* 88: 386–92, 2000.
48. Bird SP, Tarpenning KM, and Marino FE: Independent and combined effects of liquid carbohydrate/essential amino acid ingestion on hormonal and muscular adaptations following resistance training in untrained men. *Eur J Appl Physiol* 97: 225–38, 2006.
49. Bird SP, Tarpenning KM, and Marino FE: Liquid carbohydrate/essential amino acid ingestion during a short-term bout of resistance exercise suppresses myofibrillar protein degradation. *Metabolism* 55: 570–7, 2006.
50. Bird SP, Tarpenning KM, and Marino FE: Effects of liquid carbohydrate/essential amino acid ingestion on acute hormonal response during a single bout of resistance exercise in untrained men. *Nutrition* 22: 367–75, 2006.
51. Borsheim E, Tipton KD, Wolf SE, and Wolfe RR: Essential amino acids and muscle protein recovery from resistance exercise. *Am J Physiol Endocrinol Metab* 283: E648–57, 2002.

52. Tipton KD, Ferrando AA, Phillips SM, Doyle D, Jr., and Wolfe RR: Postexercise net protein synthesis in human muscle from orally administered amino acids. *Am J Physiol* 276: E628–34, 1999.
53. Tipton KD, Rasmussen BB, Miller SL, Wolf SE, Owens-Stovall SK, Petrini BE, and Wolfe RR: Timing of amino acid-carbohydrate ingestion alters anabolic response of muscle to resistance exercise. *Am J Physiol Endocrinol Metab* 281: E197–206, 2001.
54. Kooman JP, Deutz NE, Zijlmans P, van den Wall Bake A, Gerlag PG, et al.: The influence of bicarbonate supplementation on plasma levels of branched-chain amino acids in haemodialysis patients with metabolic acidosis. *Nephrol Dial Transplant* 12: 2397–401, 1997.
55. Bird SR, Wiles J, and Robbins J: The effect of sodium bicarbonate ingestion on 1500-m racing time. *J Sports Sci* 13: 399–403, 1995.
56. Kolkhorst FW, Rezende RS, Levy SS, and Buono MJ: Effects of sodium bicarbonate on VO_2 kinetics during heavy exercise. *Med Sci Sports Exerc* 36: 1895–9, 2004.
57. Matson LG, and Tran ZV: Effects of sodium bicarbonate ingestion on anaerobic performance: A meta-analytic review. *Int J Sport Nutr* 3: 2–28, 1993.
58. McNaughton L, and Thompson D: Acute versus chronic sodium bicarbonate ingestion and anaerobic work and power output. *J Sports Med Phys Fitness* 41: 456–62, 2001.
59. Price M, Moss P, and Rance S: Effects of sodium bicarbonate ingestion on prolonged intermittent exercise. *Med Sci Sports Exerc* 35: 1303–8, 2003.
60. Requena B, Zabala M, Padial P, and Feriche B: Sodium bicarbonate and sodium citrate: Ergogenic aids? *J Strength Cond Res* 19: 213–24, 2005.
61. Tiryaki GR, and Atterbom HA: The effects of sodium bicarbonate and sodium citrate on 600 m running time of trained females. *J Sports Med Phys Fitness* 35: 194–8, 1995.
62. Van Montfoort MC, Van Dieren L, Hopkins WG, and Shearman JP: Effects of ingestion of bicarbonate, citrate, lactate, and chloride on sprint running. *Med Sci Sports Exerc* 36: 1239–43, 2004.
63. Verbitsky O, Mizrahi J, Levin M, and Isakov E: Effect of ingested sodium bicarbonate on muscle force, fatigue, and recovery. *J Appl Physiol* 83: 333–7, 1997.
64. Coombes J, and Mc Naughton L: Effects of bicarbonate ingestion on leg strength and power during isokintetic knee flexion and extension. *J Strength Condition Res* 7: 241–49, 1993.
65. Heck KL, Potteiger JA, Nau KL, and Schroeder JM: Sodium bicarbonate ingestion does not attenuate the VO_2 slow component during constant-load exercise. *Int J Sport Nutr* 8: 60–9, 1998.
66. Kozak-Collins K, Burke ER, and Schoene RB: Sodium bicarbonate ingestion does not improve performance in women cyclists. *Med Sci Sports Exerc* 26: 1510–5, 1994.
67. McNaughton L, Dalton B, and Palmer G: Sodium bicarbonate can be used as an ergogenic aid in high-intensity, competitive cycle ergometry of 1 h duration. *Eur J Appl Physiol Occup Physiol* 80: 64–9, 1999.
68. Santalla A, Perez M, Montilla M, Vicente L, Davison R, Earnest C, and Lucia A: Sodium bicarbonate ingestion does not alter the slow component of oxygen uptake kinetics in professional cyclists. *J Sports Sci* 21: 39–47, 2003.
69. Stephens TJ, McKenna MJ, Canny BJ, Snow RJ, and McConell GK: Effect of sodium bicarbonate on muscle metabolism during intense endurance cycling. *Med Sci Sports Exerc* 34: 614–21, 2002.
70. Gaitanos GC, Nevill ME, Brooks S, and Williams C: Repeated bouts of sprint running after induced alkalosis. *J Sports Sci* 9: 355–70, 1991.

71. Gao JP, Costill DL, Horswill CA, and Park SH: Sodium bicarbonate ingestion improves performance in interval swimming. *Eur J Appl Physiol Occup Physiol* 58: 171–4, 1988.
72. Ball D, and Maughan RJ: The effect of sodium citrate ingestion on the metabolic response to intense exercise following diet manipulation in man. *Exp Physiol* 82: 1041–56, 1997.
73. Cox G, and Jenkins DG: The physiological and ventilatory responses to repeated 60 s sprints following sodium citrate ingestion. *J Sports Sci* 12: 469–75, 1994.
74. Parry-Billings M, and MacLaren DP: The effect of sodium bicarbonate and sodium citrate ingestion on anaerobic power during intermittent exercise. *Eur J Appl Physiol Occup Physiol* 55: 524–9, 1986.
75. van Someren K, Fulcher K, McCarthy J, Moore J, Horgan G, and Langford R: An investigation into the effects of sodium citrate ingestion on high-intensity exercise performance. *Int J Sport Nutr* 8: 356–63, 1998.
76. Hausswirth C, Bigard AX, Lepers R, Berthelot M, and Guezennec CY: Sodium citrate ingestion and muscle performance in acute hypobaric hypoxia. *Eur J Appl Physiol Occup Physiol* 71: 362–8, 1995.
77. Kowalchuk JM, Maltais SA, Yamaji K, and Hughson RL: The effect of citrate loading on exercise performance, acid-base balance and metabolism. *Eur J Appl Physiol Occup Physiol* 58: 858–64, 1989.
78. Linossier MT, Dormois D, Bregere P, Geyssant A, and Denis C: Effect of sodium citrate on performance and metabolism of human skeletal muscle during supramaximal cycling exercise. *Eur J Appl Physiol Occup Physiol* 76: 48–54, 1997.
79. McNaughton L, and Cedaro R: Sodium citrate ingestion and its effects on maximal anaerobic exercise of different durations. *Eur J Appl Physiol Occup Physiol* 64: 36–41, 1992.
80. Oopik V, Saaremets I, Medijainen L, Karelson K, Janson T, and Timpmann S: Effects of sodium citrate ingestion before exercise on endurance performance in well trained college runners. *Br J Sports Med* 37: 485–9, 2003.
81. Shave R, Whyte G, Siemann A, and Doggart L: The effects of sodium citrate ingestion on 3,000-meter time-trial performance. *J Strength Cond Res* 15: 230–4, 2001.
82. Blomqvist BI, Hammarqvist F, von der Decken A, and Wernerman J: Glutamine and alpha-ketoglutarate prevent the decrease in muscle free glutamine concentration and influence protein synthesis after total hip replacement. *Metabolism* 44: 1215–22, 1995.
83. Wernerman J, Hammarqvist F, von der Decken A, and Vinnars E: Analogues to glutamine in clinical practice. *Clin Nutr* 9: 41–3, 1990.
84. Marconi C, Sassi G, and Cerretelli P: The effect of an alpha-ketoglutarate-pyridoxine complex on human maximal aerobic and anaerobic performance. *Eur J Appl Physiol Occup Physiol* 49: 307–17, 1982.
85. Barazzoni R, Meek SE, Ekberg K, Wahren J, and Nair KS: Arterial KIC as marker of liver and muscle intracellular leucine pools in healthy and type 1 diabetic humans. *Am J Physiol* 277: E238–44, 1999.
86. Gao Z, Young RA, Li G, Najafi H, Buettger C, Sukumvanich SS, et al.: Distinguishing features of leucine and alpha-ketoisocaproate sensing in pancreatic beta-cells. *Endocrinology* 144: 1949–57, 2003.
87. van Someren KA, Edwards AJ, and Howatson G: Supplementation with beta-hydroxy-beta-methylbutyrate (HMB) and alpha-ketoisocaproic acid (KIC) reduces signs and symptoms of exercise-induced muscle damage in man. *Int J Sport Nutr Exerc Metab* 15: 413–24, 2005.
88. Buckspan R, Hoxworth B, Cersosimo E, Devlin J, Horton E, and Abumrad N: Alpha-Ketoisocaproate is superior to leucine in sparing glucose utilization in humans. *Am J Physiol* 251: E648–53, 1986.

89. Matthews DE, Harkin R, Battezzati A, and Brillon DJ: Splanchnic bed utilization of enteral alpha-ketoisocaproate in humans. *Metabolism* 48: 1555–63, 1999.
90. Yarrow J, et al.: The effects of short-term alpha-ketoisocaproic acid supplementation on exercise performance: A randomized controlled trial. *J Int Soc Sports Nutr* 4: 2007.
91. Marangon K, Devaraj S, Tirosh O, Packer L, and Jialal I: Comparison of the effect of alpha-lipoic acid and alpha-tocopherol supplementation on measures of oxidative stress. *Free Radic Biol Med* 27: 1114–21, 1999.
92. Sen CK, and Packer L: Thiol homeostasis and supplements in physical exercise. *Am J Clin Nutr* 72: 653S–69S, 2000.
93. Burke DG, Chilibeck PD, Parise G, Tarnopolsky MA, and Candow DG: Effect of alpha-lipoic acid combined with creatine monohydrate on human skeletal muscle creatine and phosphagen concentration. *Int J Sport Nutr Exerc Metab* 13: 294–302, 2003.
94. Blomstrand E, Eliasson J, Karlsson HK, and Kohnke R: Branched-chain amino acids activate key enzymes in protein synthesis after physical exercise. *J Nutr* 136: 269S–73S, 2006.
95. Matsumoto K, Mizuno M, Mizuno T, Dilling-Hansen B, Lahoz A, Bertelsen V, et al.: Branched-chain amino acids and arginine supplementation attenuates skeletal muscle proteolysis induced by moderate exercise in young individuals. *Int J Sports Med* 28: 531–8, 2007.
96. Shimomura Y, Yamamoto Y, Bajotto G, Sato J, Murakami T, Shimomura N, et al.: Nutraceutical effects of branched-chain amino acids on skeletal muscle. *J Nutr* 136: 529S–532S, 2006.
97. Blomstrand E: A role for branched-chain amino acids in reducing central fatigue. *J Nutr* 136: 544S–547S, 2006.
98. Mittleman KD, Ricci MR, and Bailey SP: Branched-chain amino acids prolong exercise during heat stress in men and women. *Med Sci Sports Exerc* 30: 83–91, 1998.
99. Blomstrand E, Hassmen P, Ek S, Ekblom B, and Newsholme EA: Influence of ingesting a solution of branched-chain amino acids on perceived exertion during exercise. *Acta Physiol Scand* 159: 41–9, 1997.
100. Struder HK, Hollmann W, Platen P, Donike M, Gotzmann A, and Weber K: Influence of paroxetine, branched-chain amino acids and tyrosine on neuroendocrine system responses and fatigue in humans. *Horm Metab Res* 30: 188–94, 1998.
101. van Hall G, Raaymakers JS, Saris WH, and Wagenmakers AJ: Ingestion of branched-chain amino acids and tryptophan during sustained exercise in man: Failure to affect performance. *J Physiol* 486 (Pt 3): 789–94, 1995.
102. Candeloro N, Bertini I, Melchiorri G, and De Lorenzo A: Effects of prolonged administration of branched-chain amino acids on body composition and physical fitness. *Minerva Endocrinol* 20: 217–23, 1995.
103. Mero A, Miikkulainen H, Riski J, Pakkanen R, Aalto J, and Takala T: Effects of bovine colostrum supplementation on serum IGF-I, IgG, hormone, and saliva IgA during training. *J Appl Physiol* 83: 1144–51, 1997.
104. Kishikawa Y, Watanabe T, Watanabe T, and Kubo S: Purification and characterization of cell growth factor in bovine colostrum. *J Vet Med Sci* 58: 47–53, 1996.
105. Kuhne S, Hammon HM, Bruckmaier RM, Morel C, Zbinden Y, and Blum JW: Growth performance, metabolic and endocrine traits, and absorptive capacity in neonatal calves fed either colostrum or milk replacer at two levels. *J Anim Sci* 78: 609–20, 2000.
106. Buckley JD, Brinkworth GD, and Abbott MJ: Effect of bovine colostrum on anaerobic exercise performance and plasma insulin-like growth factor I. *J Sports Sci* 21: 577–88, 2003.

107. Kern PA, Svoboda ME, Eckel RH, and Van Wyk JJ: Insulinlike growth factor action and production in adipocytes and endothelial cells from human adipose tissue. *Diabetes* 38: 710–7, 1989.
108. Coombes JS, Conacher M, Austen SK, and Marshall PA: Dose effects of oral bovine colostrum on physical work capacity in cyclists. *Med Sci Sports Exerc* 34: 1184–8, 2002.
109. Buckley JD, Abbott MJ, Brinkworth GD, and Whyte PB: Bovine colostrum supplementation during endurance running training improves recovery, but not performance. *J Sci Med Sport* 5: 65–79, 2002.
110. Antonio J, Sanders MS, and Van Gammeren D: The effects of bovine colostrum supplementation on body composition and exercise performance in active men and women. *Nutrition* 17: 243–7, 2001.
111. Buckley JD: Bovine colostrum: Does it improve athletic performance? *Nutrition* 18: 776–7, 2002.
112. Hofman Z, Smeets R, Verlaan G, Lugt R, and Verstappen PA: The effect of bovine colostrum supplementation on exercise performance in elite field hockey players. *Int J Sport Nutr Exerc Metab* 12: 461–9, 2002.
113. Wallace MB, Lim J, Cutler A, and Bucci L: Effects of dehydroepiandrosterone vs androstenedione supplementation in men. *Med Sci Sports Exerc* 31: 1788–92, 1999.
114. Yen SS, Morales AJ, and Khorram O: Replacement of DHEA in aging men and women. Potential remedial effects. *Ann N Y Acad Sci* 774: 128–42, 1995.
115. Villareal DT, and Holloszy JO: DHEA enhances effects of weight training on muscle mass and strength in elderly women and men. *Am J Physiol Endocrinol Metab* 291: E1003–8, 2006.
116. Cavagnini F, Invitti C, Pinto M, Maraschini C, Di Landro A, Dubini A, and Marelli A: Effect of acute and repeated administration of gamma aminobutyric acid (GABA) on growth hormone and prolactin secretion in man. *Acta Endocrinol (Copenh)* 93: 149–54, 1980.
117. Cavagnini F, Benetti G, Invitti C, Ramella G, Pinto M, Lazza M, et al.: Effect of gamma-aminobutyric acid on growth hormone and prolactin secretion in man: Influence of pimozide and domperidone. *J Clin Endocrinol Metab* 51: 789–92, 1980.
118. Cavagnini F, Pinto M, Dubini A, Invitti C, Cappelletti G, and Polli EE: Effects of gamma aminobutyric acid (GABA) and muscimol on endocrine pancreatic function in man. *Metabolism* 31: 73–7, 1982.
119. Tergau F, Geese R, Bauer A, Baur S, Paulus W, and Reimers CD: Motor cortex fatigue in sports measured by transcranial magnetic double stimulation. *Med Sci Sports Exerc* 32: 1942–8, 2000.
120. Sievenpiper JL, Arnason JT, Vidgen E, Leiter LA, and Vuksan V: A systematic quantitative analysis of the literature of the high variability in ginseng (*Panax* spp.): should ginseng be trusted in diabetes? *Diabetes Care* 27: 839–40, 2004.
121. Bucci LR: Selected herbals and human exercise performance. *Am J Clin Nutr* 72: 624S–36S, 2000.
122. Liang MT, Podolka TD, and Chuang WJ: Panax notoginseng supplementation enhances physical performance during endurance exercise. *J Strength Cond Res* 19: 108–14, 2005.
123. Kim SH, Park KS, Chang MJ, and Sung JH: Effects of Panax ginseng extract on exercise-induced oxidative stress. *J Sports Med Phys Fitness* 45: 178–82, 2005.
124. Kulaputana O, Thanakomsirichot S, and Anomasiri W: Ginseng supplementation does not change lactate threshold and physical performances in physically active Thai men. *J Med Assoc Thai* 90: 1172–9, 2007.
125. Kiefer D, and Pantuso T: Panax ginseng. *Am Fam Physician* 68: 1539–42, 2003.

126. Hsu CC, Ho MC, Lin LC, Su B, and Hsu MC: American ginseng supplementation attenuates creatine kinase level induced by submaximal exercise in human beings. *World J Gastroenterol* 11: 5327–31, 2005.
127. Vuksan V, Sievenpiper JL, Koo VY, Francis T, Beljan-Zdravkovic U, Xu Z, and Vidgen E: American ginseng (*Panax quinquefolius* L.) reduces postprandial glycemia in nondiabetic subjects and subjects with type 2 diabetes mellitus. *Arch Intern Med* 160: 1009–13, 2000.
128. Vuksan V, Stavro MP, Sievenpiper JL, Koo VY, Wong E, Beljan-Zdravkovic U, et al.: American ginseng improves glycemia in individuals with normal glucose tolerance: Effect of dose and time escalation. *J Am Coll Nutr* 19: 738–44, 2000.
129. Trimmer JK, Casazza GA, Horning MA, and Brooks GA: Autoregulation of glucose production in men with a glycerol load during rest and exercise. *Am J Physiol Endocrinol Metab* 280: E657–68, 2001.
130. Lyons TP, Riedesel ML, Meuli LE, and Chick TW: Effects of glycerol-induced hyperhydration prior to exercise in the heat on sweating and core temperature. *Med Sci Sports Exerc* 22: 477–83, 1990.
131. Goulet ED, Robergs RA, Labrecque S, Royer D and Dionne IJ: Effect of glycerol-induced hyperhydration on thermoregulatory and cardiovascular functions and endurance performance during prolonged cycling in a 25 degrees C environment. *Appl Physiol Nutr Metab* 31: 101–9, 2006.
132. Magal M, Webster MJ, Sistrunk LE, Whitehead MT, Evans RK, and Boyd JC: Comparison of glycerol and water hydration regimens on tennis-related performance. *Med Sci Sports Exerc* 35: 150–6, 2003.
133. Hitchins S, Martin DT, Burke L, Yates K, Fallon K, Hahn A, and Dobson GP: Glycerol hyperhydration improves cycle time trial performance in hot humid conditions. *Eur J Appl Physiol Occup Physiol* 80: 494–501, 1999.
134. Montner P, Stark DM, Riedesel ML, Murata G, Robergs R, Timms M, and Chick TW: Pre-exercise glycerol hydration improves cycling endurance time. *Int J Sports Med* 17: 27–33, 1996.
135. Wagner DR: Hyperhydrating with glycerol: Implications for athletic performance. *J Am Diet Assoc* 99: 207–12, 1999.
136. Coutts A, Reaburn P, Mummery K, and Holmes M: The effect of glycerol hyperhydration on olympic distance triathlon performance in high ambient temperatures. *Int J Sport Nutr Exerc Metab* 12: 105–19, 2002.
137. Latzka WA, and Sawka MN: Hyperhydration and glycerol: Thermoregulatory effects during exercise in hot climates. *Can J Appl Physiol* 25: 536–45, 2000.
138. Murray R, Eddy DE, Paul GL, Seifert JG, and Halaby GA: Physiological responses to glycerol ingestion during exercise. *J Appl Physiol* 71: 144–9, 1991.
139. Kelly GS: Clinical applications of N-acetylcysteine. *Altern Med Rev* 3: 114–27, 1998.
140. Patrick L: Nutrients and HIV: part three: N-acetylcysteine, alpha-lipoic acid, L-glutamine, and L-carnitine. *Altern Med Rev* 5: 290–305, 2000.
141. Kinscherf R, Hack V, Fischbach T, Friedmann B, Weiss C, Edler L, et al.: Low plasma glutamine in combination with high glutamate levels indicate risk for loss of body cell mass in healthy individuals: The effect of N-acetyl-cysteine. *J Mol Med* 74: 393–400, 1996.
142. Quadrilatero J, and Hoffman-Goetz L: N-acetyl-L-cysteine inhibits exercise-induced lymphocyte apoptotic protein alterations. *Med Sci Sports Exerc* 37: 53–6, 2005.
143. Quadrilatero J, and Hoffman-Goetz L: N-acetyl-l-cysteine protects intestinal lymphocytes from apoptotic death after acute exercise in adrenalectomized mice. *Am J Physiol Regul Integr Comp Physiol* 288: R1664–72, 2005.

144. Medved I, Brown MJ, Bjorksten AR, Leppik JA, Sostaric S, and McKenna MJ: N-acetylcysteine infusion alters blood redox status but not time to fatigue during intense exercise in humans. *J Appl Physiol* 94: 1572–82, 2003.
145. Medved I, Brown MJ, Bjorksten AR, and McKenna MJ: Effects of intravenous N-acetylcysteine infusion on time to fatigue and potassium regulation during prolonged cycling exercise. *J Appl Physiol* 96: 211–7, 2004.
146. Medved I, Brown MJ, Bjorksten AR, Murphy KT, Petersen AC, Sostaric S, et al.: N-acetylcysteine enhances muscle cysteine and glutathione availability and attenuates fatigue during prolonged exercise in endurance-trained individuals. *J Appl Physiol* 97: 1477–85, 2004.
147. Reid MB, Stokic DS, Koch SM, Khawli FA, and Leis AA: N-acetylcysteine inhibits muscle fatigue in humans. *J Clin Invest* 94: 2468–74, 1994.
148. McKenna MJ, Medved I, Goodman CA, Brown MJ, Bjorksten AR, Murphy KT, et al: N-acetylcysteine attenuates the decline in muscle Na+,K+-pump activity and delays fatigue during prolonged exercise in humans. *J Physiol* 576: 279–88, 2006.
149. Matuszczak Y, Farid M, Jones J, Lansdowne S, Smith MA, Taylor AA, and Reid MB: Effects of N-acetylcysteine on glutathione oxidation and fatigue during handgrip exercise. *Muscle Nerve* 32: 633–8, 2005.
150. Brekhman, II, and Dardymov IV: New substances of plant origin which increase nonspecific resistance. *Annu Rev Pharmacol* 9: 419–30, 1969.
151. Rhodiola rosea. Monograph. *Altern Med Rev* 7: 421–3, 2002.
152. Abidov M, Grachev S, Seifulla RD, and Ziegenfuss TN: Extract of *Rhodiola rosea* radix reduces the level of C-reactive protein and creatinine kinase in the blood. *Bull Exp Biol Med* 138: 63–4, 2004.
153. De Sanctis R, De Bellis R, Scesa C, Mancini U, Cucchiarini L, and Dacha M: In vitro protective effect of *Rhodiola rosea* extract against hypochlorous acid-induced oxidative damage in human erythrocytes. *Biofactors* 20: 147–59, 2004.
154. Kelly GS: Rhodiola rosea: A possible plant adaptogen. *Altern Med Rev* 6: 293–302, 2001.
155. Maslova LV, Kondrat'ev B, Maslov LN, and Lishmanov Iu B: The cardioprotective and antiadrenergic activity of an extract of *Rhodiola rosea* in stress. *Eksp Klin Farmakol* 57: 61–3, 1994.
156. Pogorelyi VE, and Makarova LM: *Rhodiola rosea* extract for prophylaxis of ischemic cerebral circulation disorder. *Eksp Klin Farmakol* 65: 19–22, 2002.
157. Shevtsov VA, Zholus BI, Shervarly VI, Vol'skij VB, Korovin YP, Khristich MP, et al.: A randomized trial of two different doses of a SHR-5 *Rhodiola rosea* extract versus placebo and control of capacity for mental work. *Phytomedicine* 10: 95–105, 2003.
158. De Bock K, Eijnde BO, Ramaekers M, and Hespel P: Acute *Rhodiola rosea* intake can improve endurance exercise performance. *Int J Sport Nutr Exerc Metab* 14: 298–307, 2004.
159. Burke ER: *D-Ribose: What You Need to Know*. Avery Publishing Group, Garden City Park, NY, 1999.
160. Hellsten Y, Skadhauge L, and Bangsbo J: Effect of ribose supplementation on resynthesis of adenine nucleotides after intense intermittent training in humans. *Am J Physiol Regul Integr Comp Physiol* 286: R182–8, 2004.
161. Kerksick C, Rasmussen C, Bowden R, Leutholtz B, Harvey T, Earnest C, et al.: Effects of ribose supplementation prior to and during intense exercise on anaerobic capacity and metabolic markers. *Int J Sport Nutr Exerc Metab* 15: 653–64, 2005.
162. Pauly DF, and Pepine CJ: D-Ribose as a supplement for cardiac energy metabolism. *J Cardiovasc Pharmacol Ther* 5: 249–58, 2000.
163. Kreider RB, Melton C, Greenwood M, Rasmussen C, Lundberg J, Earnest C, and Almada A: Effects of oral D-ribose supplementation on anaerobic capacity and

selected metabolic markers in healthy males. *Int J Sport Nutr Exerc Metab* 13: 76–86, 2003.
164. Berardi JM, and Ziegenfuss TN: Effects of ribose supplementation on repeated sprint performance in men. *J Strength Cond Res* 17: 47–52, 2003.
165. Dunne L, Worley S, and Macknin M: Ribose versus dextrose supplementation, association with rowing performance: A double-blind study. *Clin J Sport Med* 16: 68–71, 2006.
166. Op 't Eijnde B, Van Leemputte M, Brouns F, Van Der Vusse GJ, Labarque V, Ramaekers M, et al.: No effects of oral ribose supplementation on repeated maximal exercise and de novo ATP resynthesis. *J Appl Physiol* 91: 2275–81, 2001.
167. Rave U, Gallagher PM, Williamson D, Godard MP, and Trappe SW: Effect of ribose supplementation on performance during repeated high-intensity cycle sprints. *Med Sci Sport Exerc* 33(5): S44, 2001.
168. Gallagher PM, Williamson D, Godard MP, Witter J, and Trappe SW: Effects of ribose supplementation on adenine nucleotide concentration in skeletal muscle following high-intensity exercise. *Med Sci Sport Exerc* 33(5): S166, 2001.
169. Antonio J, Falk D, and Van Gammerren D: Ribose supplementation improves muscular strength and endurance in male bodybuilders. *Fed Am Soc Experiment Biol J* 15: A752, 2001.
170. Stipanuk MH: Role of the liver in regulation of body cysteine and taurine levels: A brief review. *Neurochem Res* 29: 105–10, 2004.
171. Birdsall TC: Therapeutic applications of taurine. *Altern Med Rev* 3: 128–36, 1998.
172. Huxtable RJ: Physiological actions of taurine. *Physiol Rev* 72: 101–63, 1992.
173. Petrosian AM, and Haroutounian JE: Taurine as a universal carrier of lipid soluble vitamins: A hypothesis. *Amino Acids* 19: 409–21, 2000.
174. Messina SA, and Dawson R, Jr.: Attenuation of oxidative damage to DNA by taurine and taurine analogs. *Adv Exp Med Biol* 483: 355–67, 2000.
175. Schaffer S, Takahashi K, and Azuma J: Role of osmoregulation in the actions of taurine. *Amino Acids* 19: 527–46, 2000.
176. El Idrissi A, and Trenkner E: Taurine as a modulator of excitatory and inhibitory neurotransmission. *Neurochem Res* 29: 189–97, 2004.
177. Zhang M, Izumi I, Kagamimori S, Sokejima S, Yamagami T, Liu Z, and Qi B: Role of taurine supplementation to prevent exercise-induced oxidative stress in healthy young men. *Amino Acids* 26: 203–7, 2004.
178. Dawson R, Jr., Biasetti M, Messina S, and Dominy J: The cytoprotective role of taurine in exercise-induced muscle injury. *Amino Acids* 22: 309–24, 2002.
179. Bouchama A, el Yazigi A, Yusuf A, and al Sedairy S: Alteration of taurine homeostasis in acute heatstroke. *Crit Care Med* 21: 551–4, 1993.
180. Matsuzaki Y, Miyazaki T, Miyakawa S, Bouscarel B, Ikegami T, and Tanaka N: Decreased taurine concentration in skeletal muscles after exercise for various durations. *Med Sci Sports Exerc* 34: 793–7, 2002.
181. Yatabe Y, Miyakawa S, Miyazaki T, Matsuzaki Y, and Ochiai N: Effects of taurine administration in rat skeletal muscles on exercise. *J Orthop Sci* 8: 415–9, 2003.
182. McArdle WD, Katch FI, and Katch VL: *Exercise Physiology: Energy, Nutrition, and Human Performance.* Darcy P (Ed) Lippincott Williams & Wilkins, Philadelphia, PA, 2001.
183. Parkin JM, Carey MF, Zhao S, and Febbraio MA: Effect of ambient temperature on human skeletal muscle metabolism during fatiguing submaximal exercise. *J Appl Physiol* 86: 902–8, 1999.
184. Jordan AN, Jurca R, Abraham EH, Salikhova A, Mann JK, Morss GM, et al.: Effects of oral ATP supplementation on anaerobic power and muscular strength. *Med Sci Sports Exerc* 36: 983–90, 2004.

185. Herda TJ, Ryan ED, Stout JR, and Cramer JT: Effects of a supplement designed to increase ATP levels on muscle strength, power output, and endurance. *J Int Soc Sports Nutr* 5: 3, 2008.
186. Anon. Betaine. Monograph. *Altern Med Rev* 8: 193–6, 2003.
187. Olthof MR, van Vliet T, Boelsma E, and Verhoef P: Low dose betaine supplementation leads to immediate and long term lowering of plasma homocysteine in healthy men and women. *J Nutr* 133: 4135–8, 2003.
188. Schwab U, Torronen A, Toppinen L, Alfthan G, Saarinen M, Aro A, and Uusitupa M: Betaine supplementation decreases plasma homocysteine concentrations but does not affect body weight, body composition, or resting energy expenditure in human subjects. *Am J Clin Nutr* 76: 961–7, 2002.
189. Armstrong LE, Roti MW, Hatch HL, Sutherland JW, Mahood NV, Clements JM, et al.: Rehydration with fluids containing betaine: Running performance and metabolism in a 31 C environment. *Med Sci Sports Exerc* 35: S311(abstr), 2003.
190. Roti MW, Hatch HL, Sutherland JW, Mahood NV, Clements JM, Seen AD, et al.: Homocysteine, lipid and glucose responses to betaine supplementation during running in the heat. *Med Sci Sports Exerc* 35: S271(abstr), 2003.
191. Wurtman RJ, Hefti F, and Melamed E: Precursor control of neurotransmitter synthesis. *Pharmacol Rev* 32: 315–35, 1980.
192. Zeisel SH: Choline: needed for normal development of memory. *J Am Coll Nutr* 19: 528S–531S, 2000.
193. Babb SM, Ke Y, Lange N, Kaufman MJ, Renshaw PF, and Cohen BM: Oral choline increases choline metabolites in human brain. *Psychiatry Res* 130: 1–9, 2004.
194. Spector SA, Jackman MR, Sabounjian LA, Sakkas C, Landers DM, and Willis WT: Effect of choline supplementation on fatigue in trained cyclists. *Med Sci Sports Exerc* 27: 668–73, 1995.
195. Buchman AL, Awal M, Jenden D, Roch M, and Kang SH: The effect of lecithin supplementation on plasma choline concentrations during a marathon. *J Am Coll Nutr* 19: 768–70, 2000.
196. Warber JP, Patton JF, Tharion WJ, Zeisel SH, Mello RP, Kemnitz CP, and Lieberman HR: The effects of choline supplementation on physical performance. *Int J Sport Nutr Exerc Metab* 10: 170–81, 2000.
197. Lefavi RG, Anderson RA, Keith RE, Wilson GD, McMillan JL, and Stone MH: Efficacy of chromium supplementation in athletes: emphasis on anabolism. *Int J Sport Nutr* 2: 111–22, 1992.
198. Clancy SP, Clarkson PM, DeCheke ME, Nosaka K, Freedson PS, Cunningham JJ, and Valentine B: Effects of chromium picolinate supplementation on body composition, strength, and urinary chromium loss in football players. *Int J Sport Nutr* 4: 142–53, 1994.
199. Lukaski HC, Bolonchuk WW, Siders WA, and Milne DB: Chromium supplementation and resistance training: Effects on body composition, strength, and trace element status of men. *Am J Clin Nutr* 63: 954–65, 1996.
200. Briand J, Blehaut H, Calvayrac R and Laval-Martin D: Use of a microbial model for the determination of drug effects on cell metabolism and energetics: study of citrulline-malate. *Biopharm Drug Dispos* 13: 1–22, 1992.
201. Lambert EV, Goedecke JH, Bluett K, Heggie K, Claassen A, Rae DE, et al.: Conjugated linoleic acid versus high-oleic acid sunflower oil: Effects on energy metabolism, glucose tolerance, blood lipids, appetite and body composition in regularly exercising individuals. *Br J Nutr* 97: 1001–11, 2007.
202. Gaullier JM, Halse J, Hoivik HO, Hoye K, Syvertsen C, Nurminiemi M, et al.: Six months supplementation with conjugated linoleic acid induces regional-specific fat mass decreases in overweight and obese. *Br J Nutr* 97: 550–60, 2007.

203. Syvertsen C, Halse J, Hoivik HO, Gaullier JM, Nurminiemi M, Kristiansen K, et al.: The effect of 6 months supplementation with conjugated linoleic acid on insulin resistance in overweight and obese. *Int J Obes (Lond)* 31: 1148–54, 2007.
204. Gaullier JM, Halse J, Hoye K, Kristiansen K, Fagertun H, Vik H, and Gudmundsen O: Supplementation with conjugated linoleic acid for 24 months is well tolerated by and reduces body fat mass in healthy, overweight humans. *J Nutr* 135: 778–84, 2005.
205. Bates SH, Jones RB, and Bailey CJ: Insulin-like effect of pinitol. *Br J Pharmacol* 130: 1944–8, 2000.
206. Davis A, Christiansen M, Horowitz JF, Klein S, Hellerstein MK, and Ostlund RE, Jr.: Effect of pinitol treatment on insulin action in subjects with insulin resistance. *Diabetes Care* 23: 1000–5, 2000.
207. Fonteles MC, Almeida MQ, and Larner J: Antihyperglycemic effects of 3-O-methyl-D-chiro-inositol and D-chiro-inositol associated with manganese in streptozotocin diabetic rats. *Horm Metab Res* 32: 129–32, 2000.
208. Syrov VN, and Kurmukov AG: Anabolic activity of phytoecdysone–ecdysterone isolated from Rhaponticum carthamoides (Willd.) Iljin. *Farmakol Toksikol* 39: 690–3, 1976.
209. Cai YJ, Dai JQ, Fang JG, Ma LP, Hou LF, Yang L, and Liu ZL: Antioxidative and free radical scavenging effects of ecdysteroids from Serratula strangulata. *Can J Physiol Pharmacol* 80: 1187–94, 2002.
210. Gadzhieva RM, Portugalov SN, Paniushkin VV, and Kondrat'eva, II: A comparative study of the anabolic action of ecdysten, leveton and Prime Plus, preparations of plant origin. *Eksp Klin Farmakol* 58: 46–8, 1995.
211. Kokoska L, Polesny Z, Rada V, Nepovim A, and Vanek T: Screening of some Siberian medicinal plants for antimicrobial activity. *J Ethnopharmacol* 82: 51–3, 2002.
212. Mirzaev Iu R, Syrov VN, Khrushev SA, and Iskanderova SD: Effect of ecdystene on parameters of the sexual function under experimental and clinical conditions. *Eksp Klin Farmakol* 63: 35–7, 2000.
213. Mosharrof AH: Effects of extract from *Rhapontcum carthamoides* (Willd) Iljin (Leuzea) on learning and memory in rats. *Acta Physiol Pharmacol Bulg* 13: 37–42, 1987.
214. Syrov VN, Nasyrova SS, and Khushbaktova ZA: The results of experimental study of phytoecdysteroids as erythropoiesis stimulators in laboratory animals. *Eksp Klin Farmakol* 60: 41–4, 1997.
215. Trenin DS, and Volodin VV: 20-hydroxyecdysone as a human lymphocyte and neutrophil modulator: In vitro evaluation. *Arch Insect Biochem Physiol* 41: 156–61, 1999.
216. Smith RJ: Glutamine metabolism and its physiologic importance. *JPEN J Parenter Enteral Nutr* 14: 40S–44S, 1990.
217. Coster J, McCauley R, and Hall J: Glutamine: metabolism and application in nutrition support. *Asia Pac J Clin Nutr* 13: 25–31, 2004.
218. Phillips GC: Glutamine: The nonessential amino acid for performance enhancement. *Curr Sports Med Rep* 6: 265–8, 2007.
219. van Hall G, Saris WH, van de Schoor PA, and Wagenmakers AJ: The effect of free glutamine and peptide ingestion on the rate of muscle glycogen resynthesis in man. *Int J Sports Med* 21: 25–30, 2000.
220. Bowtell JL, Gelly K, Jackman ML, Patel A, Simeoni M, and Rennie MJ: Effect of oral glutamine on whole body carbohydrate storage during recovery from exhaustive exercise. *J Appl Physiol* 86: 1770–7, 1999.
221. Buchman AL: Glutamine: commercially essential or conditionally essential? A critical appraisal of the human data. *Am J Clin Nutr* 74: 25–32, 2001.
222. Castell L: Glutamine supplementation in vitro and in vivo, in exercise and in immunodepression. *Sports Med* 33: 323–45, 2003.

223. Garcia-de-Lorenzo A, Zarazaga A, Garcia-Luna PP, Gonzalez-Huix F, Lopez-Martinez J, Mijan A, et al.: Clinical evidence for enteral nutritional support with glutamine: A systematic review. *Nutrition* 19: 805–11, 2003.
224. Novak F, Heyland DK, Avenell A, Drover JW, and Su X: Glutamine supplementation in serious illness: A systematic review of the evidence. *Crit Care Med* 30: 2022–9, 2002.
225. Kovacs EM, Westerterp-Plantenga MS and Saris WH: The effects of 2-week ingestion of (--)-hydroxycitrate and (--)-hydroxycitrate combined with medium-chain triglycerides on satiety, fat oxidation, energy expenditure and body weight. *Int J Obes Relat Metab Disord* 25: 1087–94, 2001.
226. Kriketos AD, Thompson HR, Greene H, and Hill JO: (-)-Hydroxycitric acid does not affect energy expenditure and substrate oxidation in adult males in a post-absorptive state. *Int J Obes Relat Metab Disord* 23: 867–73, 1999.
227. van Loon LJ, van Rooijen JJ, Niesen B, Verhagen H, Saris WH, and Wagenmakers AJ: Effects of acute (-)-hydroxycitrate supplementation on substrate metabolism at rest and during exercise in humans. *Am J Clin Nutr* 72: 1445–50, 2000.
228. Leonhardt M, Hrupka B, and Langhans W: Effect of hydroxycitrate on food intake and body weight regain after a period of restrictive feeding in male rats. *Physiol Behav* 74: 191–6, 2001.
229. Mattes RD, and Bormann L: Effects of (-)-hydroxycitric acid on appetitive variables. *Physiol Behav* 71: 87–94, 2000.
230. Preuss HG, Bagchi D, Bagchi M, Rao CV, Dey DK, and Satyanarayana S: Effects of a natural extract of (-)-hydroxycitric acid (HCA-SX) and a combination of HCA-SX plus niacin–bound chromium and *Gymnema sylvestre* extract on weight loss. *Diabetes Obes Metab* 6: 171–80, 2004.
231. Preuss HG, Garis RI, Bramble JD, Bagchi D, Bagchi M, Rao CV, and Satyanarayana S: Efficacy of a novel calcium/potassium salt of (-)-hydroxycitric acid in weight control. *Int J Clin Pharmacol Res* 25: 133–44, 2005.
232. Westerterp-Plantenga MS, and Kovacs EM: The effect of (-)-hydroxycitrate on energy intake and satiety in overweight humans. *Int J Obes Relat Metab Disord* 26: 870–2, 2002.
233. Lim K, Ryu S, Nho HS, Choi SK, Kwon T, Suh H, et al.: (-)-Hydroxycitric acid ingestion increases fat utilization during exercise in untrained women. *J Nutr Sci Vitaminol (Tokyo)* 49: 163–7, 2003.
234. Lim K, Ryu S, Suh H, Ishihara K, and Fushiki T: (-)-Hydroxycitrate ingestion and endurance exercise performance. *J Nutr Sci Vitaminol (Tokyo)* 51: 1–7, 2005.
235. Tomita K, Okuhara Y, Shigematsu N, Suh H, and Lim K: (-)-hydroxycitrate ingestion increases fat oxidation during moderate intensity exercise in untrained men. *Biosci Biotechnol Biochem* 67: 1999–2001, 2003.
236. Saint-John M, and McNaughton L: Octocosanol ingestion and its effects on metabolic responses to sub-maximal cycle ergometry, reaction time and chest and grip strength. *Int Clin Nutr Rev* 6: 81–87, 1986.
237. Stanko RT, and Adibi SA: Inhibition of lipid accumulation and enhancement of energy expenditure by the addition of pyruvate and dihydroxyacetone to a rat diet. *Metabolism* 35: 182–6, 1986.
238. Stanko RT, Robertson RJ, Galbreath RW, Reilly JJ, Jr., Greenawalt KD, and Goss FL: Enhanced leg exercise endurance with a high-carbohydrate diet and dihydroxyacetone and pyruvate. *J Appl Physiol* 69: 1651–6, 1990.
239. Stanko RT, Robertson RJ, Spina RJ, Reilly JJ, Jr., Greenawalt KD, and Goss FL: Enhancement of arm exercise endurance capacity with dihydroxyacetone and pyruvate. *J Appl Physiol* 68: 119–24, 1990.

240. Ebersole KT, Stout JR, Housh TJ, Eckerson JM, Evetovich TK, and Smith DB: The effect of pyruvate supplementation on critical power. *J Strength Cond Res* 14: 132–134, 2000.
241. Morrison MA, Spriet LL, and Dyck DJ: Pyruvate ingestion for 7 days does not improve aerobic performance in well-trained individuals. *J Appl Physiol* 89: 549–56, 2000.
242. Koh-Banerjee PK, Ferreira MP, Greenwood M, Bowden RG, Cowan PN, Almada AL, and Kreider RB: Effects of calcium pyruvate supplementation during training on body composition, exercise capacity, and metabolic responses to exercise. *Nutrition* 21: 312–9, 2005.
243. Stone MH, Sanborn K, Smith LL, O'Bryant HS, Hoke T, Utter AC, et al.: Effects of in-season (5 weeks) creatine and pyruvate supplementation on anaerobic performance and body composition in American football players. *Int J Sport Nutr* 9: 146–65, 1999.
244. Antonio J, Uelmen J, Rodriguez R, and Earnest C: The effects of *Tribulus terrestris* on body composition and exercise performance in resistance-trained males. *Int J Sport Nutr Exerc Metab* 10: 208–15, 2000.
245. Rogerson S, Riches CJ, Jennings C, Weatherby RP, Meir RA, and Marshall-Gradisnik SM: The effect of five weeks of *Tribulus terrestris* supplementation on muscle strength and body composition during preseason training in elite rugby league players. *J Strength Cond Res* 21: 348–53, 2007.
246. Gauthaman K, Ganesan AP, and Prasad RN: Sexual effects of puncturevine (*Tribulus terrestris*) extract (protodioscin): An evaluation using a rat model. *J Altern Complement Med* 9: 257–65, 2003.
247. Stevenson JS, Jaeger JR, Rettmer I, Smith MW, and Corah LR: Luteinizing hormone release and reproductive traits in anestrous, estrus-cycling, and ovariectomized cattle after tyrosine supplementation. *J Anim Sci* 75: 2754–61, 1997.
248. Chinevere TD, Sawyer RD, Creer AR, Conlee RK, and Parcell AC: Effects of L-tyrosine and carbohydrate ingestion on endurance exercise performance. *J Appl Physiol* 93: 1590–7, 2002.
249. Sutton EE, Coill MR, and Deuster PA: Ingestion of tyrosine: Effects on endurance, muscle strength, and anaerobic performance. *Int J Sport Nutr Exerc Metab* 15: 173–85, 2005.
250. Magill RA, Waters WF, Bray GA, Volaufova J, Smith SR, Lieberman HR, et al.: Effects of tyrosine, phentermine, caffeine D-amphetamine, and placebo on cognitive and motor performance deficits during sleep deprivation. *Nutr Neurosci* 6: 237–46, 2003.
251. Neri DF, Wiegmann D, Stanny RR, Shappell SA, McCardie A, and McKay DL: The effects of tyrosine on cognitive performance during extended wakefulness. *Aviat Space Environ Med* 66: 313–9, 1995.
252. Mahoney CR, Castellani J, Kramer FM, Young A, and Lieberman HR: Tyrosine supplementation mitigates working memory decrements during cold exposure. *Physiol Behav* 92: 575–82, 2007.
253. McCarty MF: Pre-exercise administration of yohimbine may enhance the efficacy of exercise training as a fat loss strategy by boosting lipolysis. *Med Hypotheses* 58: 491–5, 2002.
254. Galitzky J, Taouis M, Berlan M, Riviere D, Garrigues M, and Lafontan M: Alpha 2-antagonist compounds and lipid mobilization: Evidence for a lipid mobilizing effect of oral yohimbine in healthy male volunteers. *Eur J Clin Invest* 18: 587–94, 1988.
255. Ostojic SM: Yohimbine: The effects on body composition and exercise performance in soccer players. *Res Sports Med* 14: 289–99, 2006.

256. Mattila M, Seppala T, and Mattila MJ: Anxiogenic effect of yohimbine in healthy subjects: Comparison with caffeine and antagonism by clonidine and diazepam. *Int Clin Psychopharmacol* 3: 215–29, 1988.
257. Stout JR, Cramer JT, Zoeller RF, Torok D, Costa P, Hoffman JR, and Harris RC: Effects of beta-alanine supplementation on the onset of neuromuscular fatigue and ventilatory threshold in women. *Amino Acids* 32(3): 381–386, 2007.
258. Zoeller RF, Stout JR, O'Kroy J A, Torok DJ, and Mielke M: Effects of 28 days of beta-alanine and creatine monohydrate supplementation on aerobic power, ventilatory and lactate thresholds, and time to exhaustion. *Amino Acids* 33(3): 505–510, 2007.

10 Life Cycle Concerns

Peter R. J. Reaburn and Fiona E. Pelly

CONTENTS

I. INTRODUCTION

Aging across the lifecycle leads to many physical, physiological, psychosocial, and environmental changes that may affect the dietary and nutritional needs of professional, amateur, and weekend athletes. For example, between birth and 18 years of age, body mass (BM) increases approximately twentyfold. Moreover, the increase in BM is linear during childhood but accelerates during puberty and then decelerates rapidly at different rates in boys and girls. During adulthood, muscle mass is maintained, but from approximately 50 years of age, declines linearly then nonlinearly from approximately 65 years onward. These physical changes greatly affect energy and dietary requirements. Furthermore, energy and dietary requirements are affected by different levels of physical activity and exercise that are altered with both aging and lifestyle changes. The purpose of this chapter is to examine the specific lifecycle concerns as athletes age. Specifically, this chapter will examine the macro- and micronutrient needs of child and adolescent athletes, pregnant and lactating athletes, and aging athletes.

II. CHILD AND ADOLESCENT ATHLETES

A. Introduction

For child and adolescent athletes, an adequate dietary intake is crucial to maintain health and facilitate optimal growth and maturation as well as minimize injury and optimize training and competition performance. Childhood is also a period of continuous education about eating and good nutrition that lays the foundations of healthy nutrition practices for life that together with a physically active lifestyle can reduce the risk of many lifestyle-related diseases.

For the purposes of this chapter, children are defined as ages 6–11 years and adolescents as ages 12–18 years.[1]

Childhood is typically a period during which involvement in sport typically begins and adolescence a period where sport involvement is maintained or becomes limited. The dietary reference intakes (DRIs) for the United States of America and Canada, the Dietary Reference Values (DRVs) United Kingdom and the Recommended Daily Intakes (RDIs) for Australia are very similar and will be used interchangeably throughout the chapter, depending on the research being used to inform the topic being discussed. While specific dietary guidelines for normal healthy children and adolescents have been developed in Australia,[1] both the United Kingdom[2] and the United States[3] appear to include the dietary guidelines or nutrient requirements for normal healthy children and adolescents within their guidelines for adults.

There is little empirical scientific information relating to the specific dietary needs of child and adolescent athletes. However, a number of excellent reviews from leading sport and exercise scientists or sport dieticians have addressed the area.[4–9]

B. Factors Affecting Nutritional Needs

Throughout childhood (prepuberty) and adolescence (puberty), a number of factors influence nutritional needs. These include increases in body size and weight (growth), changes in the rate of attaining that body size (maturation), changes in physical activity levels, and both parental and peer influences on food intake patterns. During childhood there is an increase in both bone length and bone mass that accelerates at puberty.[10] However, there is enormous variability in the timing of this increased velocity or "growth spurt." Girls tend to start their growth spurt and attain their peak height 2 years earlier than boys.[11]

Age is generally a poor indicator of physiological maturity and nutritional requirements.[11] Intense training in childhood and adolescence, when combined with poor nutrition, can have negative effects on skeletal growth and maturation.[4] In a study by Theintz and colleagues,[12] the growth rates of prepubertal gymnasts was shown to be lower than moderately active prepubertal controls. The outcome of prolonged energy restriction could result in delayed maturation or growth retardation. Menarche (onset of menstruation) has also been shown to occur later in female athletes compared with nonathletes.[13] If growth rate is reduced, "catch-up" growth may occur. However, this may be compromised if the delay in maturation is severe.[4]

During the prepubertal period, the proportion of fat and muscle in boy and girls is similar. During puberty, boys gain proportionally more muscle mass than fat, experience a higher peak velocity in height growth, and develop a greater red blood cell mass, resulting in a more lean BM per unit of height.[11] In adolescent girls, peak weight occurs before peak height. This may cause concern for young athletes involved in sports where an emphasis is placed on a lean physique (e.g., gymnastics). Consequently, pubertal development in girls may make it difficult to achieve the ideal physique required by certain sports.[14] Regardless of gender, during puberty, adolescents need to eat frequently, and often in large amounts. Young athletes may have difficulty maintaining their weight during this period and may require high-energy liquid meal supplements and snacks.

Regular physical activity in a healthy, well-nourished child is crucial for normal skeletal and muscle growth as well as the development of cardiovascular fitness, neuromuscular coordination, and cognitive function.[15] Exercise and nutrition are independently recognized as important modifiable lifestyle factors essential for optimal bone health during growth.[16] Current evidence suggests that regular weight-bearing exercise and adequate dietary calcium intakes (around 1000 mg per day) may be required to optimize bone health; however, exercise would appear to be more important for optimizing bone strength because it has a direct loading effect on bone mass and structural properties, whereas nutritional factors appear to have an indirect effect (via hormonal factors) on bone mass.[16]

Some young athletes such as gymnasts and dancers undertaking intense physical training and consuming low-energy diets may be at risk of attenuated growth and delayed maturation, and catch-up growth may occur if training intensity is reduced and energy intake increased. For an excellent review see Bass and Inge.[4]

C. Energy Requirements

Adequate energy intake for the child and adolescent athlete is vital for not only normal growth and maturation, but BM maintenance and to meet the extra energy needs of physical training.[7] Female adolescent athletes, particularly those involved with distance running, walking, and jumping events, may be at greater risk of inadequate energy intake or disordered eating as they pursue a lighter and leaner physique.[14] However, few studies have empirically measured the energy requirements of children and adolescents performing sport. In general, because children are less economical in movement than adults, they tend to have higher energy needs than adults for the same activity. Moreover, the few studies measuring self-reported energy intakes of young athletes have shown large variability in energy intakes that are age-, sport- and gender-specific.[4,8]

In Australia and New Zealand in 2006, the National Health and Medical Research Council recommended estimated energy requirements based on gender, age, height, body mass, estimated basal metabolic rate, and physical activity levels based on six categories from bed rest through to vigorous activity (Table 10.1).[17] These guidelines are considered more appropriate than the alternative approach used in North

TABLE 10.1
Estimated Energy Requirements for Children and Adolescents (MJ/day)

Age	Male						Female					
(yr)	BMR	Sed	LA	MA	HA	VA	BMR	Sed	LA	MA	HA	VA
8	4.5	6.4	7.3	8.2	9.2	10.1	4.2	6.0	6.9	7.7	8.6	9.4
10	5.1	7.3	8.3	9.3	10.4	11.4	4.7	6.7	7.6	8.5	9.5	10.4
12	5.8	8.2	9.3	10.5	11.6	12.8	5.2	7.4	8.5	9.5	10.6	11.6
14	6.6	9.3	10.6	11.9	13.2	14.6	5.7	8.1	9.2	10.3	11.5	12.6
16	7.3	10.3	11.8	13.2	14.7	16.2	5.9	8.4	9.5	10.7	11.9	13.1
18	7.7	10.9	12.5	14.0	15.6	17.1	6.0	8.5	9.7	10.9	12.1	13.3

BMR = Basal metabolic rate; Sed = Very sedentary; LA = Light activity; MA = Moderate activity; HA = Heavy activity; VA = Vigorous activity.

1 MJ = 1,000 kJ. 4.18 kilojoules are equal to 1 kilocalorie.

Source: Adapted from NHMRC Nutrient Reference Values for Australia and New Zealand, 2006.[17]

America[18] and Britain,[2] both of which limit the number of physical activity categories compared with the Australian and New Zealand recommendations.

Chronic negative energy balance during childhood has been shown to result in short stature, delayed puberty, menstrual irregularities, poor bone health, increased incidence of injuries, and a greater risk of developing eating disorders.[4,14,19] In contrast, chronic positive energy balance may lead to overweight, obesity, and the associated negative health consequences of such conditions.[20,21]

D. Macronutrients

Extensive reviews of the literature related to metabolic and hormonal responses to exercise in children and adolescents have been conducted.[22,23] Both reviews concluded that substrate utilization during exercise differs between children and adults. They highlighted that lower respiratory exchange ratio values are often observed in young individuals during prolonged moderate exercise, suggesting that children rely more on fat oxidation than do adults. Increased free fatty acid mobilization, glycerol release, and growth hormone increases in preadolescent children also support this suggestion. Plasma glucose responses during prolonged exercise are generally comparable in children and adults. However, when glucose is ingested at the beginning of moderate exercise, plasma glucose levels are higher in children than in adults, possibly due to decreased insulin sensitivity during the peripubertal period.

Changes in energetic metabolism occurring during adolescence are also dependent on pubertal events with an increase in testosterone in boys and estrogen and progesterone in girls.[23] The profound effects of ovarian hormones on carbohydrate and fat metabolism, along with their effects on oxidative enzymes, could explain the differences in substrate metabolism observed between girls and women. Finally, although the regulatory mechanisms of fat and carbohydrate balance during exercise are quite well identified in adults, there is a lack of data specific to children and adolescents.

1. Carbohydrates

In adults, high-carbohydrate (CHO) diets have long been shown to benefit athletic performance.[24–26] In children, recent research has shown increased rates of both endogenous and exogenous CHO oxidation in children compared with adolescents and adults.[27–29] Stephens et al.[27] observed greater fat use, lower CHO use, and lower lactate concentrations in early and midpubescent boys compared with late puberty or young adult males. No differences in endogenous CHO oxidation were noted between early and midpuberty or late puberty and young adults at any cycling endurance exercise intensity, suggesting the development of an adultlike metabolic profile occurs between mid- to late puberty and is complete by the end of puberty. Timmons et al.[28] also observed an increased reliance on exogenous CHO during endurance exercise that is particularly sensitive to pubertal status, with the highest exogenous CHO oxidation rates observed in nonathletic pre- and early pubertal boys, independent of chronological age. Moreover, the exogenous CHO oxidation rate as a percentage of energy expenditure was inversely related to testosterone levels.

The limited available data suggest potential gender-related differences in energy substrate utilization even during childhood.[29] These investigators measured substrate utilization in 12-yr-old preadolescent and 14-yr-old adolescent girls who consumed flavored water or a CHO-enriched drink while cycling for 60 min at approximately 70% maximal aerobic power. They concluded that exogenous CHO influences endogenous substrate utilization in an age-dependent manner in healthy girls but that total exogenous CHO oxidation during exercise is not different between prepubertal and adolescent girls. In the same study they observed that serum estradiol levels in all girls significantly correlated with fat and endogenous CHO oxidation but not with exogenous CHO oxidation. Thus, it appears that in both males and females, hormonal influences at puberty alter substrate utilization patterns during exercise.

Glycogen stores appear lower in children than adults.[22,23] Low muscle glycogen content is possibly associated with a low activity of glycolytic enzymes and high oxidative capacity,[30] while lower levels of sympathoadrenal hormones are likely to favor lipid metabolism in children. This profile changes through adolescence.[31] Thus, due to a lack of empirical data, it remains unclear whether young athletes need CHO intakes similar to adults. However, it has been suggested that young athletes consume at least 50% of their total daily energy intake as carbohydrates.[8]

Of concern to parents, coaches, and clinicians is that simple sugars (soft drinks, sports drinks, confectionery) and acids (citrus fruits and drinks) found in common child food and drink preferences provide the substrates for enhancing acid production and threatening dental health.[32] Preventive measures to help prevent dental problems include

- Water rinsing
- Chewing sugar-free gum
- Drinking fluids through a straw or water bottle nozzle
- Chilling the drinks
- Preventing dehydration

2. Fat

Child athletes have been shown to have an increased ability to utilize fat as an energy source during exercise.[33] While this increased reliance on fat may suggest the need for increased fat intake in child athletes, the normal western diet delivers more than adequate dietary fat. High-fat diets are generally relatively low in CHO, thus negatively impacting on both training performance and recovery in child and adolescent athletes. As with adult athletes, there exists no evidence to suggest that young athletes undertaking endurance exercise may benefit from a higher fat content in their diets.[34]

For public health reasons, both the 2003 *Dietary Guidelines for Children and Adolescents in Australia*[1] and American Heart Association (2005)[3] recommend lowering total fat intake to 30% and 25–35% respectively, of total daily energy intakes with no more than 10% contribution from saturated fat.[1,3] Young athletes aiming to reduce BM or body fat may overly restrict dietary fat intake, resulting in an insufficient intake of essential fatty acids and fat-soluble vitamins A, D, E, and K.

Moreover, restricting the intake of fat in healthy, non-obese children and adolescents may impair growth and development, although it is not known whether this is due to restriction of fat intake or overall energy restriction.[35] Furthermore, restriction of foods containing high amounts of fat such as dairy products and red meat may create intake deficits of protein, calcium, iron, vitamin B_{12}, and fat-soluble vitamins A, D, E, and K that are crucial for both optimal physical growth and physical performance.

In summary, it has been suggested that young athletes consume 25–30% of their total daily energy intake as fat with young athletes' being able to possibly take in slightly higher amounts of fat than inactive children and adolescents because of their increased energy expenditure and use of fat as a substrate during physical training and performance.[8]

3. Protein

Proteins are the fundamental structural compounds of cells, antibodies, enzymes, and hormones.[36] An adequate intake of protein containing the essential amino acids is thus crucial for optimal growth and maturation in children. Moreover, protein also plays a role in satiety and constitutes the sole form of replacing nitrogen in the body.

Normal healthy children and adolescents have higher protein needs than adults to support the growth of muscles, bones, connective tissue, and organs. However, few studies have examined the protein requirements of child or adolescent athletes. In one of the few studies to examine protein utilization in children, the effects of 6 weeks of walking exercise (45–60 min/session, 5 days/week) on protein metabolism was examined in seven untrained prepubescent male and female children.[37] Whole-body protein oxidation significantly increased but protein synthesis decreased, suggesting the body adjusted to prevent a negative nitrogen balance. In a later study, the effects of 6 weeks of twice-weekly resistance training on protein utilization was examined in healthy children who maintained their normal dietary intake of energy and protein.[38] The investigators observed a significant increase in muscular strength and fat-free mass together with a significant down-regulation of protein metabolism.

Protein recommendations for children must take into account not only the maintenance of normal bodily functioning but also the increased requirements during growth spurts. In most western countries, protein intakes typically exceed protein requirements, suggesting that child and adolescent athletes from these countries consume adequate protein. Table 10.2 suggests that normal healthy Australian children are easily meeting the Australian RDIs for protein intake.

In adult athletes, protein intake recommendations (1.2–1.7 g/kg/day) are slightly higher than the DRIs for normal healthy adults, especially for athletes undertaking endurance-, sprint- or strength-oriented sports.[39,40] Thus, it might be suggested that athletic children, especially those engaged in strength and power sports (e.g., team sports, sprint swimming, running, or cycling) or endurance sports may require increased protein requirements compared with normal children, especially during growth spurts in athletes undertaking regular high-volume or intensity training such as swimmers or high-performance athletes in team sports.

TABLE 10.2
Protein Recommendations and Intakes for Australian Children and Adolescents

Group	Age (years)	RDI (g/day)	Protein Intake (g/day)
Males	4–7	18–24	64
	8–11	27–39	82
	12–15	42–60	101
	16–18	64–70	120
Females	4–7	18–24	57
	8–11	27–39	69
	12–15	44–55	74
	16–18	57	80

Source: Adapted from Baghurst, K. and Binns, C. 2003 *Dietary Guidelines for Children and Adolescents in Australia.* Canberra: National Health and Medical Research Council.[1]

In summary, the limited available data would suggest that child and adolescent athletes on a normal healthy diet that is not low in energy requirements are meeting protein intake requirements. However, during growth spurts, child athletes undertaking intense or prolonged training and possibly on negative energy balance diets, may be at risk of inadequate dietary protein intake.

E. Micronutrients

Micronutrients perform the same actions in both adult and young athletes and non-athletes. They serve as co-factors in metabolic reactions, are involved in tissue synthesis, maintenance of body fluid balance and neuromuscular facilitation.[36] Research has suggested that most child and adolescent athletes are taking in enough vitamins and minerals to meet their daily requirements except for calcium and vitamins D and E.[8] However, research from both the United Kingdom[41] and Australia[42] suggests young athletes widely use dietary supplements of vitamins and minerals, as adult athletes do, to maintain health, improve immune function, prevent illness, boost energy, correct poor dietary intake, and improve performance. While there is no research evidence to suggest the general use of such supplements, such supplementation might be suggested for young athletes with poor dietary habits, vegetarians, those following a reduced energy intake diet, amenorrheic, or diagnosed with iron deficiency.

1. Vitamins

In a healthy adult population it is widely acknowledged that if energy intakes meet energy expenditures, it is likely that vitamin needs will be met.[43] In contrast, a recent study investigated the energy, nutrient, and dietary fiber intakes of 180 healthy but nonathletic adolescent males using a 3-day food record.[44] These investigators observed that median intakes for percent energy from carbohydrate, fat, and protein

TABLE 10.3
Estimated Average Daily Requirements of Selected Vitamins Suggested for Young Athletes

Vitamin	Boys 9–13 Years	Girls 9–13 Years	Boys 14–18 Years	Girls 14–18 Years
A (μg)	445	420	630	485
Thiamine (mg)	0.7	0.7	1.0	0.9
Riboflavin (mg)	0.8	0.8	1.1	0.9
Niacin (mg)	9	9	12	11
B_6 (μg)	0.8	0.8	1.1	1.0
B_{12} (μg)	1.5	1.5	2.0	1.0
Folacin (μg)	250	250	330	330
C (mg)	39	39	63	56
E (mg)	9	9	12	12
D (μg)	5	5	5	5

Source: Adapted from Petrie, H.J., Stover, E.A., and Horswill, C.A. 2004. *Nutr.,* 20, 620–631.[8]

were within the accepted macronutrient distribution ranges, but more than 50% of subjects consumed inadequate amounts of vitamins A and B_6, and more than 75% of subjects consumed inadequate amounts of magnesium, phosphorus, and zinc. Although one of the few studies to examine energy and micronutrient intake in young nonathletic but healthy people, the results suggest the possible need for vitamin supplementation in young athletes.

An extensive review of macronutrient and micronutrient intake in young athletes[8] suggests they consume an amount of vitamins that achieves or comes close to achieving the daily requirements of their healthy but nonathletic peers. The same authors suggest that vitamin B intake may need to increase to meet the elevated demands of physical training (Table 10.3).

In adult athletes who restrict energy intakes, it is common to see vitamin intakes that are below the DRI.[45] Similarly, young athletes who follow low-energy diets (e.g., dancers, gymnasts, wrestlers) may risk suboptimal vitamin intakes with a number of studies suggesting low intake levels of folate in 12–17 year-old ballet dancers[45] and low levels of vitamin E in young gymnasts.[46] Again, these results suggest the need for child and adolescent athletes to supplement with multivitamin and mineral supplements.

2. Minerals

Research based on athletic adult populations suggests that, with the exception of minerals lost in high amounts in sweat (sodium, potassium, calcium, and magnesium), elevated metabolism through exercise does not increase mineral requirements in those adult athletes taking in a normal healthy and well-balanced diet.[8] Similarly, in children and adolescent athletes, there may be a need to increase dietary intake of sodium, potassium, calcium, and magnesium lost in athletes where high volumes of sweat are normal.

Calcium, iron, and zinc intakes are often reported to be below DRIs in the few dietary surveys conducted on child[47–49] and adolescent[50] athletes. These surveys suggest that young female athletes who may restrict their energy intake (e.g., dancers, gymnasts) tend also to restrict their dairy product intake and thus calcium intake. Dietary intake of calcium recommendations are based on the amount needed to both maintain calcium balance and promote optimum bone development. If calcium intake is low (< 400 mg/day) during childhood and adolescence, it may negatively impact bone development and overall health.[51] Crucially, approximately 26% of bone mineral is accrued during puberty[52] with exercise, particularly if started before puberty, enhancing bone mineral density.[53] Furthermore, Manore et al.[14] concluded that amenorrhea in female athletes has negative consequences on long-term mineral density. Moreover, poor bone quality has consistently been shown to increased fracture rates in both boys and girls, particularly those on low calcium intakes.[54] Thus, it appears prudent to ensure that young athletes' daily intake of calcium be encouraged at levels (1300 mg/day) suggested in an extensive review of child and adolescent athlete mineral needs summarized in Table 10.4.[8]

Young team players or child athletes undertaking intense or prolonged endurance training may be at risk of iron loss via hemolysis, gastrointestinal blood loss, and excessive sweating.[55] Again, adolescent female athletes in particular are at risk due to their menstrual losses combined with possible low consumption of dietary iron.

Finally, suboptimal zinc intakes have been observed in young female athletes.[48,49] Taken together, these finding suggest, especially in vegetarian households, the need for ensuring adequate dietary intakes on calcium, iron, and zinc in child athletes through either dietary means or supplementation.

In summary, few studies have examined the macro- or micronutrient needs of child or adolescent athletes. Those that have strongly suggest the need for increased energy intake with an emphasis on carbohydrates, especially in young athletes undertaking regular high-intensity or volume training such as swimmers, runners, and team sport players. The limited available research suggest that fat and protein intake is adequate to meet both the needs of training and growth in most young athletes.

TABLE 10.4
Estimated Average Daily Requirements of Selected Mineral Suggested for Young Athletes

Age Group	Calcium (mg)	Iron (mg)	Zinc (mg)
Males 9–13 years	1300	5.9	7
Females 9–13 years	1300	5.7	7
Males 14–18 years	1300	7.7	8.5
Females 14–18 years	1300	7.9	7.3

Source: Adapted from Petrie, H.J., Stover, E.A., and Horswill, C.A. 2004. *Nutr.*, 20, 620–631.[8]

However, during growth spurts or in young athletes undertaking regular physical training with high energy expenditures (e.g., swimming, dancing, gymnastics), protein intake should increase to ensure adequate supply of amino acids for tissue synthesis and muscle repair.

Micronutrient intake for young athletes appears adequate, except in young athletes undertaking high-volume or intensity training or who may be in at-risk groups such as distance runners, swimmers, gymnasts, and dancers who may be restricting energy intake or taking in inadequate energy. In such groups, it appears that iron and zinc needs may increase and in young female athletes with diet- or exercise-induced amenorrhea, calcium requirements may increase from 1300 mg/day to 1500 mg/day (see Table 10.4 for daily recommended intakes of calcium, iron and zinc).

In conclusion, the limited available research on the nutrient and energy needs of young athletes suggests the need for increased energy intake with an increased energy intake that emphasizes carbohydrates and, during growth spurts, increased protein intake. In recognition of these facts, Sports Dieticians Australia[56] has recommended increased intakes of cereals, vegetables, fruit, and dairy products for young athletes compared with normal healthy Australian children (Table 10.5).

F. Fluids

Compared with the available research on hydration and thermoregulation in adult athletes, relatively few studies have been conducted on children and adolescent athletes. A number of reviews[57–59] and position statements[60] have focused on the issue,

TABLE 10.5
Recommended Number of Servings of Food for Child and Adolescent Athletes

Food Group	4–7 Years	8–11 Years	12–18 Years	SDA Recommendation
Cereals	5–7	6–9	5–11	3–9+
Vegetables, legumes	2	3	3	2–5+
Fruit	1	1	3	1–2+
Milk, yogurt and cheese	2	2	3	2–3
Lean meat, fish. poultry, nuts, legumes	1	1	1	1
Extra foods (e.g., cakes, pies, soft drinks, lollies)	1–2	1–2	1–3	1–2

SDA = Sports Dieticians Australia

Source: Adapted from Baghurst, K. and Binns, C. 2003. Dietary *Guidelines for Children and Adolescents in Australia.* Canberra: National Health and Medical Research Council[1] and Sports Dietitians Australia. 2001. *Fuelling and Cooling the Junior Athlete*. Melbourne: Sports Dietitians Australia.[56]

with a recent review highlighting the differences between young and mature athletes when examining heat regulation during exercise.[61]

Children have less developed and less efficient thermoregulatory mechanisms than adults.[61] Specifically, the available research has identified the following age-related differences in thermoregulatory factors between young and mature athletes:

1. *Body size*: Children in particular and adolescents in general have a larger body surface area (BSA) to BM ratio (BSA:Mass) than adults. As a result, during exercise they generate more heat per kilogram of BM than adolescents or adults but their ability to transfer heat from the core to the skin is less effective. Moreover, they are also exposed to a faster influx of heat when the environmental temperature exceeds skin temperature, thus making it more difficult to regulate their core body temperature. Even during the puberty-related growth spurts, smaller adolescents may continue to be thermoregulatory challenged due to their greater BSA:Mass ratio compared with adults.
2. *Sweating mechanisms*: The major form of heat loss during exercise in high ambient temperatures is evaporation of sweat from the skin. Research has consistently shown that children have immature sweat mechanisms compared with adults, with children relying more on convection and radiation than evaporation to thermoregulate.[61] Children have a lower sweat rate than adults (approx. 2.5 times less) due to a lower sweat production rate per sweat gland.[62] This sweat rate is higher at the end of puberty than at the beginning.[63] Furthermore, children are at greater risk of heat-related injuries due to the sweating threshold (the core temperature when sweating starts) being higher in children than in adults.[63]
3. *Voluntary hydration*: Like adults, children and adolescents progressively dehydrate when left to drink *ad libitum*.[64] However, dehydration in children is accompanied by a more rapid rise in core temperature compared with adults, possibly due to a lower cardiac output or evaporative cooling capacity in children.[65] Recent research examining the determinants of endurance exercise capacity in the heat in prepubertal boys suggests that this more rapid rise in core temperature or brain perception (RPE), rather than circulatory insufficiency, may be the critical factors defining limits to exercise in the heat in children.[66]
4. *Drinking practices*: While water is often described as the best choice of fluid before, during, and after vigorous physical activity, a sports electrolyte-replacement drink may help children rehydrate more effectively.[67] Studies on voluntary drinking habits and flavor preferences in children after exercise also suggest that they drink more fluids to rehydrate when flavored (especially grape or orange) sports drinks are offered instead of water.[67,68] During exercise, it appears that both junior endurance athletes[64] and team players[69] may not take in adequate fluid during competition performance. For example, Dougherty and others (2006)[69] demonstrated a significant deterioration in basketball skill performance and court sprint performance accompanying 2% dehydration in skilled 12- to 15-yr-old

basketball players. In contrast, when fluid replacement was adequate and included a 6% sports drink, both basketball shooting performance and on-court sprinting significantly improved compared with taking in water alone.[69] Moreover, recent research has suggested that exogenous carbohydrate oxidation is significantly higher during exercise in pre- and early-pubertal boys, compared with pubertal boys.[29,70] Taken together, these results strongly suggest the use of sports drinks as a fluid replacement during exercise in children.

5. *Clothing*: As discussed earlier, children's and adolescents' larger BSA:Mass ratio and less well-developed sweating mechanisms compared with adults mean they rely more heavily on convection and radiation than evaporation to thermoregulate.[71] This would strongly suggest that the type (light-colored and cotton) and fit (loose) of clothing for children and adolescents exercising in the heat is important to minimize radiant heat load and increase the body's access to air currents for convective heat loss, respectively.
6. *Acclimatization*: The limited available research suggest that young athletes can improve their heat tolerance with improved aerobic fitness and acclimatization, as adults can.[72] Similar to adults, children and adolescents adapt to heat stress through lowering heart rates, lowering core and skin temperatures, increasing sweat rates, lowering the core temperature at which sweat onset occurs, and reducing the loss of electrolytes in sweat. However, the limited available research evidence suggests that the rate of acclimatization is slower in children and adolescents than in adults.[72]

In conclusion, a recent review highlighted that an optimal drink volume and composition for young people during exercise depends upon age, sweat and urine electrolyte losses, drink palatability, fat mass, stage of puberty, clothing worn, and degree of acclimatization.[61] The same researchers stated that it is thus not possible to recommend a single volume for all children and adolescents. However, maintaining adequate hydration before, during, and after exercise is crucial for the prevention of heat injuries in children and adolescents, as it is in adult athletes. The lower sweat capacity of children and adolescents compared with adults' may suggest that a smaller fluid intake during exercise may be appropriate. However, the limited research available suggests that for a given level of dehydration, children experience a greater increase in core temperature compared with adults.[65] As a result, the margin for detrimental fluid loss may be smaller. Table 10.6 outlines the Sports Medicine Australia guidelines for fluid replacement before, during, and after exercise in children and adolescents.[73]

G. Supplement Use

Adolescents are likely to use supplements to enhance performance and recovery. A survey of UK junior track and field athletes reported 62% of athletes used some type of supplement, mainly multivitamins.[41] In a survey of Australian adolescents, supplements were used for short-term health benefits, prevention of illness, improved immunity, an energy boost, better sports performance, and to rectify a poor diet.[42]

TABLE 10.6
Sports Medicine Australia Guidelines for Fluid Replacement in Children and Adolescents

Age (years)	Time (minutes)	Volume (mL)*
Approximately 15	45 (before exercise)	300–400
	20 (during exercise)	150–200
	As soon as possible after exercise	Liberal until urination
Approximately 10	45 (before exercise)	150–200
	20 (during exercise)	75–100
	As soon as possible after exercise	Liberal until urination

* In hot environments fluid intake may need to be more frequent.

Source: Adapted from Sports Medicine Australia. 1997. Guidelines for fluid replacement in children and adolescents.[73]

Currently, no evidence supports the use of supplements for enhanced growth, lean body mass, or physical performance in healthy adolescents. Young athletes generally consume more food and therefore obtain adequate amounts of vitamins and minerals from dietary sources. Adolescents with marginal intake of nutrients such as iron and calcium may benefit from use of a vitamin or mineral supplement. Young athletes who are vegetarian, on energy-restricted diets, or amenorrheic should seek medical or dietetic advice in regard to supplementation.[7]

Adolescents are particularly vulnerable to peer pressure and anecdotal stories by their sporting heroes who endorse the use of supplements. In addition, many believe that supplements available from health food stores are safe and have been scientifically tested,[74] and are unaware of any potential risks.[42] Young athletes should be made aware that supplements will not instantly improve their performance or change their physique, and may be potentially dangerous to their health.

The efficacy and potentially harmful effects of ergogenic substances have not been researched in athletes younger than 18 years.[75] Muscle-building substances such as protein powders, creatine monohydrate and β-hydroxy-β-methylbutyrate (HMB) are frequently used by young male athletes. However, the long-term safety of many of these substances is unknown. Furthermore, some ingredients in these products may be banned and may result in a positive drug test. The consensus by the American College of Sports Medicine is that creatine monohydrate should not be consumed by children under 18 years.[76] The American Academy of Pediatrics has taken a stronger stance and condemns the use of any performance-enhancing substance by children and adolescents.[75]

The increased use of energy drinks and other caffeinated beverages in children and adolescents is also of concern. In a study of Australian adolescents, those involved in sport, particularly males, reported deliberately using energy drinks as stimulants.[42] While there are no formal guidelines for caffeine consumption in children and adolescents, children who consume high levels of caffeine may experience headaches and sleep disturbances.[77] Further investigation into the use of supplements, energy drinks, and other products containing caffeine in adolescent athletes is warranted.

H. Food Habits

Few studies have been conducted on the determinants of healthy eating habits in children. One of the most extensive reviews in the area suggests a number of individual, economic, social, and environmental factors influence healthy food choice in western children.[78] These are summarized in Table 10.7.

While many factors contribute to childhood obesity and children's poor diets, food marketing affects children's food choices, preferences, diets, and health. A recent Australian study[79] examined the nature and amount of both healthy and unhealthy food sales promotion use on food packaging in selected Australian supermarkets, specifically those directed at children. The study found that within seven food categories (cookies, snack foods, confectionery, chips and savory snacks, cereals, dairy snacks, and ice cream), between 9 and 35% of food products used promotional tactics. The use of television, movie celebrities, and cartoon characters for promotion was most common, making up 75% of all promotions, with giveaways accounting for 13% of all promotions. Data from this study also confirmed that 82% of all food promotions were for unhealthy foods and only 18% were used to promote healthy foods.[79]

In support of the suggestion that food marketing is negatively affecting children's nutrition, a recent North American study assessed the nutritional quality of the foods marketed by Nickelodeon, one of the largest companies that markets food to children.[80] The study showed that of 168 television food ads, 148 (88%) were for foods of poor nutritional quality. Of 21 Nickelodeon magazine food ads, 16 (76%) were for foods of poor nutritional quality. Fifteen grocery store products were identified with Nickelodeon characters on the packaging; 9 (60%) were foods of poor nutritional quality. In addition, of the 48 possible children's meal combinations at restaurants with promotional offers tied to Nickelodeon programs, 45 (94%) were of poor nutritional quality. Taken together, these studies highlight the reason that the American Academy of Pediatrics[81] concluded that television has a negative influence on the nutritional status of children and adolescents and recommended limiting television viewing to 1–2 hours a day.

Parents, caregivers, siblings, peers, and coaches can act as role models and be major influences on children's food choices later in life.[82] The "Dietary guidelines for children and adolescents in Australia"[1] has recommended the following strategies for encouraging the adoption of good eating habits and monitoring of food intake in children and adolescents:

1. Establish routines where the child and caregiver sit down together and talk during meal times and snacks.
2. Establish habits—such as milk with a meal or water at bedtime—that will help ensure variety and nutritional adequacy.
3. Keep in the fridge or on the kitchen counter a 'snack-box' containing healthy snack foods such as fruit, vegetables, cheese and small sandwiches that children can either use independently or have offered to them.

TABLE 10.7
Factors Affecting Healthy Food Choices in Children and Youth

Determinant	Factor(s)
Individual	• Age (e.g., decreased diet quality and breakfast consumption and increased snacking with age) • Gender (females at greater nutritional risk than males) • Food preferences (taste) • Nutrition knowledge and relationship to physical activity and health (generally low among children) • Attitudes
Economic	• Income and socio-economic status • Food pricing (low income leads to poor healthy food choices) • Education (low parental education levels leads to poor health food choices) • Employment (maternal employment negatively associated with family meal frequency)
Social	• Cultural • Familial ○ parental intakes, especially maternal, strongly influence childrens' food choices ○ food exposure and availability (positive influence) ○ family-focused meal structures (positive influence) ○ authoritarian parenting style ('junk foods' as rewards or restricted for punishment are negative influences) ○ Parental knowledge and attitudes (positive influence) • Peers ○ Peer modeling a strong predictor, especially with new foods in pre-schoolers • Product marketing/mass media ○ Influence food preferences, food purchases and food requests ○ Influence knowledge and attitudes ○ Influence dieting behavior and body image problems (especially girls) ○ Television a major negative influence as it promotes less healthy foods and influences food requests.
Environmental	• Home ○ Healthy food availability and access (positive influence) • Fast-food establishment ○ Expanding food portion size (negative influence) ○ Increased energy dense but nutrient poor foods (negative influence) • School ○ Availability of healthy food (positive influence) ○ School policy (positive influence) ○ School curricula (positive influence) ○ Teacher and peer modeling (positive influence)

Source: Adapted from Taylor, J. P., Evers, S., and McKenna, M. 2005. *Can. J. Public Health.* 96 Suppl 3, S20-6, S22-9.[78]

4. Introduce the practice of including the child at mealtimes as soon as he or she is able to sit up and handle meals.
5. Do not give the child too large a serving. It is better to offer small amounts and have more available if desired.
6. Provide foods the child likes, plus new food to try. Be accepting if the child does not like particular foods, but remember that likes and dislikes change over time. Do not avoid serving a food the child dislikes but the rest of the family likes; continue to serve it, placing only a small amount on the child's plate; and accept it if it is not eaten.

Adolescents have eating behaviors that differ from adults' and children's.[83] However, to date. most research has focused on eating patterns of adults. Furthermore, there is little information on the eating behaviors of adolescent athletes. Rapid physical and cognitive development in this age group is substantial.[11] Despite their additional energy requirements, many adolescents consume diets that are not adequate to meet their developmental needs.[84,85] While most adolescents are aware of the importance of a healthy diet, their eating behaviors are heavily influenced by age-related attitudes and beliefs. Food choices are influenced by factors such as physical growth, peer group pressure, the media, and psychological factors such as body image (Table 10.8).[86]

The taste preferences of adolescents are generally for high-fat, fast, and take-away foods,[87] with snacks contributing significantly to energy intake.[4] Many adolescents cite lack of time and convenience as significant barriers to healthy eating[86] and many eat from boredom.[88] Skipping meals is also a common behavior. Breakfast intake declines as children move into adolescence, particularly in girls.[89] This may be associated with attempts to lose weight through energy restriction. There is also a decrease in frequency of meals eaten with the family as youngsters age.[86] Adolescents who eat with their family have been shown to eat more fruit and vegetables and fewer fried foods.[90]

Throughout childhood, eating habits of boys and girls are similar. As children move into adolescence, gender differences become more apparent. Female adolescents are influenced by their emotional state and are more likely to diet to lose weight.[91] Concerns with body image can translate into poor eating practices and

TABLE 10.8
Factors Affecting Adolescent Food Choices

Most Important	Secondary Importance	Less Importance
Food cravings	Food availability	Mood
Appeal of food (taste)	Parental influence	Body image
Time considerations	Perceived benefit (get energy, body shape)	Habit
Convenience	The situation (with peers, family)	Cost, Media, Vegetarian

Source: Adapted from Neumark-Sztainer, D., Story, M., Perry, C., and Casey, M. 1999. *J. Am. Diet Assoc.* 99, 929–937.[86]

TABLE 10.9
Suitable Snack Food for Adolescent Athletes

Breakfast cereal with milk
Sandwiches or bread rolls filled with cheese or meat (turkey, chicken, tuna)
Pancakes with banana and honey
Smoothies (made with milk, fruit and yogurt) or milkshakes
Homemade pizzas (made with English muffins or pita bread)
Dried fruit and nut mixes
Pita bread and hummus
Stewed fruit and yogurt sprinkled with Granola
Cereal and sports bars
Liquid meal supplements
English muffins or crumpets spread with peanut butter
Baked or microwave potato topped with salsa and grated cheese

disordered eating patterns. However, adolescent females tend to have better nutrition knowledge, and eat more fruit and vegetables and fewer foods that are high in fat and sugar than adolescent boys.[88,92]

Adolescents may obtain their nutrition information from a range of sources. Girls are more likely than boys to obtain their information from magazines.[88] Coaches, trainers, and peers have been identified as primary sources of nutrition information for the athlete.[93] Coaches, in particular, have been shown to be linked to eating habits in adolescent athletes.[94] Younger, less experienced athletes may follow the dietary advice provided by their coach, trainer, or peers when they are eating with them and modify their food intake accordingly.

In educating younger athletes, it is important to understand the various influences on food choice that can assist in providing appropriate advice to this age group. Adolescent athletes should be encouraged to consume nutritious snacks that will assist with meeting additional energy requirements (Table 10.9). As breakfast is a meal that is commonly high in carbohydrate, adolescent athletes who skip this meal may struggle to adequately meet the additional energy and carbohydrate requirements of training and competition. Young athletes should be encouraged to be responsible for their own food choices and be provided with simple information on how to choose suitable food. Parents can assist by modeling healthy eating practices and attitudes towards eating.

I. Adolescent Body Image and Weight Control

Concerns about body image are common in adolescents and can start before puberty in both boys and girls.[91] Young males tend to prefer a muscular physique, while young females prefer to be small and thin.[91] Concerns about body image may translate to restricted energy intake, poor eating practices, and disordered eating. Many young athletes who are not overweight may attempt to lose weight due to issues with body image.

Many children and adolescents are involved in sports where a lean physique is perceived to be advantageous (e.g., gymnastics, diving, rowing, boxing, wrestling, and swimming). Other sports emphasize attaining maximal muscle mass with minimal body fat (e.g., soccer, rugby, wrestling, weightlifting). Reduction in BM can also be of benefit to performance in certain sports such as distance running, rowing, and cycling.[95] Common methods used to reduce weight include food restriction, vomiting, overexercising, diet pill use, inappropriate use of prescribed stimulants or insulin, nicotine use, and voluntary dehydration.[96] These practices can impair athlete performance and increase risk of injury.[96] Medical complications may include delayed maturation, oligomenorrhea (infrequent menstruation), and amenorrhea (absence of menstruation) in females, development of eating disorders, permanent growth impairment, increased risk of infectious diseases, and changes in endocrine, gastrointestinal, renal, cardiovascular, and thermoregulatory systems and depression.[13]

Restriction of food intake is the most common way athletes attempt to lose weight.[95,96] Many studies have shown that young athletes, in particular female athletes involved in weight sensitive sports, have low energy intakes.[97]

Young athletes may overly restrict dietary fat intake to control their weight. This may result in an insufficient intake of essential fatty acids and fat-soluble vitamins A, D, E, and K. Elimination of fat may also result in an inadequate intake of protein-rich foods.[8] This may cause a negative nitrogen balance and be insufficient for adequate growth. Young athletes should be counseled on nutritional requirements for their age, including calcium and Vitamin D and the benefits of regular weight-bearing exercise for bone health.[13] Food restriction may develop into disordered eating behaviors such as fasting, bingeing, and purging.

J. Disordered Eating

Female adolescents who participate in sports where there is emphasis on a lean physique may be at increased risk of disordered eating.[14] Some young athletes develop clinical eating disorders such as anorexia nervosa, bulimia nervosa, or eating disorders not otherwise specified. Eating disorders appear to peak in prevalence and severity during adolescence and may be related to physiological, psychological, and social changes that occur during this time.[89]

Restrictive eating in young females can impair reproductive and skeletal health. The interrelationship between energy availability, menstrual function, and bone mineral density is described as the female athlete triad.[13] Most negative effects occur when energy availability is below 30 $kcal.kg^{-1}$ of fat-free mass per day. Menstrual dysfunction or functional hypothalamic amenorrhea (secondary amenorrhea) can result in low peak bone density (z-score of –1.0 to –2.0 below the expected range for age).[13] Poor bone density and menstrual irregularity is associated with increased rate of stress fractures.[98] The prevalence of delayed menarche (primary amenorrhea) has been shown to be 22% in adolescent female athletes[99] in comparison with 1% of the general population.[100] Secondary amenorrhea (loss of menstruation) has been shown to be higher (67%) in female runners of less than 15 years of gynecological age compared with their older counterparts (9%).[101] Young athletes who have been identified with the female athlete triad will require multidisciplinary treatment including a physician, a mental health practitioner, and a dietician. The younger the athlete, the greater the need for family involvement in the treatment.[13]

K. Summary

The nutrition needs of child and adolescent athletes are crucial for their overall health, growth and maturation, and sporting performance. As with adult athletes, a well-nourished and hydrated athlete will play better and for longer, stay more mentally alert, and recover more quickly from training and competition. In contrast, young athletes who are undernourished through not eating well or too little may suffer poor bone growth, delayed maturation, and poor sports performance.

Sports Dietitians Australia[56] has developed a fact sheet for fueling and cooling junior athletes during sporting events and recovery from training and competition.

- During day-long events
- Take food and drinks to events including simple and quick snacks (see Table 10.10).
- Include two water bottles per athlete, one of water, the other a flavored drink e.g., sports drink, cordial or juice. Encourage the continual sipping of the drinks.
- If conditions are hot, include frozen fruit juices.
- If there is less than 1 hour before or between events, priority is carbohydrate-rich fluids or jelly confectionery for quick energy boosts.
- If there is 1–2 hours between events, have fluids and a light snack (Table 10.10) such as energy bars, cereal bars, fresh or canned fruit, bread with honey or jam, low-fat dairy product, or a small number of jelly lollipops.
- If there is longer than 2 hours between events, offer sandwiches, bread rolls, toast, crumpets and honey, baked beans, spaghetti, noodles, cereal and milk, creamy rice and fruit, or pancakes. If nerves are a problem, try liquid meals such as a smoothie instead of solid foods.
- If the break is longer than 3 hours, consume a larger meal.
- Eating for recovery after day-long events
- Canned, frozen and packet products that are high carbohydrate foods (rice, pasta).

TABLE 10.10
Simple and Quick Snacks Recommended for Children and Adolescent Athletes

Pancakes/scones/muffins	Flavored dairy foods (yogurt/milk)
Muesli/cereal bars	Smoothies/milk shakes
Fruit—canned/fresh/dried	Baked bean snack paks
Jellied fruit packs	Canned noodles/spaghetti
Fruit juice	Dairy desserts
Fruit buns/fruit loaf	Boiled potato/sweet corncobs
Breakfast cereal	Honey/jam/cheese sandwich
Bread/rolls/crumpets	Cracker biscuits with cheese and spread

- Salad bars at restaurants.
- High-carbohydrate, low-fat dessert.
- After sport meals
- Drink lots of fluids.
- Carbohydrate-rich foods such as fruit or juice, crackers with cheese, toast, bread, or crumpets, muffins, fruit bread, rice or pasta with stir fry meat and vegetables, canned beans and salad, mashed potatoes and salad.

III. PREGNANT AND LACTATING ATHLETES

A. Introduction

A number of potential health benefits exist for women who continue a regular exercise program throughout pregnancy. These include prevention of gestational diabetes, less subcutaneous fat deposition, facilitation of labor, and reduced stress.[102]

Currently, few studies have investigated the specific nutritional requirements of athletes who continue to engage in regular high-intensity exercise throughout pregnancy. Dietary advice for pregnant women is commonly focused on preventing low infant birth weight, decreasing the risk of neural tube defects, and preventing fetal alcohol syndrome. However, a number of diet-related complications may occur during pregnancy that require specific advice from a nutrition expert. These include nausea and vomiting, heartburn, constipation and hemorrhoids, edema, gestational diabetes, and pregnancy-induced hypertension.[102] The physiological effects of pregnancy that are most likely to impact on nutrient requirements in the athlete are an increase in blood volume, cardiac output, oxygen requirements, slowing of the gastrointestinal system, and alterations to thermoregulatory control.[102,103] Pregnant athletes can benefit from specific nutrition advice that can meet the changing physiological needs and dietary-related complications of pregnancy, and a concurrent exercise regime.

Birth weight is correlated with infant mortality and morbidity. Low birth weight (< 2500g) and very low birth weight (< 1500g) are major factors in perinatal mortality.[104] Newborns who are small for gestational age are at risk of hypertension, obesity, glucose intolerance, and cardiovascular disease.[104] There have been reports that suggest a link between women who engage in strenuous physical activities and lower-birth-weight babies.[105] However, other studies have failed to confirm this association.[106,107] The guidelines of the American College of Obstetricians and Gynecologists for exercise during pregnancy and postpartum period state that "it appears that birth weight is not affected by exercise in women who have adequate energy intake" (p. 8).[103] Conversely, the additive energy requirements of exercise and pregnancy when combined with poor maternal weight gain may lead to fetal growth restriction.[103] Furthermore, birth weight has been shown to be substantially lower in women exercised at or above 50% of preconception levels compared with nonexercisers.[108] This suggests that female athletes should not attempt to increase the intensity or duration of their training during pregnancy. Maternal size and pregnancy weight gain have been correlated to infant birth weight.[102] Weight gain in pregnant athletes may be less than for the sedentary women. This has been attributed to decreased neonatal fat mass.[108]

TABLE 10.11
Dietary Reference Intake Values for Energy during Pregnancy and Lactation

Pregnancy

Age (years)	Stage of Pregnancy	Estimated Energy Requirement (EER)[a] kcal (kJ)
14–18	1st trimester	2368 (9898)
	2nd trimester	2708 (11319)
	3rd trimester	2820 (11788)
19–50	1st trimester	2403 (10045)[b]
	2nd trimester	2743 (11466)[b]
	3rd trimester	2855 (11934)[b]

Lactation

Age (years)	Stage of lactation	Estimated Energy Requirement (EER)[a] kcal (kJ)
14–18	1st 6 months	2698 (11278)
	2nd 6 months	2768 (11570)
19–50	1st 6 months	2733 (11424)[b]
	2nd 6 months	2803 (11717)[b]

[a] The intake meets that meets the average energy expenditure of individuals at the reference height, weight and age.

[b] Subtract 7 kcal/d (29.3kJ/d) for each year above 19 years.

Source: Adapted from the Institute of Medicine, Food and Nutrition Board, 2002. *Dietary Reference Intakes for Energy, Carbohydrate, Fiber, Fat, Fatty Acids, Cholesterol, Protein and Amino Acids.*[18]

B. Energy Requirements

Additional energy is required to meet the needs of the developing fetus and the metabolic needs of pregnancy. Energy requirements increase with increase in weight.[103] There is an increase in requirements of 340 to 360 kcal/day (1421 to 1505 kJ/day) during the second trimester and an additional 112 kcal/d (470 kJ/day) in the third trimester.[102] See Table 10.11.

Overall energy requirements will increase with increased physical activity. The female athlete who has trained up until pregnancy and is in energy balance will have an energy intake matched to her current level of activity. As her training level is likely to decrease in the second and third trimesters, it is unlikely that the athlete will need to significantly increase her energy intake beyond the additional needs of pregnancy. However, some female athletes are restrictive eaters who limit their energy intake to control their weight.[13] Excessive exercise with inadequate energy intake may lead to suboptimal intake and poor fetal growth.[103] The impact of restrictive energy intakes in recreational or elite athletes who continue to exercise throughout pregnancy and the effect on fetal growth and development has not been addressed in the literature. Female athletes who have previously been diagnosed with disordered eating should be carefully monitored throughout pregnancy.

C. Carbohydrate Requirements

Carbohydrate is an important fuel source for the developing fetus; particularly during the second and third trimester of pregnancy.[109] Pregnant athletes require adequate carbohydrate to meet the concurrent demands of exercise and pregnancy. Furthermore, there is evidence that pregnant women may use carbohydrate at a greater rate both at rest and during exercise than nonpregnant women. Soultanakis et al.[110] found that 1 hour of continuous prolonged exercise at 55% of maximal oxygen consumption resulted in a significantly faster decline in blood glucose to a lower level post exercise in pregnant women compared with nonpregnant women. Artal et al.[111] did not find any significant difference in blood glucose before and after 15 minutes of a low-intensity exercise bout, suggesting that the intensity and duration of the exercise impacts on the ability to maintain blood glucose in pregnancy. However, research on substrate use during exercise in pregnant athletes is limited. Further studies investigating the use of carbohydrate as a fuel source during pregnancy are needed before any conclusive recommendations on carbohydrate intake can be made.

D. Protein Requirements

Protein requirements increase during gestation and are greatest in the third trimester. However, increase in protein requirements are usually met by a subsequent increase in total energy intake.[102] Athletes also have increased requirement for protein depending on the type, intensity, and duration of exercise. Provided sufficient additional energy is consumed to meet the needs of exercise and pregnancy, protein requirements will in most circumstances be adequate to meet additional needs.

E. Iron Requirements

Increase in the maternal blood supply increases the demand for dietary iron. Iron requirements increase substantially during pregnancy (an additional 700–800 mg throughout the pregnancy), although a higher rate of absorption also compensates for this increase.[112] Athletes also have higher iron requirements and potentially higher losses than nonathletes.[36] Pregnant or lactating athletes have very high iron requirements, despite no menstrual blood loss, and are unlikely to meet these needs from their dietary intake. Iron supplementation may be necessary to meet the physiological needs of pregnancy and exercise. If the athlete continues training through pregnancy, hemoglobin and hematocrit should be measured every 6 to 8 weeks and 2 to 3 weeks postpartum. A level of hemoglobin less than 12g/dL has been suggested to impede training in the pregnant athlete.[113] Iron deficiency anemia is commonly treated with 60–120 mg of ferrous iron throughout the day.[102] Once hemoglobin levels return to normal, 30 mg/d may be continued. Excessive doses of iron are not recommended in pregnancy as they have been linked to the pathogenesis of preeclampsia and gestational diabetes.[102] For women of childbearing age who become pregnant, the importance of eating foods high in heme-iron or iron-rich foods or iron-fortified foods with an enhancer of iron absorption such as vitamin C-rich foods is highlighted as one of the key recommendations of the 2005 *Dietary Guidelines for Americans*.[114]

F. Folic Acid Requirements

Folic acid requirements increase throughout pregnancy and are particularly important in the early stages for the prevention of neural tube defects. The recommended daily allowance (RDA) for folic acid in non-pregnant women is 400 mcg/d.[115] This increases during pregnancy and lactation to 600 mcg/d. The Institute of Medicine, Food and Nutrition Board,[115] recommends that 400 mcg come from folate-fortified foods or supplements in additional to dietary folate, and suggests that women should commence taking additional folate prior to conception. The importance of this to women of childbearing age who become pregnant and those in the first trimester of pregnancy is highlighted as one of the key recommendations of the 2005 *Dietary Guidelines for Americans.*[114] Specifically, these women should consume adequate synthetic folic acid daily from fortified foods or supplements in addition to food forms (mushrooms, green vegetables, peanuts, legumes, citrus fruits) of folate from a varied diet. Female athletes who are trying to conceive are advised to take a folic acid supplement.

G. Other Considerations

1. Thermoregulation

During pregnancy, heat production is increased due to an increase in basal metabolic rate. Data on the effect of exercise on core temperature during pregnancy is limited. An increase in maternal core temperature of more than 1.5°C during formation of the embryo can cause congenital malformations.[102] Maintenance of euhydration and blood volume is clearly of importance to the pregnant woman to ensure heat dissipation to prevent a rise in core temperature. Pregnant women should exercise caution when exercising in hot, humid conditions. Particular attention should be paid to ensuring regular fluid consumption before, during, and after exercise sessions.

2. Caffeine

Caffeine may be harmful in pregnancy. Intakes above 300 mg/day (four average-sized cups or three average-sized mugs of instant coffee or six average-sized cups of tea) may be associated with low birth weight and miscarriage.[116] Pregnant athletes should be made aware of the risks of caffeine consumption above this amount. This may be particularly relevant to athletes who have previously used caffeine as an ergogenic aid in addition to habitual consumption.

3. Adolescent Athletes and Pregnancy

Adolescents have a higher risk of low-birth-weight infants.[102] Many enter pregnancy with a suboptimal nutrient intake due to poor eating habits. Pregnant adolescent athletes need specific nutrition counseling to ensure adequate weight gain throughout pregnancy. Special attention should be paid to at-risk nutrients, in particular low iron, calcium, and folic acid intake.

4. Postpartum

Exercise regimes should be gradually resumed, as many of the physiological changes of pregnancy persist for 4 to 6 weeks after delivery.[103] Some detraining will have occurred and therefore resumption should be gradual. Some athletes may be anxious to regain their pre-pregnancy weight. Moderate weight reduction is encouraged. Decreased milk reduction in breastfeeding women may be attributed to inadequate fluid consumption or insufficient energy intake for training.

Athletes may want to regain their pre-pregnancy weight as soon as possible after pregnancy. Athletes who are breastfeeding should be reminded that exclusively breastfeeding with no reduction in energy intake will support the loss of body fat. Lean women may compromise milk production if they restrict their energy intake.[102] Breastfeeding before exercise may avoid any potential problem associated with increased acidity of milk due to lactic acid build-up.[103] Athletes should be encouraged to breastfeed due to the potential long-term health benefits for the baby, which may include better weight stability, decreased risk of Type 2 diabetes mellitus, and decreased incidence of infectious disease. The mother may also benefit by decreased risk of breast and ovarian cancer, improved bone health, and earlier return to pre-pregnancy weight.[117]

H. Recommendations

Exercise has minimal risks and definite benefits for most women during pregnancy.[103] However, there is minimal research on athletes who continue an intensive training regime throughout pregnancy. The American College of Obstetricians and Gynecologists (ACOG) recommends that pregnant athletes require closer supervision than routine pregnancies.[103] The overall health, obstetric, and medical risks should be assessed before an athlete is prescribed an exercise program. Once engaging in a regular training program, the nutritional, cardiovascular, and musculoskeletal condition of the athlete should be assessed regularly. The additional energy and nutrient requirements of pregnant athletes need careful planning. Advice should be sought from a sports dietitian to ensure they are obtaining sufficient energy for both pregnancy and their training regime. The athlete should be informed that she will not be able to reach the same performance levels as before pregnancy and she should not attempt to increase either intensity or duration of training. Special attention needs to be given to nutrients such as iron and folate. Pregnant adolescent athletes will need specialized nutrition care with a focus on iron, calcium, and folic acid intake.

Due to a decreased thermoregulatory response, particular attention should be paid to hydration status. Pregnant athletes should ensure that they consume adequate fluid throughout the day and drink regularly throughout training to replace fluid losses. Fluid balance can be monitored by weighing pre- and post-exercise. Carbohydrate-electrolyte drinks (sports drinks) may be of benefit during exercise due to the concurrent supply of carbohydrate and fluid. The carbohydrate may attenuate the negative effects of decreased blood glucose. It is clearly evident that further research is needed on the pregnant female athlete before specific nutrient recommendations can be made.

IV. THE AGING ATHLETE

A. INTRODUCTION

During recent decades there has been an increase in the number of older individuals engaging in regular physical activity and exercise for the health benefits of decreasing both morbidity and all-cause mortality.[118,119] Many of these physically active older individuals are increasingly becoming recreational or competitive athletes focused on sports performance. For example, the inaugural World Masters Games held in Toronto, Ontario had 8305 participants across 22 sports; the 2002 Melbourne, Australia World Masters Games 24,886 participants across 26 sports, and the 2009 World Masters Games being held in Sydney, Australia anticipating the biggest mass participation (30,000), multinational, multisport (28 sports) festival in the world.[120]

Recommendations for nutrition in aging athletes should focus on both the nutritional requirements of the aging process[121,122] and the nutrient needs of the aging exerciser.[123–131] Individuals age at greatly differing rates for genetic, environmental, lifestyle, and cultural reasons. Furthermore, aging athletes participate in sports ranging from bowling to ironman triathlon and vary from the physically dependent to the physically elite. Moreover, aging athletes compete for a wide variety of reasons with enjoyment, health and fitness benefits, social, and competition appearing to be the primary drivers for involvement.[132,133]

Compared with younger athletes, aging athletes display an age-related decline in training intensity and volume, and, as they age, appear to move from strength, speed, and power events to endurance-oriented events.[134–137] For the health professional, consideration of the above factors is further complicated by the fact that 85% of the elderly population suffers from some type of chronic degenerative disease requiring medication(s) that may have potential drug–nutrient interactions. Such interactions may affect the intake, digestion, absorption, and utilization of several nutrients.[138,139] Indeed, a number of reports have suggested that between 14% and 25% of participants in masters sport have a preexisting medical condition (primarily hypertension, asthma, coronary heart disease), with up to 34% taking medication (cardiovascular, respiratory, non-steroidal anti-inflammatory).[136,140]

Recently, nutrition research has shifted from a focus on alleviating nutrient deficiencies to also stressing chronic disease prevention in aging individuals.[141–145] Thus, the motivations, training practices, presence of chronic disease and medication usage patterns, and variety of sports or activities participated in by aging athletes make generic guidelines for nutrition in this group a challenge for the health practitioner.

The aging process, at least in sedentary individuals, is accompanied by many physiological changes that may affect nutritional needs. These include loss of muscle mass, less efficient immune system, gastric atrophy, decreased sensitivity to taste and smell, poor dental health, a loss of thirst sensitivity, decreased cardiovascular health, and decreased bone density. Whether these declines are the result of the aging process per se or the inactivity that accompanies the aging process remains to be conclusively evaluated. However, a number of empirical studies appear to suggest that some of these factors do decline with age, even in aging athletes.[146,147] For example, several studies have shown that muscle mass declines in aging endurance athletes[148,149] Thus, the health practitioner must be aware that aging athletes present with a wide range of motivations, training backgrounds, physiology, medical conditions, and dietary practices that must be considered together when giving individualized advice.

DRIs for the general population rarely include recommendations for athletes or active individuals young or old. Furthermore, the oldest age group for which many recommendations have only recently been developed is 51 to 70 years and, for only several nutrients, greater than 70 years.[150] These age ranges are very large and make little allowance for the metabolic and physiological changes that occur during aging or the activity levels or health status of aging individuals. While the limited available evidence[151,152] suggests that both men and women with higher cardiovascular fitness consume diets more closely approaching national dietary recommendations than their less fit peers, the DRIs may not be a valid means of evaluating the nutritional needs of the aging athlete in physical training of different modes, intensities, frequencies, and durations.

While several investigations have examined the dietary[153–157] and nutritional supplementation practices[158] of various aging athletic populations, only recently have a number of reviews attempted to examine the nutritional needs of an aging athletic population.[127,129,131]

B. Factors Affecting Nutritional Needs

A number of physiological changes occur in the aging athlete that may affect not only training and competition performance, but nutritional recommendations. Table 10.12 summarizes the major changes that may affect the nutritional requirements of aging athletes.

C. Energy Requirements

The daily energy requirements of an aging population decrease due to age-related decreases in each of the components of energy expenditure: resting metabolic rate (RMR), the thermic effect of food, and daily energy expenditure.[159–161] For example, Elia et al.[159] demonstrated that, in a healthy but sedentary aging population, decreased physical activity levels explained 46% of the variance in decreased daily energy expenditure with age, with decreased basal metabolic rate (44% variance) and decreased thermogenesis (10% variance) explaining the balance. Studies on male and female masters athletes have suggested that the age-related decline in RMR is attenuated in older females who remain physically active[162] and maintained at levels similar to younger athletes in male masters athletes who maintain training volumes and energy intakes.[151]

In 2002, the Institute of Medicine estimated daily energy requirements for older adults of various age groups who are physically active (Table 10.13).[18]

An age-related decrease in daily energy expenditure, in both nonathletes and physically active men training for endurance events more than three times a week, is primarily due to both age-related decreases in fat-free mass (FFM) and decreases in physical activity or training volume levels.[137,151,163,164] However, research evidence

TABLE 10.12
Age-Related Changes That May Influence Nutrient Requirements of Aging Athletes

Age-Related Change	Nutritional Implication
Decreased muscle mass	Decreased energy requirement
Decreased aerobic capacity	Decreased energy requirement
Decreased bone density	Increased need for calcium and vitamin D
Decreased immune function	Increased need for vitamins B_6, E and zinc
Decreased gastric acid	Increased need for vitamin B_{12}, folic acid, calcium, iron and zinc
Decreased skin capacity for Vitamin D synthesis	Increased need for vitamin D
Decreased calcium bioavailability	Increased need for calcium and vitamin D
Increased oxidative stress status	Increased need for carotenoids, vitamins C and E
Increased levels of homocysteine	Increased need for folate and vitamins B6 and B_{12}
Decreased thirst perception	Increased fluid needs
Decreased kidney function	Increased fluid needs

Source: Modified from Reaburn, P. 2006. Nutrition and the aging athlete, in Burke, L. and Deakin, V. (Eds.) *Clinical Sports Nutrition*, 3rd ed., p. 636. Sydney: McGraw-Hill.[129]

from sedentary populations suggests that body composition (fat mass versus FFM) changes dramatically with aging with an approximate doubling of body fat between 20 and 50–60 years of age and a fall in body fat after 70 years of age.[165,166] Similar observations of decreased FFM are also observed in older male and female endurance runners, except that the body fat levels increase only marginally with age.[151,167]

A number of studies examining the energy intakes of older athletes suggested that older athletes undertaking regular physical training have higher energy intakes

TABLE 10.13
Estimated Energy Requirements for Older Adults Who Are Active

Age Group (yr)	Males		Females	
	kcal/day	kJ/day	kcal/day	kJ/day
50–59	2757	11579	2186	9181
60–69	2657	11159	2116	8887
70–79	2557	10739	2046	8593
80–89	2457	10319	1967	8261

Source: Adapted from Intitute of Medicine. 2002. *Dietary Reference Intakes for Energy, Carbohydrates, Fiber, Fat, Protein and Amino Acids (Macronutrients).* Washington, DC: National Academy Press.[18]

than those of age-matched sedentary but healthy controls,[154,155,168] especially when matched for energy intake per kilogram of body mass.[151] Furthermore, the energy intakes of these older athletes appear higher than those suggested for their respective age groups or gender in the DRIs.[154–156] For example, energy intakes ranging between 10,336 kJ/d[155] and 11,549 kJ/d[156] have been reported by older (55–75 years) male endurance athletes, with a mean intake of 8663 kJ/d reported by 65–84-year-old female endurance athletes undertaking physical training of at least 1 hour per day.[154]

In general, the reported energy intakes of older athletes are lower than those observed in similarly trained younger athletes.[151,169,170] This may be due to an age-related decrease in active muscle mass previously observed in aging athletes,[148,149] reduced training volumes (frequency, intensity, duration) that has previously been observed in older athletes,[134–136] or reduced leisure time activity levels commonly reported in older populations.[171] Some evidence suggests that aging athletes who maintain high-intensity training at levels similar to those of younger athletes also appear to experience an age-related decline in resting energy expenditure and dietary energy requirement relative to younger athletes, but both factors are higher than those of sedentary age-matched controls.[151] This finding would suggest that the more competitive aging athlete who maintains high-volume and high-intensity training into older age may have the same percent energy and dietary requirements as a younger athlete but greater absolute needs than sedentary controls of the same age.

D. Macronutrients

Carbohydrate, fat, and protein intakes are essential for meeting not only the energy requirements of an individual, but to ensure normal bodily functioning through the associated intake of fiber, vitamins, and minerals.[172] Age-related decreases in the intakes of these macronutrients have been observed in a sedentary aging population.[161,163] The Food and Nutrition Board of the Institute of Medicine in the United States has set a macronutrient distribution range for healthy diets at 45–65% CHO, 10–35% protein, and 20–35% fat.[18] The American College of Sports Medicine (ACSM), American Dietetic Association (ADA) and the Dieticians of Canada (DC) Joint Position Statement[173] suggests that athletes will obtain adequate macronutrient intakes by consuming a body weight maintenance diet that provides energy as 55–58% CHO, 12–15% protein, and 25–30% fat.

Few studies have examined the macronutrient intake of aging athletes.[151,168] Beshgetoor and Nichols[168] examined 4-day diet records of 25 female masters cyclists and runners aged 50.4 years who used or didn't use dietary supplements. They observed 52–55% CHO, 17–20% protein, and 28% fat intake in their cohort, values that are within the guidelines for both healthy adults and athletes. Brodney et al.[152] examined nutrient intakes of 7959 men and 2453 women aged 20–87 years in low, moderate, and highly aerobically fit cohorts. They observed significantly higher percent CHO and lower percent fat intakes and in both men and women in the high fitness group compared with the low or moderate fit groups. However, the CHO intake of the high fit group was lower (48% men, 51% women) and higher for fat intake (33% men, 31% women) than that recommended by the ACSM, ADA, and DC for athletes. Taken together, these studies suggest the need for increased CHO intake and lower fat intake in aging athletes, for both performance and health reasons.

1. Carbohydrates

For athletes, CHO is the primary fuel source for working muscles and is stored within the liver and muscle as glycogen.[36] In older endurance athletes, glycogen storage per unit of muscle is lower than in similarly trained younger runners, while glycogen utilization per unit of energy expenditure appears higher during submaximal exercise.[174] However, following regular endurance training, older individuals are able to increase muscle glycogen storage and restore glycogen stores post-exercise at rates similar to younger athletes.[174,175]

The recommended CHO intake for athletes is similar to that of the general population, and therefore is similar for older athletes because CHO absorption and utilization remain intact with a physically active lifestyle and nutritious diet in aging persons.[176,177] Thus, the older athlete should consume at least 55% of energy intake as CHO obtained from a variety of food sources and the bulk of the CHO-containing foods consumed should be those rich in complex CHOs and with a low glycemic index.[24] A high percentage of this intake should be starchy CHO (bread, cereals, rice, pasta, potato), which also provides protein, vitamin, mineral, and fiber intake.

Thus, apart from the physical benefits (enhanced performance and recovery) gained by a high-CHO diet of 5–12 g/kg/d[24–26], an older athlete can also derive great health benefits that may lower all-cause mortality and morbidity. Based on this data, Table 10.14 shows the suggested daily carbohydrate needs of older athletes undertaking various types of training.

2. Fat

Dietary fat is ncessary as a source of essential fatty acids, fat-soluble vitamins (A, D, E, and K),[172] and as an energy source during low-intensity or prolonged exercise at below 70% of maximal aerobic power.[178] The optimal daily intake of fat need only be 25–30% of daily energy intake in both a young and older sedentary or exercising populations.[173] It appears that older populations are meeting this recommendation as the 1995 Australian National Nutrition Survey (NNS) showed that the mean percent energy intake for persons aged 25–65 years and over was approximately 32% for males and 33% for females, with no difference between young and older groups.[171]

TABLE 10.14
Suggested Daily Carbohydrate Needs of Older Athletes

Type of Training	CHO Needs (g/kg/d)
General training	5–7
Regular moderate intensity/Endurance	7–10
Ultraendurance	10–12

Similarly, the most recent British National Diet and Nutrition Survey of adults aged 19–64 years showed that approximately 35% of energy intake was from fats.[179]

An aging population retains the ability to digest, absorb, and utilize fat.[176,180] Furthermore, older athletes and highly aerobically fit individuals appear to consume more fat relative to total energy than the recommended population targets or than healthy sedentary age-matched controls.[152,154,156,168,181] Older athletes consuming more than 30% of daily energy intake as fat may compromise cardiovascular health. As in younger athletes, older athletes on a low-energy diet should consume between 20–25% of daily energy intake from fat sources for more energy to be derived from CHO and protein.[182] While research has shown that low-fat diets neither positively or negatively affect performance,[173] daily energy intake containing less than 20% fat may compromise the absorption of fat-soluble vitamins (A, D, E, K) and decrease satiety between meals.

3. Protein

Protein is continually being degraded and synthesized within the human body so that a dietary supply of amino acids is necessary to offset protein losses. Amino acids are used in the synthesis of structural proteins (e.g., connective tissue, muscle tissue), functional proteins (e.g., enzymes, antibodies, hemoglobin), and as an energy source in the absence of adequate glucose or fatty acids.[36]

The current U.S. DRI for protein for adults of all ages is 0.8 g/kg/d[18] and the Australian RDI is 0.75 g/kg/d.[150] An athlete's protein needs are even greater than those of a nonathlete because of increased use of protein during physical activity for gluconeogenesis, amino acid oxidation, and the tissue breakdown accompanying both training and competing.[183,184] Furthermore, within an athletic population, the DRIs for protein may vary depending on exercise intensity, CHO availability, exercise mode, energy balance, gender, training age, timing of macronutrient intake, and age.[173,183,184]

Insufficient energy intakes are also associated with a negative nitrogen balance and protein loss, given that there is a well-defined interaction between total energy intake and protein need.[185] Moreover, increased protein requirements have been observed with high- versus low-intensity exercise[186] and long- versus short-duration exercise.[187] Thus, it has been suggested that younger endurance-trained athletes in regular training consume about 1.2–1.4 g/kg BM/d (150% of current U.S. DRI) and young strength-trained athletes consume about 1.2–1.7 g/kg BM/d (200% of current U.S. DRI).[173,183]

Older endurance or power athletes may have lower protein requirements than suggested for younger athletes for a number of reasons. First, the aging process is accompanied by a decline in muscle mass in both healthy active individuals[188] and older athletes[148,149] secondary to an age-related decrease in both whole-body protein turnover and protein synthesis.[189,190] Second, older athletes appear not to train with the same intensity or volume as younger athletes.[134,136,137,191] Third, although not conclusively investigated, there may be an age-related reduction in the absorptive capacity of the gut for amino acids and peptide.[176] Fourth, due to a number of underlying problems (dietary recall problems, inadequate equilibration periods or inadequate energy intakes given by researchers in nitrogen-balance studies), the protein requirements suggested in the DRIs may have been overestimated.[126] Taken together, the above factors suggest that older athletes may require a lower daily protein intake than those suggested by Lemon[192] and the ACSM, ADA, DC[173] for younger athletes.

Thus, although the protein needs of different aged athletic populations has yet to be investigated, it has previously been suggested that aging exercisers may require 0.8–1.0 g/kg BM/d,[126] with Evans[193] suggesting older exercisers may require 1.0–1.25 g/kg BM/d to maintain or promote a positive nitrogen balance. Recently, Lucas and Heiss[194] suggested that an intake of between 1.0–1.3 g/kg BM/d for older adults engaged in resistance training, provided that their overall energy needs are being met.

The customary diets of both younger and older athletes have been shown to provide enough protein to adequately meet need, especially when the diets contain sufficient energy and include complete sources of protein (e.g., diary, meats, eggs, and fish).[151,195] However, adjustments may have to be made for illness, chronic disease, or suboptimal total energy intakes. The recommended figure of 1.0–1.3 g/kg BM/d approximates the reported protein intakes of 1.25–1.45 g/kg BM/d previously observed in older athletes and regular exercisers from a variety of training backgrounds.[151,156,164,168] However, older athletes in heavy training, particularly those involved with strength and power sports, may require increased intakes[192,195] because resistance exercise increases muscle protein synthesis in both elderly and young individuals.[196,197]

Previous data suggest that exogenous amino acids may stimulate protein synthesis in an elderly male population.[198,199] However, other studies have observed either no anabolic effect of high-protein diets[200] or no relationship between protein intake (adjusted for BM and physical activity) and appendicular muscle mass. These data suggest that protein intake above the DRI is not linked to preservation of muscle mass in older populations.[164,196] However, recent research strongly suggests that protein supplemention (0.3 g/kg), particularly when combined with creatine supplementation (5g/day), immediately before or after resistance training sessions in aging individuals may be important for creating an anabolic environment important for both muscle growth and strength gains.[201–203]

E. Micronutrients

Vitamins and minerals are essential for efficient nutrient metabolism and numerous bodily functions affecting sports performance.[36] A large proportion of older adults do not consume sufficient amounts of many micronnutrients from foods alone.[204] While supplements compensate to some extent, only an estimated half of people over 51 years of age in the United States use them daily.[204] Fewer than 50% of both supplement users and nonusers met the estimated average requirement for folate, vitamin E, and magnesium from food sources alone. After accounting for the contribution of supplements, 80% or more of users met the estimated average requirement for vitamins A, B_6, B_{12}, C, and E; folate; iron; and zinc; but not magnesium. However, some supplement users, particularly men, exceeded the tolerable upper intake levels for iron and zinc and a small percentage of women exceeded the tolerable upper intake level for vitamin A.[204]

The intensity, duration, and frequency of the sport or training session and the overall energy and nutrient intakes of the individual athlete increases an athlete's requirements for vitamins and minerals above recommended levels.[43] This increased need may be the result of many factors, including losses via sweat, urine, and feces; decreased gastrointestinal absorption; increased degradation rates; increased needs for muscle and connective tissue maintenance and repair; increased metabolic rates at rest and during exercise; and the stress of early bodily adaptation to heavy training loads.[205] Research has shown that a linear relationship exists between overall energy intake and vitamin and mineral intake.[169,206] High-energy intakes are required by both younger[170] and older athletes[154–156,168] to meet the energy demands of physical training and competition. It would thus be expected that the micronutrient intake in both these groups should be in excess of the DRIs, assuming that a well-balanced diet is chosen.

Numerous studies examining the dietary practices of younger athletes have shown that dietary intakes of the minerals zinc, iron, magnesium, copper and calcium, together with the vitamins B_6, B_{12}, and D, are below the DRIs.[170,182] The few studies that have examined nutritional intakes of older endurance athletes suggest low intakes of the minerals calcium, iron, zinc, and magnesium, and vitamins D and E, despite consuming energy intakes that were well above the DRIs.[154–156,168]

Athletes, in general, have increased losses of many micronutrients, especially minerals, compared with nonathletes, as a result of losses through sweat and urine,[207] especially during endurance activities.[205] When associated with low dietary intakes, the body stores of these micronutrients can be reduced,[173] resulting in a deficiency state which negatively affects performance.[205] Furthermore, the risk of micronutrient deficiency may be higher in older athletes who have very low energy intakes or chronic medical conditions, or take medications that may impair micronutrient absorption or utilization.[138] This review examined in detail the area of food–drug interactions and highlighted that more than 50% of non-institutionalized Americans aged over 65 years or over use five or more medications, and 12% use 10 or more. More importantly, 25% take prescribed drugs from one or two therapeutic classes, more than 20% from three classes, 30% from four or five classes, and over 15% from six or more classes. This highlights the issue of polypharmacy in older individuals and the importance of the health practitioner in screening for such usage when working with the aging athlete. A number of previous reports have suggested that between 14% and 25% of participants in masters sport have a preexisting medical condition (primarily hypertension, asthma, coronary heart disease), with up to 34% taking medication (cardiovascular, respiratory, non-steroidal anti-inflammatory).[136,140]

Older athletes may be at a greater risk of micronutrient deficiencies than younger athletes. Possible reasons for this increased risk are age-related gut impairment associated with reduced nutrient absorption,[176] different nutrient requirements between individuals, use of medication (Table 10.15), and the presence of chronic disease states.

TABLE 10.15
Drug–Nutrient Interactions That May Affect Nutrient Requirements

Drug	Effect	Nutrients Affected
Diuretics (e.g., *Aldactone, Chlotoride, Lasix*)	Alterations in renal tubular function	Loss of sodium, potassium and magnesium
Antipsychotic / psychoactives	Disinterest in food	Protein and calories intake reduced
Cardiac glycosides (e.g., *Digoxin*)	Anorexia, nausea, vomiting, disinterest in food	Protein and calories intake reduced
Anticonvulsants (e.g., *Phenytoin, Dilantin, Phenobarbitone*)	Induction of liver enzymes	Altered vitamin D metabolism Folic acid
	Reduced absorption of folic acid	
Salicyclate (e.g., *Aspirin, Voltaren, Nurofen, Orudis*)	Gastrointestinal blood loss	Iron deficiency
Corticosteroids (e.g., *Prednisone, Prednisolone, Cortisone*)	Inhibition of calcium absorption, alterations in glucose metabolism and electrolyte imablance	Calcium imbalance (osteoporosis), hyperglycemia, sodium retention and potassium deficiency Vitamin C
	Increased excretion of vitamin C	
Antacids	Decreased absorption of phosphate	Phosphate
Tetracycline	Increased excretion of vitamin C	Vitamin C
Bile acid sequesters	Malabsorption of fat-soluble vitamins	Vitamins A, D, E and K
Mineral oil laxatives (e.g., *Agarol*)	Inhibition of fat-soluble vitamins absorption	Vitamins A, D, E and K malabsorption
	Depletion of Potassium	Potassium

Sources: Adapted from Basu, T. K. and Dickerson, J. W. 1974. *Chem Biol Interact* 8, 193–206[208]; Roe, D. A. 1994. *Prim Care* 21, 135–47[209]; and Thomas, J. A. and Burns, R. A. 1998. *Drugs Aging* 13, 199–209.[210]

1. Vitamins

a. *Vitamin A*

Vitamin A (retinol) is essential for vision, growth, maintenance of epithelial tissues, and the integrity of the immune system.[172] Together with ß-carotene, vitamin A's precursor, this vitamin has been suggested as an antioxidant and thus helps prevent tissue damage and facilitate tissue repair.[172] In a healthy aging population, the renal and liver clearance of vitamin A is decreased by about 50% compared with younger adults. This suggests that the current DRIs for retinol, of 900 and 700 μg/d for older males and females respectively, may be too high.

Thus, aging athletes should focus on consuming vitamin A precursors, the carotenoids from food sources, as suggested in the *Dietary Guidelines for Older Australians,*[211] to take advantage of the antioxidant and immune system benefits of vitamin A. Healthy sources of Vitamin A include broccoli, carrot, pumpkin, tomato, spinach, brussels sprouts, and cabbage.

b. *Vitamin B_6*

Vitamin B_6 is a coenzyme involved in amino acid and glycogen metabolism. It aids in the formation of hemoglobin and myoglobin and thus plays an important role in an athlete's diet.[172] The requirement for vitamin B_6 increases as the intake of protein increases because of vitamin B_6's role in amino acid metabolism.[212] Because vitamin B_6 and protein tend to occur together in foods (meat, fish, poultry, cereals, vegetables, whole grains), dietary adequacy of this vitamin is usually satisfactory in individuals eating the normal western diet.

The current U.S. DRI for vitamin B_6 is 1.7 and 1.5 mg/d for elderly (> 51 years) males and females respectively, and does not differ significantly from the recommendation for younger adults 19–50 years of 1.3 mg/d.[18] However, most dietary intake surveys have confirmed that the intake of vitamin B_6 in inactive elderly persons is inadequate to meet the DRIs.[213] Furthermore, evidence from depletion and repletion studies suggests that the amount of vitamin B_6 needed to obtain balance in older persons is greater than the U.S. DRI.[214]

In older exercisers, as in younger ones, there is increased loss of vitamin B_6 through urinary 4-PA excretion,[215] thus suggesting increased need for vitamin B_6 in aging exercisers. Furthermore, in an aging population, the serum concentrations of vitamin B_6 appear to decrease and there appears to be a greater amount of the vitamin needed to ensure immune system functioning in elderly individuals.[216,217] Finally, vitamin B_6 plays a crucial role in converting homocysteine to cystathionine. High levels of homocysteine are a risk factor for cardiovascular disease.[218] Thus, for health and physical performance reasons, it has been suggested that the DRI for vitamin B_6 be increased in aging athletes to 2.0 mg/d.[126]

c. *Vitamin B_{12}*

Vitamin B_{12}, required for hematopoiesis, acts as a coenzyme in nucleic acid metabolism and thus plays an important role in an athlete's physiology.[172] The major dietary intakes of vitamin B_{12} come from red and organ meats. However, older people may eat less red meat in an attempt to keep cholesterol and fat intakes down, thus limiting their intake of B_{12}. Moreover, strict vegetarians may not meet the DRI for vitamin B_{12} of 2.4 μg/d as B_{12} is found only in animal food sources.

A decrease in the overall energy intake of older athletes relative to younger athletes[154–156,168] might suggest a decrease in the need for thiamin and niacin. The incidence of pernicious anemia, as a result of malabsorption and deficiency of B_{12}, increases in aging individuals. This type of anemia is linked to an age-related atrophic gastritis seen in approximately 30% of those over 60 years of age[219] and the subsequent decrease in stomach acid and intrinsic factor secretion.[220]

Despite the suggestion that older athletes may have an increased need for vitamin B_{12} for hematopoiesis, the only published studies to date that have examined vitamin B_{12} intakes in older endurance athletes on a mixed diet showed intake of this vitamin was above the DRI.[156,168] However, it has been suggested that the vitamin B_{12} and folate requirements necessary to prevent anemia in older persons may be less than that required to maintain low homocysteine levels necessary for cardiovascular health.[221] Thus, it has been suggested that the DRI for vitamin B_{12} be increased in older people to 150% of the current U.S. DRI (2.4 μg/d) in order to prevent deficiency symptoms.[213] Moreover, one of the key recommendations of the *Dietary Guidelines for Americans*[114] is the need for people over 50 years of age to consume vitamin B_{12} in its crystalline form as a supplement or in fortified foods. It has also been suggested that a further increase of the DRI to 2.8 μg B_{12} per day may be needed for older persons undertaking regular exercise, particularly those who are vegetarians or have atrophic gastritis.[126]

d. *Vitamin C*

The antioxidant properties of vitamin C play a role in the protection of connective tissue damage, enhancing tissue repair, and may, therefore, enhance recovery from physical training and competition.[222,223] Moreover, vitamin C enhances iron absorption from foods and acts as a cofactor in some hydroxylation reactions such as converting dopamine to noradrenaline.[172] Importantly, for an older population more at risk of chronic disease, diets rich in antioxidants have also been linked to reduced risk of cancer, cardiovascular disease, and cataracts.[224–226] Major sources of vitamin C include citrus fruits, tomatoes, capsicums, and salad greens including broccoli, brussels sprouts, cabbage, and spinach.

At present, there is no evidence to suggest that vitamin C absorption or utilization is impaired with aging[227] or that dietary intakes in an aging sedentary population[228] or aging athletes[154–156,168] are lower than the current U.S. DRI of 75 and 90 mg/d for females and males over the age of 51 years, respectively. While vitamin C requirements may be increased in hot climates, by smoking cigarettes (increase intake by 35 mg/d), or heavy pollution, there appears to be no suggestion to encourage supplementation of vitamin C in older athletes.[126,213] Importantly, for an older population with increased prevalence of chronic disease, megadoses of vitamin C (> 1000 mg/d) have been shown to cause side negative effects. Kidney stone formation, gout (in those predisposed to this disease), impairment of copper absorption, and destruction of B_{12} have been reported with megadoses of vitamin C.[229] Vitamin C supplements in megadoses have also been associated with "runners diarrhea."[230]

e. *Vitamin D*

Vitamin D, together with calcium, phosphorus, and protein, is widely regarded as promoting growth and mineralization of bones, as well as enhancing the absorption of calcium.[172] Importantly for athletes undertaking heavy training loads, vitamin D is also a modulator of mononuclear phagocyte and lymphocyte functioning,[231] which is important to the body's immune response. Apart from dietary intake of vitamin D (fortified cereals and margarines, and eggs), most vitamin D is manufactured in the liver and, to a lesser extent, in the kidney, and by the action of UV light on a vitamin D precursor in the skin.

Adequate intakes of vitamin D appear crucial for older individuals, given its importance in maintenance of bone integrity. However, there appears to be an age-related decrease in the capacity of aging skin to synthesize vitamin D precursors.[232] Vitamin D production may also be compromised by seasonal variations in light, latitude, clothing, and sunscreens.[233] Moreover, there appears to be an age-related reduction in the renal production of activated vitamin D_3[234] and a decreased dietary intake and absorption of vitamin D in healthy but sedentary aging populations.[176,235]

The United States National Research Council[236] reported that about 75% of elderly Americans (> 51 years) met two thirds of the then-DRI for vitamin D of 5 μg/d. Moreover, the Australian National Nutrition Survey of 1995[171] also showed that the dietary intakes of vitamin D were inadequate in aging Australians. In light of the importance of vitamin D in calcium absorption and bone mineralization and thus osteoporosis prevention, these findings suggested that the U.S. DRI should increase to 10 μg/d in males and females over 51 years of age and 15 μg/d in those over 70 years of age.[18] Thus, that vitamin D supplementation may be warranted in older persons, including athletes who have difficulty meeting recommendations by dietary means, have dark skin, or have little exposure to sunlight, is highlighted as one of the key recommendations of the 2005 *Dietary Guidelines for Americans*.[114]

f. Vitamin E

Vitamin E is another antioxidant that has a protective role similar to vitamins C and A. Vitamin E is thought to protect tissues against lipid peroxidation that can result from prolonged or eccentric exercise (e.g., running, cycling, weight training).[237,238] A recent study observed a significant association between low serum concentrations of vitamin E and a decline in physical function in the elderly, strongly suggesting the need for supplementation in an aged population.[239] Elderly populations have been shown to benefit from vitamin E supplementation through improved immune function,[240] and reduced incidence of cataracts,[241] cancers[242] and cardiovascular disease.[243]

No evidence of vitamin E deficiency has been observed in older male athletes or female endurance athletes who take supplements,[154–156,168] with a previous study of 18 older male endurance athletes suggesting a more than adequate intake of vitamin E.[156] However, more recent evidence from female masters endurance runners and cyclists suggests that aging female endurance athletes who do not use supplements may have lower than the DRI for vitamin E.[168] The current U.S. DRI for vitamin E was increased from 10 and 8 mg/day for males and females, respectively, to 15 mg/d for both genders and all age groups over 14 years of age.[18] This requirement may increase with increasing intakes of polyunsaturated fat in diets, which are more susceptible to lipid peroxidation than diets higher in saturated fat.

Vitamin E is found in vegetable oils, unprocessed cereal grains, nuts and seeds, green leafy vegetables, meats, and wheat germ, and no negative side effects have been observed with supplementation of up to and over 700 mg TE/d.[244] Sachek and Roubenoff,[126] in a review of nutrition for elderly exercisers, suggested that older individuals undertaking endurance training who were concerned about cardiovascular problems may consider a vitamin E supplement of 100–200 mg TE/d.

g. *Riboflavin*

Riboflavin, or vitamin B_2, is a major constituent of two coenzymes involved with energy metabolism and, as such, is of importance to athletes,[172] particularly those embarking on a new training program, increasing the intensity of physical activity, or dieting.[215] The current U.S. DRI for riboflavin is 1.3 and 1.1 mg/d for elderly males and females, respectively.[18]

Older athletes, particularly those exercising 2.5 or more hours a week, dieting, or increasing training volume or intensity, may have a greater need for riboflavin than the present DRI,[215] although the only study to examine riboflavin intake in aging athletes has shown deficiency.[168] However, a 1992 study identified that 14 older women (aged 50–67 years) undertaking an exercise program and having a riboflavin intake equal to the U.S. DRI had a decrease in urinary riboflavin excretion, which may be indicative of riboflavin depletion.[245] In a classic paper examining the vitamin needs of the elderly, it was suggested that the nutrient recommendation for riboflavin for older persons be the same as for younger persons (1.3 mg/d for males and 1.1 mg/d for females).[213] Selected food sources of riboflavin include organ meats, milk, bread, and fortified cereals.

h. *Folate*

Folate is a coenzyme for both nucleic acid and amino acid metabolism and red blood cell formation.[172] Although aging does not appear to affect folate absorption or use, low folate status is a risk factor for cognitive decline associated with older age.[246] Results from the 1995 National Nutrition Survey (NNS) of Australians suggested that older persons consuming a western diet are not likely to be at risk of folate deficiency.[171] In Australia in 1995, folate was allowed to be added to some commercial foods, for example, breakfast cereal, bread, and fruit juice. Folate-rich foods include nuts, seeds, dark green leafy vegetables, legumes, meats, milk products, and now the fortified products. However, in older athletes with gastric atrophy so common in elderly persons,[219] the associated decrease in stomach acid production may lead to decreased folate absorption.[247] An earlier review of nutrition for older exercisers suggested that exercising older individuals consume at least 200 μg/d of folate, as long as vitamin B_{12} intake is adequate, because high levels of folate can mask vitamin B_{12} deficiency.[126] However, more recently, the Institute of Medicine of the National Academies has increased the DRI for folate to 400 μg/d for adults over 30 years of age and to 500 and 600 μg/d for lactating and pregnant women, respectively, given folate's importance in preventing neural tube defects in the fetus.[18] Major sources of folic acid include green leafy vegetables (eg. spinach and broccoli), fortified cereals, mushrooms, peas, asparagus, peas, and beetroot.

2. Minerals

a. *Calcium*

Calcium is essential for neuromuscular transmission, blood coagulation, muscular contraction, and bone health.[172] Calcium becomes even more important with aging, given that there is an age-related loss of bone minerals in both males and females as a result of bone resorption's predominating over bone formation, particularly postmenopause.[248] Although weight-bearing exercise promotes bone density, older athletes who already have low bone density and poor dietary intakes of calcium are likely to be at high risk of stress fractures when undertaking repetitive impact activities.[249] Moreover, such repetitive impact activities (e.g., running), particularly in a hot or humid environment, may lead to significant calcium loss via sweating.[250] Thus, calcium is an important dietary mineral in older athletes, particularly perimenopausal and postmenopausal women, to help maintain long-term bone health. However, research has consistently shown that a large percentage of older males and females from industrialized countries have calcium intakes below the DRI.[161,179,251]

Aging is accompanied by an overall decrease in calcium absorption, particularly in postmenopausal women. This decrease, together with suboptimal calcium intakes reported in some older athletes[154,156,168] increases the requirements for calcium. This increase is reflected by the higher DRI for older (> 51 years) males and females (1200 mg/day) compared with younger populations (1000 mg/day).

Calcium bioavailability is also affected by atrophic gastritis, which is common in older persons as a result of decreased stomach acid's decreasing the dissociation of calcium from food complexes.[252] Calcium absorption is dependent on activated vitamin D. Vitamin D status, as suggested earlier, may be suboptimal in older people. A deterioration in renal function, where active vitamin C is manufactured, has been attributed to the age-related decrease in circulating active vitamin D and thus the decreases in calcium absorption.

The RDI for calcium, as recommended by the Institute of Medicine of the National Academies, is 1000 and 1200 mg/d for males and females 19–50 years and > 51 years, respectively. However, calcium balance studies have suggested intakes of 1000 mg/d for estrogen-treated postmenopausal females and as high as 1500 mg/d for untreated females.[253,254] It wou'd appear prudent to suggest calcium intakes at the higher end of these recommended ranges for older athletes who lose sweat profusely, as substantial amounts of calcium can be lost through sweat.[250] In older (> 65 years) healthy females, mean calcium intakes from the 1995 Australian NNS[171] were only 68% of the DRI, a major concern given the etiology of osteoporosis, risks of fall fractures, and the role of calcium in bone mineralization. This finding of lower than recommended intakes of calcium appears consistent, with Wakimoto and Block[161] observing that only 5% of older women and 10% of older men consuming the DRI of 1200 mg/d of calcium.

In older athletes, both exercise and calcium-enriched diets have been shown to have independent effects on bone mineral density in postmenopausal women.[255,256] The majority of available evidence from studies of older athletes suggests that older persons in regular physical training are not consuming enough calcium in the diet.[154,156,168,257] Calcium supplements may be warranted in those people who are lactose intolerant, dislike milk and dairy products, are allergic to milk, or cannot meet these calcium requirements through other dietary means. Supplements of calcium citrate malate are better absorbed than calcium carbonate supplements in postmenopausal women with low dietary intakes of calcium, and appear more effective than calcium carbonate in reducing bone demineralization and lowering bone fracture rates. [254]

b. Iron

In athletes of any age, particularly those involved with endurance exercise, iron is an integral component of the oxygen-carrying capacity of both hemoglobin in the blood and myoglobin within muscle. Moreover, iron is also found within the mitochondrial cytochrome complex and thus is crucial for aerobic metabolism.[36]

Iron deficiency anemia has been shown to reduce performance capacity and maximal aerobic power in younger athletes[258] and is commonly observed in both younger endurance athletes, particularly those who are female and vegetarian.[259] It also appears that weight-bearing endurance athletes such as runners are more prone to iron deficiency, because iron losses occur with excessive sweating,[260] gastrointestinal bleeding,[261] and hemolysis.[262] The iron losses of older athletes have not been examined, although a study of 25 middle-aged female endurance cyclists and runners showed iron intake to more than adequately meet the DRI of 8 mg.[168]

Although losses of iron in younger endurance athletes may be as high as 18 mg/d,[207] iron losses have not been studied in older athletes undertaking similar levels of physical activity. Iron stores usually increase with aging in both males and females.[263] Older people, therefore, usually need less dietary iron than younger people. In a male sedentary older population, nutritional iron deficiency is rare and any observed anemia is most commonly associated with chronic illness that may decrease or interfere with iron absorption.[264] However, an Australian survey suggested that up to 30–45% of adult females had estimated dietary intakes of iron below the DRI.[171] The U.S. DRI for both elderly males and females, assuming 75% of DRI is from heme iron sources, is 8 mg/d for males over 19 years of age and 18 and 8 mg/d for females 19–50 years and over > 51 years, respectively, and should be adequate for aging athletes adhering to the *Dietary Guidelines for Older Australians*.[211] The Institute of Medicine of the National Academies recommends pregnant women consume 27 mg/d and lactating women 9 mg/d.[18] However, older athletes who are female or vegetarian involved with intense endurance running in thermally stressful environments might benefit by consuming up to 15 mg iron/d.[126]

Selected food sources of iron include fruits, vegetables, fortified cereals and grain products such as cereal (non-heme iron sources), and meat and poultry (heme iron sources). Non-heme iron absorption is lower for vegetarians than meat-eaters. Therefore, the Institute of Medicine of the National Academies suggests that the iron requirement for vegetarians is approximately twofold greater than those consuming a nonvegetarian diet.[18]

c. *Zinc*

Dietary zinc is an important mineral in older individuals because of its role in tissue repair and immune function,[265] particularly in an aging population.[266] Zinc is also an essential component of a large number of enzymes that synthesize and degrade CHOs, fats, proteins, and nucleic acids.[267] Zinc is primarily lost through urine, feces, and sweating[268,269] and may thus be compromised in athletes training in hot, humid environments. There is also a suggestion that zinc has a higher turnover in anaerobic exercise.[270,271] This might suggest increased zinc requirements for older power athletes, team players, or endurance athletes undertaking high-intensity interval training. However, there is no evidence to suggest that the zinc balance is different between young and older populations on a similar type of diet. While there is evidence of decreased zinc absorption in elderly persons, there is evidence that zinc excretion is also diminished, thus zinc balance is better maintained.[272]

The 1995 Australian NNS revealed that the average zinc intake for older males (> 65 years) was borderline but was below the DRI of 12 mg/d for the same cohort of women.[171] The same study observed poor dietary zinc intakes, with the finding that 30–69% of Australian adults had intakes less than the DRI. [171] This finding was more recently confirmed in the United States, where researchers observed 75% of women aged 50 to 69 years and 90% of men over 70 years do not consume the DRI for zinc, with 25% of older women and 10% of older men consuming 5 mg/d or less.[161] Suboptimal or borderline dietary intakes of zinc are also reported in older athletes.[168]

High intake of foods containing phytates (e.g., cereals and grains) reduces the bioavailability of zinc from these and other zinc-rich foods.[273] Moreover, the bioavailability of zinc can be further compromised in athletes taking calcium or iron supplements with food.[274] Thus, athletes on high-CHO diets (e.g., vegetarians), who have small amounts of meat or seafood (good sources of zinc), and are on iron or calcium supplements, may be at risk of zinc deficiency. These athletes may warrant supplementation. The Institute of Medicine of the National Academies has recommended DRIs of 11 and 8 mg/d for all males and female adults over 19 years of age with increased values of 11 and 12 mg/d for pregnant and lactating women, respectively.[18] As with iron intake, zinc absorption may be lower in vegetarians than meat-eaters. It is thus recommended that vegetarians take in a twofold greater intake versus meat-eaters.[18]

In summary, zinc depletion may be a problem in an aging population or for older endurance athletes with high sweat rates and older atheletes consuming high-CHO diets with a high phytate content. It may be of benefit to increase dietary zinc intake to 15 mg/d for both males and females in this cohort.

F. Fluids

Fluids are lost from the body via respiratory loss, feces, urine, and sweating.[172] The limited research examining the hydration status of healthy older adults suggests they maintain water input, output, and balance at levels comparable to those of younger adults and have no apparent changes in hydration status.[275] In young adult athletes, particularly those involved in endurance sports, sweat losses of up to 2 L/h have been reported during long-duration, high-intensity exercise in hot and humid conditions.[276] For an athlete of any age, even modest fluid losses (< 2% BW) have led to decreased athletic performance.[277]

The older athlete may be more susceptible than younger athletes to hydration problems. This suggestion was highlighted by Ainslie et al.,[278] who examined the effect of age on hydration, energy balance, metabolism, and performance in young (24 ± 3 yr) versus older (56 ± 3 yr) walkers undertaking strenuous hill walking over 10 consecutive days. While they observed maintained BM over the 10 days of walking between 10 and 35 km/day, the older walkers exhibited a twofold increase in urine osmolarity compared with a maintained urine osmolarity in the younger group, strongly suggesting that the older walkers became progressively dehydrated.

The aging process is associated with a number of age-related changes that may explain this increased rise.[279–282] These include age-related decreases in total body protein leading to an age-related decrease in total body water, renal antidiuretic hormone receptors losing their efficiency leading to increased water excretion by the kidneys, an age-related reduction in thirst sensation caused by a decrease in osmoreceptors that are sensitive to blood concentrations of fluid-regulating hormones and electrolytes, an age-related decrease in sweat production, and a delay in the onset of the sweat response. However, it has been reported that lifelong aerobic exercise may retard the age-related decrease in peripheral sweat production reported in earlier studies.[283] Taken together, these age-related changes strongly suggest that aging athletes may have problems with heat exchange and fluid balance, and should be cautious about fluid intake during exercise, particularly during prolonged endurance exercise in thermally stressful environments. Older competitors should be encouraged to experiment with different hydration strategies during training and competition.

Numerous studies examining fluid replacement in young adults have shown that, due mainly to the presence of sodium, carbohydrate-electrolyte drinks are more effective than water in stimulating fluid intake, restoring plasma volume, maintaining fluid and electrolyte balance, and attenuating core body temperature during exercise in thermally stressful environments.[284,285] Similar results were observed in 27 older male ($n = 13$) and female ($n = 14$) recreational exercisers aged 54–70 years who undertook four bouts of 15 minutes of moderate intensity cycling at 65% of VO_{2max} followed by 15 minutes of rest at 30°C and 50% relative humidity.[286] Subjects drank either carbohydrate-electrolyte solutions or water *ad libitum* during the rest breaks. While the older adults drank enough to maintain fluid balance, the carbohydrate-electrolyte solution promoted greater voluntary fluid intake and restored plasma volume losses faster than water. In addition, the older women drank more water than the men during interval exercise in the heat, possibly putting the smaller women at an increased risk of developing hyponatremia than the older men.

G. Supplement Use

It is well recognized that physically active persons eating well-balanced diets and following standard recommended dietary guidelines such as those recommended

TABLE 10.16
Dietary Guidelines for Older Australians

1.	Enjoy a wide variety of nutritious foods.
2.	Keep active to maintain muscle strength and a healthy body weight.
3.	Eat plenty of vegetables (including legumes) and fruit.
4.	Eat plenty of cereals, breads, and pastas.
5.	Eat a diet low in saturated fat.
6.	Drink adequate amounts of water and/or other fluids.
7.	If you drink alcohol, limit your intake.
8.	Choose foods low in salt and use salt sparingly.
9.	Include foods high in calcium.
10.	Use added sugars in moderation.
11.	Eat at least three meals every day.
12.	Care for your food: prepare and store it correctly.

Source: Adapted from Binns, C. 1999. *Dietary Guidelines for Older Australians*. Canberra: National Health and Medical Research Council.[211]

for older Australians (Table 10.16) may not need to take vitamin supplements. Moreover, most experts agree there is little harm in taking multivitamin/multimineral (MVMM) capsule(s) containing the recommended quantity of each vitamin or mineral, particularly in those with marginal intakes.[206]

Athletes in physical training tend to increase food and energy intake and thus meet macronutrient and micronutrient recommendations. Moreover, vitamin and mineral supplementation appears to have no effect on performance when standard dietary guidelines for older persons, such as those in Table 10.16 are met. However, supplementation may be recommended in older athletes with low-energy intakes, high-energy outputs, or excessive sweat losses, specific diseases affecting micronutrient requirements, a diagnosed micronutrient deficiency, or with poor dietary practices.

In the National Health and Nutrition Examination Survey (NHANES) 1999–2000, 52% of adults reported taking a dietary supplement in the past month, and 35% reported regular use of a MVMM product. NHANES III data indicate an overall prevalence of dietary supplement usage of 40%, with prevalence rates of 35% in NHANES II and 23% in NHANES I. Women (versus men), older age groups, non-Hispanic whites (versus nonHispanic blacks or Mexican Americans), and those with a higher education level, lower BM index, higher physical activity level, and more frequent consumption of wine had a greater likelihood of reporting use of MVMM supplements in NHANES 1999–2000.[287,288]

Three studies have examined supplement use in older athletes.[158,168] Streigel et al.[158] examined supplement use in 598 male and female masters athletes competing in the World Masters Indoor Athletic Championships in 2004. They observed that 60.5% of all participants used supplements, with the predominant substances being vitamins (35.4%) and minerals (29.9%). In contrast to younger elite athletes, who use such supplements for performance enhancement,[290] the masters athletes in this study used these substances predominantly for health reasons that were linked to health professionals' advice.[158] Other findings of interest from this study were that:

- Only 0.4% used illicit drugs or doping substances.
- Supplement users tended to train with a higher frequency than nonusers.
- Supplement users compared with nonusers showed no differences for age, gender, family status, education, disciplines, training years, or use of alcohol.
- The most frequent reasons for using supplements included injuries (25.5%), health reasons (19.9%), success in sports (18.3%), increased endurance and performance (17.3%), and increased strength (10.3%).

An earlier study compared the dietary intakes of supplementing (n = 16) and nonsupplementing (n = 9) female masters cyclists and runners with a mean age of 50.4 years.[168] They observed no differences in energy intakes between the groups but did observe that, despite both groups meeting the DRIs for all micronutrients except calcium and vitamin E, that the supplement group had greater intakes than the nonsupplement group for calcium, magnesium, vitamin C, and vitamin E. They concluded that female masters athletes may need to rely on dietary supplements rather than nutrient-dense foods to provide daily nutritional needs.

It has previously been suggested that a daily MVMM supplement that provides no more than 100% of the U.S. DRI may be recommended for aging exercisers involved in regular physical training. Furthermore, the same authors suggested that single-nutrient supplements should be limited to calcium and vitamins B_6, B_{12}, D, and E, depending on an individual's risk for certain diseases and food consumption patterns.[126]

Finally, while anecdotal evidence and popular myth suggest the use of micronutrient supplements to benefit cardiovascular, cancer, eye health, immune, and cognitive functions, the widespread enthusiasm for the use of these supplements, especially antioxidants, as anti-aging treatments or as treatments for specific diseases of aging is not supported by the currently available scientific literature. [291,292]

H. Medication–Nutrient Interactions

There are many nutrient–nutrient interactions, such as the relationship between calcium intake, protein intake, vitamin D, and sodium intake in the prevention or cause of osteoporosis. With up to 85% of older persons having at least one chronic medical condition,[293] the aged population uses more medications than younger persons. There also appears to be a high rate of chronic illness in masters athletes (primarily hypertension, asthma, and coronary heart disease) and thus it is not surprising that up to 34% of masters athletes take medication (primarily cardiovascular, respiratory, and non-steroidal anti-inflammatory),[136,140] figures similar to those observed in a normal population.[138]

The number of medications used is an important predictor of the adverse nutrient interactions that may occur, because the number of reactions increases exponentially with the number of drugs used.[294] These interactions are further complicated by an age-related decrease in endocrine function, prescriptive dietary restrictions, and the pathophysiologic changes that occur with aging. While prescribing drugs with a meal is an effective means of reminding older persons to take their medication, the interaction of food and drug may not maximize ingestion of either.[295] For example, anticholinergics may change gastrointestinal tract motility, and antacids may alter the pH within the same tract.[295]

Certain drugs can affect nutritional status and may lead to over- or under-nutrition. Table 10.15 summarizes the major medication–nutrient interactions that may affect older athletes. In summary, the mechanisms by which nutritional status can be affected is by a decrease or increase in appetite, malabsorption of nutrients, stimulation of basal metabolic rate, and changes in the glycemic level of food.[211] Given the complexity of the drug–nutrient interaction, it is important that the health professional work closely with a sports physician in maximizing both nutrient and drug effectiveness or refer to the excellent reviews available in this area.[138,296]

I. Summary

Nutritional recommendations for older athletes must consider the following important factors:

1. Age-related changes in physiology
2. Dietary changes that occur with exercise
3. The type of exercise (power, endurance)
4. Training volumes (frequency, intensity, duration)
5. The presence of chronic illness or disease
6. Nutrient–medication interactions
7. The goals and motivations of the older athlete (competitive, health and fitness, or recreational)

It appears the limited amount of available research examining the nutritional practices of older athletes or exercising older adults suggests the need for older athletes to monitor intakes of vitamins B_6, B_{12}, D, and E, folate and the minerals calcium, iron, and zinc. This should be achieved through eating a wide variety of lower-energy, nutrient-dense or fortified fiber-containing foods; adequate fluid intake; and the possible need for supplementation; especially of calcium, vitamin D, and vitamin B_{12}. Moreover, older athletes should become aware of guidelines such as the *Dietary Guidelines for Older Australians*[211] that emphasize the need for maintaining energy balance through selection of a wide variety of foods high in vegetables (including legumes) and fruit, cereals, breads, and pastas and low in saturated fat. Finally, the paucity of studies examining the interactive effects of diet, exercise, and the presence of chronic disease, strongly suggests the need for more research related to the highly trained aging athlete.

V. CONCLUSIONS

The issues facing coaches and athletes as they mature from childhood through adolescence and adulthood to older age are multifaceted. Physical and physiological changes, lifestyle influences, cultural, environmental, and training factors (type, intensity, duration, and frequency) all influence the dietary requirements of athletes as they age. Into older age, the issues of chronic disease and drug interactions also appear to influence dietary needs.

Despite the complex issues faced by health professionals individualizing nutrient needs of athletes as they age, the importance of a healthy diet that meets the recommended dietary guidelines for healthy eating, together with the unique demands of athletes compared with their sedentary peers is paramount. Specifically, it appears that the carbohydrate and protein needs of athletes of all ages are greater, as is the requirement for the micronutrients calcium, iron, zinc. Furthermore, it appears that multivitamin and mineral supplements are recommended for athletes of all ages, with an emphasis on the B-group and vitamins D and E. More research is suggested regarding the specific nutrient needs of the specific populations in specific types of sports.

VI. FUTURE RESEARCH

Based on the preceding extensive review of the literature, the following potential areas of research are suggested:

1. Determination of the macro- and micronutrient needs of general and specific endurance, speed and power, and team sports of child and adolescent athletes
2. Determination of the energy requirements of general and specific endurance, speed and power, and team sports of child and adolescent athletes
3. The use of supplements, energy drinks, and caffeinated drinks by child and adolescent athletes
4. Eating patterns of child and adolescent athletes
5. The impact of restrictive energy intakes on fetal growth and development in pregnant recreational and elite athletes maintaining physical training
6. Energy and macronutrient requirements of pregnant and lactating athletes
7. Substrate use during exercise of various exercise intensities during pregnancy in recreational and elite female athletes
8. The interaction between prescriptive drugs, exercise intensities, and diet in recreational and elite aging speed and power and endurance athletes
9. The food and eating habits of aging recreational and elite speed, power, and endurance athletes
10. Substrate usage patterns at various exercise intensities in aging endurance athletes
11. The dietary habits (macro- micronutrient) of recreational and elite aging speed, power, and endurance athletes

REFERENCES

1. Baghurst, K. and Binns, C., *Food for health: Dietary Guidelines for Children and Adolescents in Australia.* National Health and Medical Research Council, Canberra, 2003.
2. British Nutrition Foundation: Teenagers. http://www.nutrition.org.uk/home.asp?siteid=43§ionid=397. Accessed 04/15/2008.

3. Gidding, S. S., Dennison, B. A., Birch, L. L., Daniels, S. R., Gillman, M. W., Lichtenstein, A. H., et al., Dietary recommendations for children and adolescents: A guide for practitioners. Consensus statement from the American Heart Association, *Circulation* 112, 2061–75, 2005.
4. Bass, S. and Inge, K., Nutrition for special populations: Children and young athletes, in *Clinical Sports Nutrition.* Burke, L. and Deakin, V. Eds. 3rd ed, Sydney, McGraw-Hill, 2006, pp.589–632.
5. Bar–Or, O., Nutritional considerations for the child athlete, *Can. J. Appl. Physiol.* 26 Suppl, S186–91, 2001.
6. Cotunga, N., Vickery, C. E., and McBee, S., Sports nutrition for young athletes, *J. Sch. Nurs.* 21, 323–8, 2005.
7. Meyer, F., O'Connor, H., and Shirreffs, S. M., Nutrition for the young athlete, *J. Sports. Sci.* 25, 2007.
8. Petrie, H. J., Stover, E. A., and Horswill, C. A., Nutritional concerns for the child and adolescent competitor, *Nutrition* 20, 620–31, 2004.
9. Unnithan, V. B. and Goulopoulou, S., Nutrition for the pediatric athlete, *Curr. Sports. Med. Rep.* 3, 206–11, 2004.
10. Preece, M. A., Pan, H., and Ratcliffe, S. G., Auxological aspects of male and female puberty, *Acta Paediatr. Suppl.* 383, 11–3; discussion 14, 1992.
11. Spear, B., Adolescent growth and development, *J. Am. Diet. Assoc.* 102, S23–S29, 2002.
12. Theintz, G., Endocrine adaptations to intensive physical training during growth, *Clin. Endocrinol.* 41, 267, 1994.
13. American College of Sports Medicine, The female athlete triad, *Med. Sci. Sports Exerc.* 39, 1867–1882, 2007.
14. Manore, M. M., Kam, L. C., and Loucks, A. B., The female athlete triad: Components, nutrition issues, and health consequences, *J. Sports Sci.* 25, 2007.
15. Malina, R. M., Physcial activity and training: Effects on stature and the adolescent growth spurt, *Med. Sci. Sports Exerc.* 26, 759–766, 1994.
16. Specker, B. and Vukovich, M., Evidence for an interaction between exercise and nutrition for improved bone health during growth, *Med. Sport. Sci.* 51, 50–63, 2007.
17. National Health and Medical Research Council. *Nutrient Reference Values*. Canberra: National Health and Medical Research Council. 2006.
18. Institute of Medicine, *Dietary Reference Intakes for Energy, Carbohydrate, Fiber, Fat, Fatty Acids, Cholesterol, Protein and Amino Acids* National Academy Press, Washington DC, 2002.
19. Thompson, J. L., Energy balance in young athletes, *Int. J. Sport. Nutr.* 8, 160–74, 1998.
20. Lee, I. M., Blair, S. N., Allison, D. B., Folsom, A. R., Harris, T. B., Manson, J. E., and Wing, R. R., Epidemiologic data on the relationships of caloric intake, energy balance, and weight gain over the life span with longevity and morbidity, *J. Gerontol. A Biol. Sci. Med. Sci.* 56 Spec No 1, 7–19, 2001.
21. Olds, T., Obesity wars, *Sport Health* 24, 6–10, 2007.
22. Boisseau, N. and Delamarche, P., Metabolic and hormonal responses to exercise in children and adolescents, *Sports Med.* 30, 405–22, 2000.
23. Aucouturier, J., Baker, J. S., and Duche, P., Fat and carbohydrate metabolism during submaximal exercise in children, *Sports Med.* 38, 213–38, 2008.
24. Burke, L. M., Kiens, B., and Ivy, J. L., Carbohydrates and fat for training and recovery, *J. Sports Sci.* 22, 15–30, 2004.
25. Cook, C. M. and Haub, M. D., Low-carbohydrate diets and performance, *Curr. Sports Med. Rep.* 6, 225–9, 2007.

26. Erlenbusch, M., Haub, M., Munoz, K., MacConnie, S., and Stillwell, B., Effect of high-fat or high-carbohydrate diets on endurance exercise: A meta-analysis, *Int. J. Sport Nutr. Exerc. Metab.* 15, 1–14, 2005.
27. Stephens, B. R., Cole, A. S., and Mahon, A. D., The influence of biological maturation on fat and carbohydrate metabolism during exercise in males, *Int. J. Sport Nutr. Exerc. Metab.* 16, 166–79, 2006.
28. Timmons, B. W., Bar-Or, O., and Riddell, M. C., Influence of age and pubertal status on substrate utilization during exercise with and without carbohydrate intake in healthy boys, *Appl. Physiol Nutr. Metab.* 32, 416–25, 2007.
29. Timmons, B. W., Bar-Or, O., and Riddell, M. C., Energy substrate utilization during prolonged exercise with and without carbohydrate intake in preadolescent and adolescent girls, *J. Appl. Physiol.* 103, 995–1000, 2007.
30. Kaczor, J. J., Ziolkowski, W., Popinigis, J., and Tarnopolsky, M. A., Anaerobic and aerobic enzyme activities in human skeletal muscle from children and adults, *Pediatr. Res.* 57, 331–5, 2005.
31. Haralambie, G., Enzyme activities in skeletal muscle of 13–15 year old adolescents, *Bull. Eur. Physiopathol. Respir.* 18, 65–74, 1982.
32. Sank, L., Dental nutrition, *Nutr. Issues Abstracts* 19, 1–2, 1999.
33. Delamarche, P., Monnier, M., Gratas-Delamarche, A., Koubi, H. E., Mayet, M. H., and Favier, R., Glucose and free fatty acid utilization during prolonged exercise in prepubertal boys in relation to catecholamine responses, *Eur. J. Appl. Physiol. Occup. Physiol.* 65, 66–72, 1992.
34. Burke, L. M., Millet, G., and Tarnopolsky, M. A., Nutrition for distance events, *J. Sports Sci.* 25, S29–S38, 2007.
35. Butte, N. F., Fat intake of children in relation to energy requirements, *Am. J. Clin. Nutr.* 72, 1246S–1252S, 2000.
36. Wilmore, J. H., Costill, D. L., and Kenney, W. L., *Physiology of Sport and Exercise*, 4th ed. Human Kinetics, Champaign, IL, 2008.
37. Bolster, D. R., Pikosky, M. A., McCarthy, L. M., and Rodriguez, N. R., Exercise affects protein utilization in healthy children, *J. Nutr.* 131, 2659–63, 2001.
38. Pikosky, M., Faigenbaum, A., Westcott, W., and Rodriguez, N., Effects of resistance training on protein utilization in healthy children, *Med. Sci. Sports. Exerc.* 34, 820–7, 2002.
39. Tarnopolsky, M., Protein and amino acid needs for training and bulking up, In Burke, L. and Deakin, V. Eds. 3rd ed, Sydney, McGraw-Hill, 2006. pp.73–111.
40. Tipton, K. D. and Witard, O. C., Protein requirements and recommendations for athletes: Relevance of ivory tower arguments for practical recommendations, *Clin. Sports. Med.* 26, 17–36, 2007.
41. Nieper, A., Nutritional supplement practices in UK junior national track and field athletes, *Br. J. Sports Med.* 39, 645–9, 2005.
42. O'Dea, J. A., Consumption of nutritional supplements among adolescents: Usage and perceived benefits, *Health. Educ. Res.* 18, 98–107, 2003.
43. Volpe, S. L., Micronutrient requirements for athletes, *Clin. Sports Med.* 26, 119–30, 2007.
44. Schenkel, T. C., Stockman, N. K., Brown, J. N., and Duncan, A. M., Evaluation of energy, nutrient and dietary fiber intakes of adolescent males, *J. Am. Coll. Nutr.* 26, 264–71, 2007.
45. Benson, J., Gillien, D. M., Bourdet, K., and Loosli, A. R., Inadequate nutrition and chronic calorie restriction in adolescent ballerinas, *Phys. Sportsmed.* 13, 79–80; 83–87;90, 1985.
46. Loosli, A. R., Benson, J., Gillien, D. M., and Bourdet, K., Nutrition habits and knowledge in competitive adolescent female gymnasts, *Phys. Sportsmed.* 14, 118–120; 129–130, 1986.

47. Benardot, D., Schwarz, M., and Heller, D. W., Nutrient intake in young, highly competitive gymnasts, *J. Am. Diet. Assoc.* 89, 401–3, 1989.
48. Loosli, A. R. and Benson, J., Nutritional intake in adolescent athletes, *Ped. Clin. North Amer.* 37, 1143–1152, 1990.
49. Rankinen, T., Fogelholm, M., Kujala, U., Rauramaa, R., and Uusitupa, M., Dietary intake and nutritional status of athletic and nonathletic children in early puberty, *Int. J. Sport. Nutr.* 5, 136–50, 1995.
50. D'Alessandro, C., Morelli, E., Evangelisti, I., Galetta, F., Franzoni, F., Lazzeri, D., et al., Profiling the diet and body composition of subelite adolescent rhythmic gymnasts, *Pediatr. Exerc. Sci.* 19, 215–27, 2007.
51. Lanou, A. J., Berkow, S. E., and Barnard, N. D., Calcium, dairy products, and bone health in children and young adults: A reevaluation of the evidence, *Pediatrics* 115, 736–43, 2005.
52. Bailey, D. A., McKay, H. A., Mirwald, R. L., Crocker, P. R., and Faulkner, R. A., A six–year longitudinal study of the relationship of physical activity to bone mineral accrual in growing children: the university of Saskatchewan bone mineral accrual study, *J. Bone Miner. Res* 14, 1672–9, 1999.
53. MacKelvie, K. J., Khan, K. M., and McKay, H. A., Is there a critical period for bone response to weight-bearing exercise in children and adolescents? A systematic review, *Br. J. Sports Med.* 36, 250–7, 2002.
54. Goulding, A., Risk factors for fractures in normally active children and adolescents, *Med. Sport. Sci.* 51, 102–20, 2007.
55. Rowland, T. W., Black, S. A., and Kelleher, J. F., Iron deficiency in adolescent endurance athletes, *J. Adolesc. Health Care* 8, 322–6, 1987.
56. Fueling and cooling the junior athlete Sports Dietitians Australia Website, http://www.sportsdietitians.com.au/www/html/1931-fuelling-and-cooling-the-junior-athlete.asp. Accessed 04/17/08.
57. Armstrong, L. E. and Maresh, C. M., Exercise-heat tolerance of children and adolescents, *Ped. Exerc. Sci.* 7, 239–252, 1995.
58. Falk, B., Effects of thermal stress during rest and exercise in the paediatric population, *Sports Med.* 25, 221–40, 1998.
59. Inoue, Y., Kuwahara, T., and Araki, T., Maturation- and aging-related changes in heat loss effector function, *J. Physiol. Anthropol. Appl. Human Sci.* 23, 289–94, 2004.
60. American Academy of Pediatrics, Climatic heat stress and the exercising child and adolescent, *Pediatrics* 106, 2000.
61. Naughton, G. A. and Carlson, J. S., Reducing the risk of heat-related decrements to physical activity in young people, *J. Sci. Med. Sport* 11, 58–65, 2008.
62. Inbar, O., Morris, N., Epstein, Y., and Gass, G., Comparison of thermoregulatory responses to exercise in dry heat among prepubertal boys, young adults and older males, *Exp. Physiol.* 89, 691–700, 2004.
63. Falk, B., Bar-Or, O., and MacDougall, J. D., Thermoregulatory responses of pre-, mid-, and late-pubertal boys to exercise in dry heat, *Med. Sci. Sports Exerc.* 24, 688–94, 1992.
64. Iuliano, S., Naughton, G., Collier, G., and Carlson, J., Examination of the self-selected fluid intake practices by junior athletes during a simulated duathlon event, *Int. J. Sport Nutr.* 8, 10–23, 1998.
65. Bar-Or, O., Temperature regulation during exercise in children and adolescents. In *Perspectives in Exercise Science and Sports Medicine: Youth, Exercise and Sport*, Gisolfi, C., Lamb, D., Eds. Benchmark Press, Indianapolis, 1989, pp. 335–367.
66. Rowland, T., Garrison, A., and Pober, D., Determinants of endurance exercise capacity in the heat in prepubertal boys, *Int. J. Sports Med.* 28, 26–32, 2007.

67. Meyer, F. and Bar-Or, O., Fluid and electrolyte loss during exercise. The pediatric angle, *Sports Med.* 18, 4–9, 1994.
68. Bar-Or, O. and Wilk, B., Water and electrolyte replenishment in the exercising child, *Int. J. Sport Nutr.* 6, 93–9, 1996.
69. Dougherty, K. A., Baker, L. B., Chow, M., and Kenney, W. L., Two percent dehydration impairs and six percent carbohydrate drink improves boys basketball skills, *Med. Sci. Sports. Exerc.* 38, 1650–8, 2006.
70. Timmons, B. W., Bar-Or, O., and Riddell, M. C., Oxidation rate of exogenous carbohydrate during exercise is higher in boys than in men, *J. Appl. Physiol.* 94, 278–84, 2003.
71. Delamarche, P., Bittel, J., Lacour, J. R., and Flandrois, R., Thermoregulation at rest and during exercise in prepubertal boys, *Eur. J. Appl. Physiol. Occup. Physiol.* 60, 436–40, 1990.
72. Inbar, O., Bar-Or, O., Dotan, R., and Gutin, B., Conditioning versus exercise in heat as methods for acclimatizing 8- to 10-yr-old boys to dry heat, *J. Appl. Physiol.* 50, 406–11, 1981.
73. Guidelines for fluid replacement in children and adolescents. Sports Medicine Australia. http://www.ausport.gov.au/_data/assets/pdf_file/0010/144937/hey_cool_kid.pdf Accessed 04/25/08
74. Massad, S., Shier, N., Koceja, D., and Ellis, N., High school athletes and nutritional supplements: A study of knowledge and use, *Int. J. Sports Nutr.* 5, 232–245, 1995.
75. American Academy of Pediatrics. Use of performance-enhancing substances. *Pediatrics* 115, 1103–1106, 2005.
76. American College of Sports Medicine, Roundtable on the physiological and health effects of oral creatine supplementation, *Med. Sci. Sports Exerc.* 32, 706–717, 2000.
77. Winston, A. P., Hardwick, E., and Jaberi, N., Neuropsychiatric effects of caffeine, *Adv. Psychiat. Treat.* 11, 432–439, 2005.
78. Taylor, J. P., Evers, S., and McKenna, M., Determinants of healthy eating in children and youth, *Can. J. Pub. Health* 96 Suppl 3, S20–6, S22–9, 2005.
79. Chapman, K., Nicholas, P., Banovic, D., and Supramaniam, R., The extent and nature of food promotion directed to children in Australian supermarkets, *Health Promot. Int.* 21, 331–9, 2006.
80. Batada, A. and Wootan, M. G., Nickelodeon markets nutrition-poor foods to children, *Am. J. Prev. Med.* 33, 48–50, 2007.
81. American Academy of Pediatrics: Children, adolescents, and television, *Pediatrics* 107, 423–6, 2001.
82. Koivisto Hursti, U. K., Factors influencing children's food choice, *Ann. Med.* 31 Suppl 1, 26–32, 1999.
83. Stang, J., Nutrition in Adolescence. In *Krause's Food and Nutrition Therapy*, Mahan, K. L. and Escott-Stump, S. Eds. Saunders Elsevier, Missouri, 2008, pp. 246–268.
84. Magarey, A., Daniels, L. A., and Smith, A., Fruit and vegetable intakes of Australians aged 2–18 years: An evaluation of the 1995 National Nutrition Survey data, *Aust. New Zeal. J. Pub. Health* 25, 155–161, 2001.
85. Harnack, L., Walters, S., and Jacobs, D., Dietary intake and food sources of whole grains among US children and adolescents: Data from the 1994–1996 Continuing Survey of Food Intakes by Individuals, *J. Am. Diet. Assoc.* 103, 1015–1019, 2003.
86. Neumark-Sztainer, D., Story, M., Perry, C., and Casey, M., Factors influencing food choices of adolescents: Findings from focus-group discussions with adolescents, *J. Am. Diet. Assoc.* 99, 929–937, 1999.
87. Tuttle, C. and Truswell, S., Children and adolescence, in *Essentials of Human Nutrition* Mann, J. and Truswell, S. Oxford University Press, 1998, pp. 481–490.

88. Nowak, M. and Speare, R., Gender differences in food-related concerns, beliefs and behaviours of North Queensland Adolescents, *J. Paed. Child Health* 32, 424–427, 1996.
89. Lytle, L., Nutritional issues for adolescents, *J. Am. Diet. Assoc.* 102, S8–S12, 2002.
90. Gillam, M., Family dinner and diet quality among older children and adolescents, *Arch. Family Med.* 9, 235, 2000.
91. O'Dea, J., Body image and nutritional status amongst adolescents and adults—A review of the literature, *Aust. J. Nutr. Diet.* 52, 56–67, 1995.
92. Story, M., Neumark-Sztainer, D., and French, S., Individual and environmental influences on adolescent eating behaviors, *J. Am. Diet. Assoc.* 102, S40–S51, 2002.
93. Burns, R. D., Schiller, M. R., Merrick, M. A., and Wolf, K. N., Intercollegiate student athlete use of nutritional supplements and the role of athletic trainers and dietitians in nutrition counseling, *J. Am. Diet. Assoc.* 104, 246–249, 2004.
94. Updegrove, N. A. and Achterberg, C. L., The conceptual relationship between training and eating in high school distance runners, *J. Nutr. Educ.* 23, 18, 1990.
95. O'Connor, H., Olds, T., and Maughan, R., Physique and performance for track and field events, *J. Sports Sci.* 25, S49–S60, 2007.
96. American Academy of Pediatrics, Promotion of healthy weight-control practices in young athletes, *Pediatrics* 116, 1557–1564, 2005.
97. Brownell, K. D. and Rodin, J., Prevalence of eating disorders in athletes. In *Eating Body Weight and Performance in Athletes: Disorders of Modern Society*, Brownell, K. D., Rodin, J., and Wilmore, J. H., Eds. Lea & Febiger, Philadelphia, 1992, pp. 128–145.
98. Bennell, K., Matheson, G., Meeuwisse, W., and Brukner, P., Risk factors for stress fractures, *Sports Med.* 28, 91–122, 1999.
99. Beals, K. A. and Manore, M. M., Disorders of the female athlete triad among collegiate athletes, *Int. J. Sports Nutr. Exerc. Metab.* 12, 281–293, 2002.
100. Chumlea, W. C., Shurbert, C. M., Roche, A. F., Kulin, H. E., Lee, P. A., Himes, J. H., and Sun, S. S., Age at menarche and racial comparisons in US girls, *Pediatrics* 111, 110–113, 2003.
101. Baker, E. R., Mathur, R. S., Kirk, R. F., and Williamson, H. O., Female runners and secondary amenorrhea: Correlation with age, parity, mileage, and plasm hormonal and sex-hormone-binding globulin concentrations, *Fert. Steril.* 36, 183–187, 1981.
102. Ericks, M., Nutrition during pregnancy and lactation. In *Krause's Food and Nutrition Therapy* Mahan, K. L. and Escott-Stump, S., Eds. Elsevier, Missouri, 2008, pp. 160–198.
103. Artal, R. and O'Toole, M., Guidelines of the American College of Obstetricians and Gynecologists for exercise during pregnancy and the postpartum period, *Br. J. Sports Med.* 37, 6–12, 2003.
104. Gibson, A. T., Outcome following preterm birth, *Best Pract. Res. Clin. Obstet. Gynaecol.* 21, 869–82, 2007.
105. Launer, L. H., Villar, J., and Kestler, E., The effect of maternal work on fetal growth and duration of pregnancy: A prospective study, *Br. J. Obst. Gyn.* 97, 62–70, 1990.
106. Kardel, K. R. and Kase, T., Training in pregnant women: Effects on fetal development and birth, *Am. J. Obst. Gyn.* 178, 280–286, 1998.
107. Magann, E. F., Evans, S. F., and Newnham, J. P., Employment, exertion, and pregnancy outcome: Assessment by kilocalories expended each day, *Am. J. Obst. Gyn.* 175, 182–187, 1996.
108. Clapp, J. F. and Capeless, E. L., Neonatal morphometrics after endurance exercise during pregnancy, *Am. J. Obst. Gyn* 163, 1805–1811, 1990.
109. Battaglia, F. C. and Meschia, G., Principle substrates of fetal metabolism, *Physiol. Rev.* 58, 499–527, 1978.

110. Soultanakis, H. N., Artal, R., and Wiswell, R. A., Prolonged exercise in pregnancy: Glucose homeostatis, ventilatory and cardiovascular responses, *Sem. Perinat.* 20, 315–327, 1996.
111. Artal, R., Platt, L. D., and Sperling, M., Exercise in pregnancy: I. Maternal cardiovascular and metabolic responses in normal pregnancy, *Am. J. Obst. Gyn.* 140, 123–127, 1981.
112. Deakin, V., Clinical sports nutrition, in *Clinical Sports Nutrition* 3rd edition, Burke, L. and Deakin, V. McGraw-Hill, Sydney 2006, pp. 263–312.
113. Hale, R. W. and Milne, L., The elite athlete and exercise in pregnancy, *Sem. Perinat.* 20, 277–284, 1996.
114. US Department of Health and Human services, *Dietary Guidelines for Americans*, 6th ed. US Government Printing Office, Washington DC, 2005.
115. Institute of Medicine, *Dietary Reference Intakes for Thiamin, Riboflavin, Niacin, Vitamin B_6, Folate, Vitamin B_{12}, Pantothenic Acid, Biotin, and Choline.* National Academy Press, Washington DC, 1998.
116. Parazzini, F., Chiaffarino, F., Chatenoud, L., Tozzi, L., Cipriani, S., Chiantera, V., and Fedele, L., Maternal coffee drinking in pregnancy and risk of small for gestational age birth, *Eur. J. Clin. Nutr.* 59, 299–301, 2005.
117. American Academy of Pediatrics, Breastfeeding and the use of human milk, *Pediatrics* 115, 496–506, 2005.
118. Paterson, D. H., Jones, G. R., and Rice, C. L., Ageing and physical activity: Evidence to develop exercise recommendations for older adults, *Can. J. Public Health* 98 Suppl 2, S69–108, 2007.
119. Sui, X., LaMonte, M. J., Laditka, J. N., Hardin, J. W., Chase, N., Hooker, S. P., and Blair, S. N., Cardiorespiratory fitness and adiposity as mortality predictors in older adults, *JAMA* 298, 2507–16, 2007.
120. Holm, I., Personal Communication. 2008.
121. Steen, B., Preventive nutrition in old age—A review, *J. Nutr. Health Aging* 4, 114–9, 2000.
122. Lichtenstein, A. H., Rasmussen, H., Yu, W. W., Epstein, S. R., and Russell, R. M., Modified *MyPyramid* for Older Adults, *J. Nutr.* 138, 5–11, 2008.
123. Evans, W. J., Exercise, nutrition and aging, *J. Nutr.* 122, 796–801, 1992.
124. Kendrick, Z. V., Nelson-Steen, S., and Scafidi, K., Exercise, aging, and nutrition, *South Med. J.* 87, S50–60, 1994.
125. Evans, W. J., Effects of aging and exercise on nutrition needs of the elderly, *Nutr. Rev.* 54, S35–9, 1996.
126. Sacheck, J. M. and Roubenoff, R., Nutrition in the exercising elderly, *Clin. Sports Med.* 18, 565–84, 1999.
127. Campbell, W. W. and Geik, R. A., Nutritional considerations for the older athlete, *Nutrition* 20, 603–8, 2004.
128. Candow, D. G., The impact of nutritional and exercise strategies for aging bone and muscle, *Appl. Physiol. Nutr. Metab.* 33, 181–3, 2008.
129. Reaburn, P., Nutrition and the aging athlete, in *Clinical Sports Nutrition.* Burke, L. and Deakin, V. Eds. 3rd ed, Sydney, McGraw-Hill, 2006, pp. 633–676.
130. Rivlin, R. S., Keeping the young-elderly healthy: Is it too late to improve our health through nutrition? *Am. J. Clin. Nutr.* 86, 1572S–6S, 2007.
131. Rosenbloom, C. A. and Dunaway, A., Nutrition recommendations for masters athletes, *Clin. Sports Med.* 26, 91–100, 2007.
132. Kolt, G. S., Driver, R. P., and Giles, L. C., Why older Australians participate in exercise and sport, *J. Aging Phys. Act.* 12, 2004.
133. Tantrum, M. and Hodge, K., Motives for participating in masters swimming, *NZ J. Health Phys. Ed. Rec.* 26, 3–7, 1993.

134. Walter, S. D., Hart, L. E., Sutton, J. R., McIntosh, J. M., and Gaud, M., Training habits and injury experience in distance runners: Age- and sex-related factors. *Phys. Sportsmed.* 16, 101–104;109–113, 1988.
135. Kavanagh, T. and Shephard, R. J., Can regular sports participation slow the aging process? Data on Masters athletes, *Phys. Sportsmed.* 18, 94–104, 1990.
136. Reaburn, P. R. J., Gillespie, A., and Lowe, J., *The World Masters Games (1994) Injury Study*. Report to Australian Sports Commission, 1995.
137. Weir, P. L., Kerr, T., Hodges, N. J., McKay, S. M., and Starkes, J. L., Master swimmers: how are they different from younger elite swimmers? An examination of practice and performance patterns, *J. Aging Phys. Act.* 10, 41–63, 2002.
138. McCabe, B. J., Prevention of food–drug interactions with special emphasis on older adults, *Curr. Opin. Clin. Nutr. Metab. Care* 7, 21–6, 2004.
139. Jette, A. M. and Branch, L. G., The Framingham Disability Study: II. Physical disability among the aging, *Am. J. Public. Health* 71, 1211–6, 1981.
140. Farquarson, T., Masters Medicine—SA Style. Report to Sports Medicine Australia, Canberra, 1990.
141. Darnton-Hill, I., Nishida, C., and James, W. P., A life course approach to diet, nutrition and the prevention of chronic diseases, *Public Health Nutr.* 7, 101–21, 2004.
142. Keep fit for life: Meeting the nutritional needs of older persons, http://www.who.int/nutrition/publications/olderpersons/en/index.html. Accessed 03/25/08.
143. Kennedy, E. T., Evidence for nutritional benefits in prolonging wellness, *Am. J. Clin. Nutr.* 83, 410S–414S, 2006.
144. Baker, H., Nutrition in the elderly: Hypovitaminosis and its implications, *Geriatrics* 62, 22–6, 2007.
145. Ljubuncic, P., Globerson, A., and Reznick, A. Z., Evidence-based roads to the promotion of health in old age, *J. Nutr. Health Aging* 12, 139–43, 2008.
146. Hawkins, S. A., Wiswell, R. A., and Marcell, T. J., Exercise and the Master athlete—A model of successful aging?, *J. Gerontol.—A Biol. Sci. Med. Sci.* 58, 1009–1011, 2003.
147. Tanaka, H. and Seals, D. R., Invited Review: Dynamic exercise performance in Masters athletes: Insight into the effects of primary human aging on physiological functional capacity, *J. Appl. Physiol.* 95, 2152–62, 2003.
148. Proctor, D. N. and Joyner, M. J., Skeletal muscle mass and the reduction of VO_{2max} in trained older subjects, *J. Appl. Physiol.* 82, 1411–5, 1997.
149. Klitgaard, H., Mantoni, M., Schiaffino, S., Ausoni, S., Gorza, L., Laurent-Winter, C., et al., Function, morphology and protein expression of aging skeletal muscle: A cross-sectional study of elderly men with different training backgrounds, *Acta Physiol. Scand.* 140, 41–54, 1990.
150. Trumbo, P., Schlicker, S., Yates, A., and Poos, M., Dietary Reference Intakes for energy, carbohydrate, fiber, fat, fatty acids, cholesterol, protein and amino acids, *J. Am. Diet. Assoc.* 102, 1621– 1630, 2002.
151. van Pelt, R. E., Dinneno, F. A., Seals, D. R., and Jones, P. P., Age-related decline in RMR in physically active men: Relation to exercise volume and energy intake, *Am. J. Physiol. Endocrinol. Metab.* 281, E633–9, 2001.
152. Brodney, S., McPherson, R. S., Carpenter, R. S., Welten, D., and Blair, S. N., Nutrient intake of physically fit and unfit men and women, *Med. Sci. Sports Exerc.* 33, 459–67, 2001.
153. Rock, C. L., Nutrition of the older athlete, *Clin. Sports Med.* 10, 445–57, 1991.
154. Butterworth, D. E., Nieman, D. C., Perkins, R., Warren, B. J., and Dotson, R. G., Exercise training and nutrient intake in elderly women, *J. Am. Diet. Assoc.* 93, 653–7, 1993.

155. Hallfrisch, J., Drinkwater, D. T., Muller, D. C., Fleg, J., Busby-Whitehead, M. J., Andres, R., and Goldberg, A., Physical conditioning status and diet intake in active and sedentary older men, *Nutr. Res.* 14, 817–827, 1994.
156. Chatard, J. C., Boutet, C., Tourny, C., Garcia, S., Berthouze, S., and Guezennec, C. Y., Nutritional status and physical fitness of elderly sportsmen, *Eur. J. Appl. Physiol. Occup. Physiol.* 77, 157–63, 1998.
157. Maharam, L. G., Bauman, P. A., Kalman, D., Skolnik, H., and Perle, S. M., Masters athletes: Factors affecting performance, *Sports Med.* 28, 273–85, 1999.
158. Striegel, H., Simon, P., Wurster, C., Niess, A. M., and Ulrich, R., The use of nutritional supplements among Master athletes, *Int. J. Sports Med.* 27, 236–41, 2006.
159. Elia, M., Ritz, P., and Stubbs, R. J., Total energy expenditure in the elderly, *Eur. J. Clin. Nutr.* 54 Suppl 3, S92–103, 2000.
160. Starling, R. D., Energy expenditure and aging: Effects of physical activity, *Int. J. Sport Nutr. Exerc. Metab.* 11 Suppl, S208–17, 2001.
161. Wakimoto, P. and Block, G., Dietary intake, dietary patterns, and changes with age: An epidemiological perspective, *J. Gerontol. A Biol. Sci. Med. Sci.* 56 Spec No 2, 65–80, 2001.
162. Van Pelt, R. E., Jones, P. P., Davy, K. P., Desouza, C. A., Tanaka, H., Davy, B. M., and Seals, D. R., Regular exercise and the age-related decline in resting metabolic rate in women, *J. Clin. Endocrinol. Metab.* 82, 3208–12, 1997.
163. Flynn, M. A., Nolph, G. B., Baker, A. S., and Krause, G., Aging in humans: A continuous 20-year study of physiologic and dietary parameters, *J. Am. Coll. Nutr.* 11, 660–72, 1992.
164. Starling, R. D., Ades, P. A., and Poehlman, E. T., Physical activity, protein intake, and appendicular skeletal muscle mass in older men, *Am. J. Clin. Nutr.* 70, 91–6, 1999.
165. Going, S. B., Williams, D. P., Lohman, T. G., and Hewitt, M. J., Aging, body composition, and physical activity: A review, *J. Aging Phys. Act.* 2, 38–66, 1994.
166. Villareal, D. T., Apovian, C. M., Kushner, R. F., and Klein, S., Obesity in older adults: Technical review and position statement of the American Society for Nutrition and NAASO, The Obesity Society, *Am. J. Clin. Nutr.* 82, 923–34, 2005.
167. Pollock, M. L., Foster, C., Knapp, D., Rod, J. L., and Schmidt, D. H., Effect of age and training on aerobic capacity and body composition of master athletes, *J. Appl. Physiol.* 62, 725–31, 1987.
168. Beshgetoor, D. and Nichols, J. F., Dietary intake and supplement use in female master cyclists and runners, *Int. J. Sport. Nutr. Exerc. Metab.* 13, 166–72, 2003.
169. van Erp-Baart, A. M., Saris, W. M., Binkhorst, R. A., Vos, J. A., and Elvers, J. W., Nationwide survey on nutritional habits in elite athletes. Part II. Mineral and vitamin intake, *Int. J. Sports Med.* 10 Suppl 1, S11–6, 1989.
170. Burke, L. M., Gollan, R. A., and Read, R. S., Dietary intakes and food use of groups of elite Australian male athletes, *Int. J. Sport Nutr.* 1, 378–94, 1991.
171. McLennan, W. and Podger, A., *National Nutrition Survey: Nutrient Intakes and Physical Measurements*. Australian Bureau of Statistics and Department of Health and Family Services, Australian Government Press, Canberra, 1998.
172. McArdle, W. D., Katch, F. I., and Katch, V. L., *Sport and Exercise Nutrition*, 3rd ed. Lippincott Williams Wilkins, New York, 2008.
173. American College of Sports Medicine, American Dietetic Association, and Dietitians of Canada, Joint Position Statement: Nutrition and athletic performance. *Med. Sci. Sports Exerc.* 32, 2130–45, 2000.
174. Meredith, C. N., Frontera, W. R., Fisher, E. C., Hughes, V. A., Herland, J. C., Edwards, J., and Evans, W. J., Peripheral effects of endurance training in young and old subjects, *J. Appl. Physiol.* 66, 2844–9, 1989.

175. Tarnopolsky, M. A., Bosman, M., Macdonald, J. R., Vandeputte, D., Martin, J., and Roy, B. D., Post-exercise protein-carbohydrate and carbohydrate supplements increase muscle glycogen in men and women, *J. Appl. Physiol.* 83, 1877–83, 1997.
176. Saltzman, J. R. and Russell, R. M., The aging gut. Nutritional issues, *Gastroenterol. Clin. North Am.* 27, 309–24, 1998.
177. Elahi, D. and Muller, D. C., Carbohydrate metabolism in the elderly, *Eur. J. Clin. Nutr.* 54 Suppl 3, S112–20, 2000.
178. Romijn, J. A., Coyle, E. F., Sidossis, L. S., Rosenblatt, J., and Wolfe, R. R., Substrate metabolism during different exercise intensities in endurance-trained women, *J. Appl. Physiol.* 88, 1707–14, 2000.
179. Marriott, H. and Buttriss, J., Key points from the National Diet and Nutrition Survey of adults aged 19–64 years, *Nutr. Bull.* 28, 355–363, 2003.
180. Toth, M. J. and Tchernof, A., Lipid metabolism in the elderly, *Eur. J. Clin. Nutr.* 54 Suppl 3, S121–5, 2000.
181. Boon, H., Jonkers, R. A., Koopman, R., Blaak, E. E., Saris, W. H., Wagenmakers, A. J., and van Loon, L. J. C., Substrate source use in older, trained males after decades of endurance training, *Med. Sci. Sports Exerc.* 39, 2160–70, 2007.
182. Economos, C. D., Bortz, S. S., and Nelson, M. E., Nutritional practices of elite athletes. Practical recommendations, *Sports Med.* 16, 381–99, 1993.
183. Tipton, K. D. and Wolfe, R. R., Protein and amino acids for athletes, *J. Sports Sci.* 22, 65–79, 2004.
184. Phillips, S. M., Dietary protein for athletes: From requirements to metabolic advantage, *Appl. Physiol. Nutr. Metab.* 31, 647–54, 2006.
185. Cheng, A. H., Gomez, A., Bergan, J. G., Lee, T. C., Monckeberg, F., and Chichester, C. O., Comparative nitrogen balance study between young and aged adults using three levels of protein intake from a combination wheat-soy-milk mixture, *Am. J. Clin. Nutr.* 31, 12–22, 1978.
186. Lemon, P. W., Nagle, F. J., Mullin, J. P., and Benevenga, N. J., In vivo leucine oxidation at rest and during two intensities of exercise, *J. Appl. Physiol.* 53, 947–54, 1982.
187. Haralambie, G. and Berg, A., Serum urea and amino nitrogen changes with exercise duration, *Eur. J. Appl. Physiol. Occup. Physiol.* 36, 39–48, 1976.
188. Lexell, J., Taylor, C. C., and Sjostrom, M., What is the cause of the aging atrophy? Total number, size and proportion of different fiber types studied in whole vastus lateralis muscle from 15– to 83–year–old men, *J. Neurol. Sci.* 84, 275–94, 1988.
189. Nair, K. S., Muscle protein turnover: Methodological issues and the effect of aging, *J. Gerontol. A Biol. Sci. Med. Sci.* 50 Spec No, 107–12, 1995.
190. Morais, J. A., Gougeon, R., Pencharz, P. B., Jones, P. J., Ross, R., and Marliss, E. B., Whole-body protein turnover in the healthy elderly, *Am. J. Clin. Nutr.* 66, 880–9, 1997.
191. Trappe, S. W., Costill, D. L., Fink, W. J., and Pearson, D. R., Skeletal muscle characteristics among distance runners: A 20-yr follow-up study, *J. Appl. Physiol.* 78, 823–9, 1995.
192. Lemon, P. W., Effects of exercise on dietary protein requirements, *Int. J. Sport Nutr.* 8, 426–47, 1998.
193. Evans, W. J., Exercise, nutrition, and aging, *Clin. Geriatr. Med.* 11, 725–34, 1995.
194. Lucas, M. and Heiss, C. J., Protein needs of older adults engaged in resistance training: A review, *J. Aging Phys. Act.* 13, 223–36, 2005.
195. Lemon, P. W., Beyond the zone: Protein needs of active individuals, *J. Am. Coll. Nutr.* 19, 513S–521S, 2000.
196. Campbell, W. W., Trappe, T. A., Wolfe, R. R., and Evans, W. J., The recommended dietary allowance for protein may not be adequate for older people to maintain skeletal muscle, *J. Gerontol. A Biol. Sci. Med. Sci.* 56, M373–80, 2001.

197. Yarasheski, K. E., Welle, S., and Nair, K. S., Muscle protein synthesis in younger and older men, *JAMA* 287, 317–8, 2002.
198. Volpi, E., Ferrando, A. A., Yeckel, C. W., Tipton, K. D., and Wolfe, R. R., Exogenous amino acids stimulate net muscle protein synthesis in the elderly, *J. Clin. Invest.* 101, 2000–7, 1998.
199. Rasmussen, B. B., Wolfe, R. R., and Volpi, E., Oral and intravenously administered amino acids produce similar effects on muscle protein synthesis in the elderly, *J. Nutr. Health Aging* 6, 358–62, 2002.
200. Welle, S. and Thornton, C. A., High-protein meals do not enhance myofibrillar synthesis after resistance exercise in 62- to 75-yr-old men and women, *Am. J. Physiol.* 274, E677–83, 1998.
201. Candow, D. G., Chilibeck, P. D., Facci, M., Abeysekara, S., and Zello, G. A., Protein supplementation before and after resistance training in older men, *Eur. J. Appl. Physiol.* 97, 548–56, 2006.
202. Candow, D. G. and Chilibeck, P. D., Timing of creatine or protein supplementation and resistance training in the elderly, *Appl. Physiol. Nutr. Metab.* 33, 184–90, 2008.
203. Tarnopolsky, M. A. and Safdar, A., The potential benefits of creatine and conjugated linoleic acid as adjuncts to resistance training in older adults, *Appl. Physiol. Nutr. Metab.* 33, 213–27, 2008.
204. Sebastian, R. S., Cleveland, L. E., Goldman, J. D., and Moshfegh, A. J., Older adults who use vitamin/mineral supplements differ from nonusers in nutrient intake adequacy and dietary attitudes, *J. Am. Diet. Assoc.* 107, 1322–32, 2007.
205. Chen, J., Vitamins: Effects of exercise on requirements, in *Nutrition in Sport. Volume 7 of the Encyclopaedia of Sports Medicine*, Chen, J. Blackwell Science Ltd, Oxford, 2000, pp. 281–291.
206. Fogelholm, M., Micronutrients: interaction between physical activity, intakes and requirements, *Public Health Nutr.* 2, 349–56, 1999.
208. Haymes, E. M. and Lamanca, J. J., Iron loss in runners during exercise. Implications and recommendations, *Sports Med.* 7, 277–85, 1989.
209. Basu, T. K. and Dickerson, J. W., Inter-relationships of nutrition and the metabolism of drugs, *Chem. Biol. Interact* 8, 193–206, 1974.
210. Roe, D. A., Medications and nutrition in the elderly, *Prim. Care* 21, 135–47, 1994.
211. Thomas, J. A. and Burns, R. A., Important drug–nutrient interactions in the elderly, *Drugs Aging* 13, 199–209, 1998.
212. Binns, C., Dietary guidelines for older Australians, National Health and Medical Research Council, 1999. http://www.nhmrc.gov.au/publications/synopses/withdrawn/n23.pdf. Accessed 02/12/09.
212. Miller, L. T. and Linkswiler, H., Effect of protein intake on the development of abnormal tryptophan metabolism by men during vitamin B6 depletion, *J. Nutr.* 93, 53–9, 1967.
213. Russell, R. M. and Suter, P. M., Vitamin requirements of elderly people: An update, *Am. J. Clin. Nutr.* 58, 4–14, 1993.
214. Ribaya-Mercado, J. D., Russell, R. M., Sahyoun, N., Morrow, F. D., and Gershoff, S. N., Vitamin B-6 requirements of elderly men and women, *J. Nutr.* 121, 1062–74, 1991.
215. Manore, M. M., Effect of physical activity on thiamine, riboflavin, and vitamin B-6 requirements, *Am. J. Clin. Nutr.* 72, 598S–606S, 2000.
216. Meydani, S. N., Ribaya-Mercado, J. D., Russell, R. M., Sahyoun, N., Morrow, F. D., and Gershoff, S. N., Vitamin B-6 deficiency impairs interleukin 2 production and lymphocyte proliferation in elderly adults, *Am. J. Clin. Nutr.* 53, 1275–80, 1991.
217. Meydani, S. N., Meydani, M., and Blumberg, J. B., Antioxidants and the aging immune response, *Adv. Exp. Med. Biol.* 262, 57–67, 1990.

218. Selhub, J., Bagley, L. C., Miller, J., and Rosenberg, I. H., B vitamins, homocysteine, and neurocognitive function in the elderly, *Am. J. Clin. Nutr.* 71, 614S–620S, 2000.
219. Krasinski, S. D., Russell, R. M., Samloff, I. M., Jacob, R. A., Dallal, G. E., McGandy, R. B., and Hartz, S. C., Fundic atrophic gastritis in an elderly population. Effect on hemoglobin and several serum nutritional indicators, *J. Am. Geriatr. Soc.* 34, 800–6, 1986.
220. Russell, R. M., Micronutrient requirements of the elderly, *Nutr. Rev.* 50, 463–6, 1992.
221. Ubbink, J. B., Vermaak, W. J., van der Merwe, A., and Becker, P. J., Vitamin B-12, vitamin B-6, and folate nutritional status in men with hyperhomocysteinemia, *Am. J. Clin. Nutr.* 57, 47–53, 1993.
222. Jakeman, P. and Maxwell, S., Effect of antioxidant vitamin supplementation on muscle function after eccentric exercise, *Eur. J. Appl. Physiol. Occup. Physiol.* 67, 426–30, 1993.
223. Kanter, M., Free radicals, exercise and antioxidant supplementation, *Proc. Nutr. Soc.* 57, 9–13, 1998.
224. Frei, B., Ascorbic acid protects lipids in human plasma and low-density lipoprotein against oxidative damage, *Am. J. Clin. Nutr.* 54, 1113S–1118S, 1991.
225. Jacques, P. F. and Chylack, L. T., Jr., Epidemiologic evidence of a role for the antioxidant vitamins and carotenoids in cataract prevention, *Am. J. Clin. Nutr.* 53, 352S–355S, 1991.
226. Simon, J. A., Hudes, E. S., and Browner, W. S., Serum ascorbic acid and cardiovascular disease prevalence in U.S. adults, *Epidemiology* 9, 316–21, 1998.
227. Blanchard, J., Conrad, K. A., Mead, R. A., and Garry, P. J., Vitamin C disposition in young and elderly men, *Am. J. Clin. Nutr.* 51, 837–45, 1990.
228. Garry, P. J., Goodwin, J. S., Hunt, W. C., and Gilbert, B. A., Nutritional status in a healthy elderly population: Vitamin C, *Am. J. Clin. Nutr.* 36, 332–9, 1982.
229. Herbert, V., Jacob, E., and Wong, K. T., Destruction of vitamin B_{12} by vitamin C, *Am. J. Clin. Nutr.* 30, 297–9, 1977.
230. Hoyt, C. J., Diarrhea from vitamin C, *JAMA* 244, 1674, 1980.
231. Manolagas, S. C., Hustmyer, F. G., and Yu, X. P., Immunomodulating properties of 1,25-dihydroxyvitamin D_3, *Kidney Int. Suppl.* 29, S9–16, 1990.
232. MacLaughlin, J. and Holick, M. F., Aging decreases the capacity of human skin to produce vitamin D3, *J. Clin. Invest.* 76, 1536–8, 1985.
233. Holick, M. F., Environmental factors that influence the cutaneous production of vitamin D, *Am. J. Clin. Nutr.* 61, 638S–645S, 1995.
234. Tsai, K. S., Heath, H., 3rd, Kumar, R., and Riggs, B. L., Impaired vitamin D metabolism with aging in women. Possible role in pathogenesis of senile osteoporosis, *J. Clin. Invest.* 73, 1668–72, 1984.
235. Barragry, J. M., France, M. W., Corless, D., Gupta, S. P., Switala, S., Boucher, B. J., and Cohen, R. D., Intestinal cholecalciferol absorption in the elderly and in younger adults, *Clin. Sci. Mol. Med.* 55, 213–20, 1978.
236. National Academy of Sciences report on diet and health, *Nutr. Rev.* 47, 142–9, 1989.
237. Packer, L., Protective role of vitamin E in biological systems, *Am. J. Clin. Nutr.* 53, 1050S–1055S, 1991.
238. Rokitzki, L., Logemann, E., Sagredos, A. N., Murphy, M., Wetzel-Roth, W., and Keul, J., Lipid peroxidation and antioxidative vitamins under extreme endurance stress, *Acta Physiol. Scand.* 151, 149–58, 1994.
239. Bartali, B., Frongillo, E. A., Guralnik, J. M., Stipanuk, M. H., Allore, H. G., Cherubini, A., et al., Serum micronutrient concentrations and decline in physical function among older persons, *JAMA* 299, 308–15, 2008.

240. Meydani, S. N., Barklund, M. P., Liu, S., Meydani, M., Miller, R. A., Cannon, J. G., Morrow, F. D., Rocklin, R., and Blumberg, J. B., Vitamin E supplementation enhances cell-mediated immunity in healthy elderly subjects, *Am. J. Clin. Nutr.* 52, 557–63, 1990.
241. Robertson, J. M., Donner, A. P., and Trevithick, J. R., Vitamin E intake and risk of cataracts in humans, *Ann. N Y Acad. Sci.* 570, 372–82, 1989.
242. Knekt, P., Aromaa, A., Maatela, J., Aaran, R. K., Nikkari, T., Hakama, M.,et al., Vitamin E and cancer prevention, *Am. J. Clin. Nutr.* 53, 283S–286S, 1991.
243. Rimm, E. B., Stampfer, M. J., Ascherio, A., Giovannucci, E., Colditz, G. A., and Willett, W. C., Vitamin E consumption and the risk of coronary heart disease in men, *N. Engl. J. Med.* 328, 1450–6, 1993.
244. Meydani, S. N., Meydani, M., Blumberg, J. B., Leka, L. S., Pedrosa, M., Diamond, R., and Schaefer, E. J., Assessment of the safety of supplementation with different amounts of vitamin E in healthy older adults, *Am. J. Clin. Nutr.* 68, 311–8, 1998.
245. Winters, L. R., Yoon, J. S., Kalkwarf, H. J., Davies, J. C., Berkowitz, M. G., Haas, J., and Roe, D. A., Riboflavin requirements and exercise adaptation in older women, *Am. J .Clin. Nutr.* 56, 526–32, 1992.
246. Kado, D. M., Karlamangla, A. S., Huang, M. H., Troen, A., Rowe, J. W., Selhub, J., and Seeman, T. E., Homocysteine versus the vitamins folate, B_6, and B_{12} as predictors of cognitive function and decline in older high-functioning adults: MacArthur Studies of Successful Aging, *Am. J. Med.* 118, 161–7, 2005.
247. Rosenberg, I. H. and Miller, J. W., Nutritional factors in physical and cognitive functions of elderly people, *Am. J. Clin. Nutr.* 55, 1237S–1243S, 1992.
248. Lewis, R. D. and Modlesky, C. M., Nutrition, physical activity, and bone health in women, *Int. J. Sport Nutr.* 8, 250–84, 1998.
249. Heaney, R. P., Calcium needs of the elderly to reduce fracture risk, *J. Am. Coll. Nutr.* 20, 192S–197S, 2001.
250. Bullen, D. B., O'Toole, M. L., and Johnson, K. C., Calcium losses resulting from an acute bout of moderate-intensity exercise, *Int. J. Sport Nutr.* 9, 275–84, 1999.
251. Bates, C. J., Benton, D., Biesalski, H. K., Staehelin, H. B., van Staveren, W., Stehle, P., et al., Nutrition and aging: A consensus statement, *J. Nutr. Health Aging* 6, 103–16, 2002.
252. Eastell, R., Yergey, A. L., Vieira, N. E., Cedel, S. L., Kumar, R., and Riggs, B. L., Interrelationship among vitamin D metabolism, true calcium absorption, parathyroid function, and age in women: evidence of an age–related intestinal resistance to 1,25-dihydroxyvitamin D action, *J. Bone Miner. Res.* 6, 125–32, 1991.
253. Heaney, R. P. and Weaver, C. M., Newer perspectives on calcium nutrition and bone quality, *J. Am. Coll. Nutr.* 24, 574S–81S, 2005.
254. Dawson-Hughes, B., Dallal, G. E., Krall, E. A., Sadowski, L., Sahyoun, N., and Tannenbaum, S., A controlled trial of the effect of calcium supplementation on bone density in postmenopausal women, *N. Engl .J. Med.* 323, 878–83, 1990.
255. Nelson, M. E., Fiatarone, M. A., Morganti, C. M., Trice, I., Greenberg, R. A., and Evans, W. J., Effects of high-intensity strength training on multiple risk factors for osteoporotic fractures. A randomized controlled trial, *JAMA* 272, 1909–14, 1994.
256. Nelson, M. E., Fisher, E. C., Dilmanian, F. A., Dallal, G. E., and Evans, W. J., A 1-y walking program and increased dietary calcium in postmenopausal women: Effects on bone, *Am. J. Clin. Nutr.* 53, 1304–11, 1991.
257. Beshgetoor, D., Nichols, J. F., and Rego, I., Effect of training mode and calcium intake on bone mineral density in female master cyclist, runners, and non-athletes, *Int. J. Sport Nutr. Exerc. Metab.* 10, 290–301, 2000.
258. Celsing, F., Blomstrand, E., Werner, B., Pihlstedt, P., and Ekblom, B., Effects of iron deficiency on endurance and muscle enzyme activity in man, *Med. Sci. Sports Exerc.* 18, 156–61, 1986.

259. Spodaryk, K., Czekaj, J., and Sowa, W., Relationship among reduced level of stored iron and dietary iron in trained women, *Physiol. Res.* 45, 393–7, 1996.
260. Waller, M. F. and Haymes, E. M., The effects of heat and exercise on sweat iron loss, *Med. Sci. Sports Exerc.* 28, 197–203, 1996.
261. Stewart, J. G., Ahlquist, D. A., McGill, D. B., Ilstrup, D. M., Schwartz, S., and Owen, R. A., Gastrointestinal blood loss and anemia in runners, *Ann. Intern. Med.* 100, 843–5, 1984.
262. Hunding, A., Jordal, R., and Paulev, P. E., Runner's anemia and iron deficiency, *Acta Med. Scand.* 209, 315–8, 1981.
263. Casale, G., Bonora, C., Migliavacca, A., Zurita, I. E., and de Nicola, P., Serum ferritin and aging, *Age Aging* 10, 119–22, 1981.
264. Yip, R. and Dallman, P. R., The roles of inflammation and iron deficiency as causes of anemia, *Am. J. Clin. Nutr.* 48, 1295–300, 1988.
265. Mann, J. and Truswell, A. S., *Essentials of Human Nutrition*, 2nd ed. Oxford University Press, Oxford, 2002.
266. Chandra, R. K., Impact of nutritional status and nutrient supplements on immune responses and incidence of infection in older individuals, *Ageing Res. Rev.* 3, 91–104, 2004.
267. Sandstrom, B., Bioavailability of zinc, *Eur. J. Clin. Nutr.* 51 Suppl 1, S17–9, 1997.
268. Anderson, R. A., Polansky, M. M., and Bryden, N. A., Strenuous running: Acute effects on chromium, copper, zinc, and selected clinical variables in urine and serum of male runners, *Biol. Trace Elem. Res.* 6, 327–336, 1984.
269. Couzy, F., Lafargue, P., and Guezennec, C. Y., Zinc metabolism in the athlete: Influence of training, nutrition and other factors, *Int. J. Sports Med.* 11, 263–6, 1990.
270. Krotkiewski, M., Gudmundsson, M., Backstrom, P., and Mandroukas, K., Zinc and muscle strength and endurance, *Acta Physiol. Scand.* 116, 309–11, 1982.
271. Lukaski, H. C., Magnesium, zinc, and chromium nutrition and athletic performance, *Can. J. Appl. Physiol.* 26 Suppl, S13–22, 2001.
272. Turnlund, J. R., Durkin, N., Costa, F., and Margen, S., Stable isotope studies of zinc absorption and retention in young and elderly men, *J. Nutr.* 116, 1239–47, 1986.
273. Solomons, N. W. and Cousins, R. J., Zinc, in *Absorption and malabsorption of mineral nutrients*, Solomons, N. W., Rosenberg, I. H., Eds. Alan R Liss, New York, 1984, pp. 125–197.
274. Wood, R. J. and Zheng, J. J., High dietary calcium intakes reduce zinc absorption and balance in humans, *Am. J. Clin. Nutr.* 65, 1803–9, 1997.
275. Bossingham, M. J., Carnell, N. S., and Campbell, W. W., Water balance, hydration status, and fat–free mass hydration in younger and older adults, *Am. J. Clin. Nutr.* 81, 1342–50, 2005.
276. Sawka, M. N. and Pandolf, K. B., Effects of fluid loss on physiological function and exercise performance, in *Fluid Homeostasis during Exercise*, Gisolfi, C. V. and Lamb, D. R., Eds. Benchmark Press, Carmel, IN, 1990, pp. 1–38.
277. Barr, S. I., Effects of dehydration on exercise performance, *Can. J. Appl. Physiol.* 24, 164–72, 1999.
278. Ainslie, P. N., Campbell, I. T., Frayn, K. N., Humphreys, S. M., MacLaren, D. P., Reilly, T., and Westerterp, K. R., Energy balance, metabolism, hydration, and performance during strenuous hill walking: the effect of age, *J. Appl. Physiol.* 93, 714–23, 2002.
279. Van Someren, E. J., Raymann, R. J., Scherder, E. J., Daanen, H. A., and Swaab, D. F., Circadian and age-related modulation of thermoreception and temperature regulation: Mechanisms and functional implications, *Ageing Res. Rev.* 1, 721–78, 2002.
280. Kenney, W. L. and Munce, T. A., Invited review: Aging and human temperature regulation, *J. Appl. Physiol.* 95, 2598–603, 2003.

281. Allison, S. P. and Lobo, D. N., Fluid and electrolytes in the elderly, *Curr. Opin. Clin. Nutr. Metab. Care* 7, 27–33, 2004.
282. Mentes, J., Oral hydration in older adults: Greater awareness is needed in preventing, recognizing, and treating dehydration, *Am. J. Nurs.* 106, 40–9; quiz 50, 2006.
283. Buono, M. J., McKenzie, B. K., and Kasch, F. W., Effects of aging and physical training on the peripheral sweat production of the human eccrine sweat gland, *Age Aging* 20, 439–41, 1991.
284. Coyle, E. F., Fluid and fuel intake during exercise, *J. Sports Sci.* 22, 39–55, 2004.
285. Shirreffs, S. M., Armstrong, L. E., and Cheuvront, S. N., Fluid and electrolyte needs for preparation and recovery from training and competition, *J. Sports Sci.* 22, 57–63, 2004.
286. Baker, L. B., Munce, T. A., and Kenney, W. L., Sex differences in voluntary fluid intake by older adults during exercise, *Med. Sci. Sports Exerc.* 37, 789–96, 2005.
287. Murphy, S. P., White, K. K., Park, S. Y., and Sharma, S., Multivitamin-multimineral supplements' effect on total nutrient intake, *Am. J. Clin. Nutr.* 85, 280S–284S, 2007.
288. Rock, C. L., Multivitamin-multimineral supplements: Who uses them? *Am. J. Clin. Nutr.* 85, 277S–279S, 2007.
289. Striegel, H., Simon, P., Wurster, C., Niess, A. M., and Ulrich, R., The use of nutritional supplements among master athletes, *Int. J. Sports Med.* 27, 236–241, 2006.
290. Millman, R. B. and Ross, E. J., Steroid and nutritional supplement use in professional athletes, *Am. J. Addict.* 12 Suppl 2, S48–54, 2003.
291. El-Kadiki, A. and Sutton, A. J., Role of multivitamins and mineral supplements in preventing infections in elderly people: systematic review and meta-analysis of randomised controlled trials, *BMJ* 330, 871, 2005.
292. Dangour, A. D., Sibson, V. L., and Fletcher, A. E., Micronutrient supplementation in later life: limited evidence for benefit, *J. Gerontol. A Biol. Sci. Med. Sci.* 59, 659–73, 2004.
293. Webster, J. A., Key to healthy aging: Exercise, *J. Gerontol. Nurs.* 14, 9–15, 1988.
294. Stewart, R. B. and Cooper, J. W., Polypharmacy in the aged. Practical solutions, *Drugs Aging* 4, 449–61, 1994.
295. Thomas, J. A., Drug–nutrient interactions, *Nutr. Rev.* 53, 271–82, 1995.
296. Akamine, D., Filho, M. K., and Peres, C. M., Drug–nutrient interactions in elderly people, *Curr. Opin. Clin. Nutr. Metab. Care* 10, 304–10, 2007.

Index

A

D

E

I

K

L

R

S

T

U

V

W

X

Y

Z